Pocket Journal Club
Essential Articles in General Surgery

Laura M. Mazer, MD MS
Stanford University School of Medicine
Stanford, California

Kiran Lagisetty, MD
University of Michigan
Ann Arbor, Michigan

Kathryn L. Butler, MD
Massachusetts General Hospital
Boston, Massachusetts

New York / Chicago / San Francisco / Athens / London /Madrid /
Mexico City / Milan / New Delhi / Singapore / Sydney / Toronto

Pocket Journal Club: Essential Articles in General Surgery

1 2 3 4 5 6 7 8 9   DOC   21 20 19 18 17 16

ISBN 978-1-259-58758-0
MHID 1-259-58758-4

This book was set in Adobe Jenson Pro by Cenveo® Publisher Services.
The editors were Brian Belval and Regina Y. Brown.
The production supervisor was Richard Ruzycka.
Production management was provided by Jyotsna Ojha of Cenveo Publisher Services.
The cover designer was Dreamit, Inc.
RR Donnelley was printer and binder.

This book is printed on acid-free paper.

Catalog-in-Publication Data is on file for this title at the Library of Congress.

This book is dedicated to Mita Darius.

Brief Contents

Contents

Contributors

Rima Ahmad, MBBS
Massachusetts General Hospital
Boston, MA

Rachel E. Beard, MD
Beth Israel Deaconess Medical Center
Boston, MA

Kathryn L. Butler, MD
Massachusetts General Hospital
Boston, MA

Matthew A. Corriere, MD, MS
Wake Forest University School of Medicine
Winston-Salem, NC

Ara Feinstein, MD, MPH
Banner University Medical Center Phoenix
University of Arizona College of Medicine
Phoenix, AZ

Amy G. Fiedler, MD
Massachusetts General Hospital
Boston, MA

Jared Forrester, MD
Stanford University School of Medicine
Stanford, CA

Denise W. Gee, MD
Massachusetts General Hospital
Boston, MA

Alex Haynes, MD
Massachusetts General Hospital
Boston, MA

Dre M. Irizarry, MD
Beth Israel Deaconess Medical Center
Boston, MA

Hadiza Kazure, MD
Stanford University School of Medicine
Stanford, CA

Tara S. Kent, MD
Beth Israel Deaconess Medical Center
Boston, MA

Cindy Kin, MD, MS
Stanford University School of Medicine
Stanford, CA

James N. Lau, MD, MSCR
Stanford University School of Medicine
Stanford, CA

Dana Lin, MD
Stanford University School of Medicine
Stanford, CA

Laura M. Mazer, MD, MS
Stanford University School of Medicine
Stanford, CA

Andrea Merrill, MD
Massachusetts General Hospital
Boston, MA

John T. Mullen, MD
Massachusetts General Hospital
Boston, MA

Raja Narayan, MD
Stanford University School of Medicine
Stanford, CA

Stephen R. Odom, MD
Beth Israel Deaconess Medical Center
Boston, MA

Laura A. Peterson, MD, MS
Wake Forest University School of Medicine
Winston-Salem, NC

Upahvan Rai, BA
Massachusetts General Hospital
Boston, MA

Blake Read, MD
Stanford University School of Medicine
Stanford, CA

Laura Rosenberg, MD
Massachusetts General Hospital
Boston, MA

Vicki Sein, MD
Banner University Medical Center Phoenix
University of Arizona College of Medicine
Phoenix, AZ

Michelle Specht, MD
Massachusetts General Hospital
Boston, MA

Christopher Stave, MLS
Stanford University
Stanford, CA

Christina R. Vargas, MD
Case Western Reserve University
Cleveland, OH

D. Dante Yeh, MD
Massachusetts General Hospital
Boston, MA

Yulia Zak, MD
Massachusetts General Hospital
Boston, MA

Preface

For centuries, new physicians have recited the Hippocratic Oath as they embark on their journey as clinicians. The Oath famously urges physicians to "do no harm," an edict that remains at the forefront of medical practice. The first mandate in the Oath, however, pertains not to patients, but to fellow practitioners. Hippocrates charges new physicians to pass their knowledge on to the next generation.

In the current era, medical practitioners face a novel problem. While Hippocrates raised concerns about the scarcity of teaching and potential loss of information, the rapid expansion of medical knowledge and enhanced availability through electronic media threatens to overwhelm trainees with content. New textbook titles accumulate almost weekly, hundreds of journals siphon articles directly onto our cellular phones, and easily accessible databases promise answers at our fingertips. Physicians can no longer concern themselves with dissemination only, but instead must focus on distillation, sifting for meaning amid an overwhelming volume of information.

Anyone who has worked in a surgical department understands the clinical repercussions of this embarrassment of riches. Dogma contests data. When studies conflict, some physicians change their practice, and some respond with stalwart adherence to tradition and routine. The conflicting practice patterns that result are a challenge for trainees. A resident may learn about prescribing Gastrografin to shorten the duration of an adhesive small-bowel obstruction from one attending surgeon, only to be chastised for suggesting the same treatment to another. One hospital routinely gives octreotide for pancreatic fistulae, while another does not keep the drug on formulary. In the operating room, is a pylorus-preserving Whipple procedure oncologically equivalent? What margins are necessary for a thin melanoma? Uncertainty infiltrates even minor decisions: Why is a surgeon adamant about the superiority of chromic gut over monocryl for skin closure? Why is IV acetaminophen preferred over ketorolac for postoperative pain? In some cases, the rationale behind these decisions is rooted in preference; in others, anecdote; and in still others, careful review of the literature.

During residency, surgical trainees develop habits that will guide them throughout their professional careers. More important than adopting any one preference over another is the method by which we choose our preferences. The data are not always conclusive, and studies are not always well designed. But surgical trainees must learn to discern among the conflicting influences of tradition and evidence in order to make clinical decisions.

This book is not intended as a textbook, or a surgical journal. This book is meant to guide you toward a practice grounded in evidence, and to enhance your ability to find and evaluate new information. Reach for this book before starting a new rotation. Reference it when asked to discuss an article at a journal club or lunchtime talk. Most importantly, remember it when you're asked to prescribe a medication, use a specific technique, or choose a certain procedure "because that's the way we do it here." Use it to determine, for yourself, the best care possible, and use it to continually challenge those decisions as you encounter new data throughout your career.

Introduction to Evidence-Based Surgery

Finding the Answers

Christopher Stave

OVERVIEW

A comprehensive literature review is essential for understanding and applying evidence-based medicine. This chapter seeks to equip the busy surgeon with a core set of techniques to efficiently retrieve and manage clinical information, and to interpret such data within the context of the greater body of surgical literature. More specifically, this chapter will provide (1) succinct database and search engine descriptions with advice for best search strategies, (2) a guide to two popular reference management applications, and (3) descriptions of tools for remaining current with the latest clinical research. To understand the importance of the literature search, the chapter begins with some relevant clinical scenarios.

Scenario 1

A 42-year-old male is admitted to the intensive care unit with refractory septic shock secondary to perforated peptic ulcer. Treatment consists of antibiotics, intravenous fluid support, and norepinephrine. The intensivist wants to know whether evidence exists to support the addition of vasopressin, and asks you to locate articles on the topic, in particular articles that have significantly impacted clinical practice.

Locate High-Impact/Seminal Articles: One quick-and-easy method for identifying high-impact articles in a particular clinical domain is to rank papers by "times cited," which is simply the number of times that an article was cited in other works (typically, other journal articles). Two tools for determining times cited are Google Scholar (free) and SCOPUS (subscription-only). Google Scholar ranks its results using a relevance weighting algorithm that, among other things, adds greater relevance to a search result that is frequently cited. SCOPUS, on the other hand, allows searchers to simply sort results from most to least cited (or vice versa).

Other tools such as Faculty of 1000 and NEJM Journal Watch use an actual cadre of subject experts rather than algorithms to identify noteworthy articles. However, both of these are subscription services.

Searching Google Scholar: As the name implies, Google Scholar is a resource for locating scholarly information, including academic articles, patents, books, court opinions, and theses. One of the key benefits of Google Scholar is the ability to search the full text of an item, not just the titles, abstracts, and supplemental keywords found in traditional literature databases such as PubMed, SCOPUS, and Web of Science. Search terms that might not appear in a standard reference (eg, an obscure lab method, a psychometric test, a health statistic) *are* potentially discoverable in the full text.

As mentioned previously, the number of times that an article is cited plays a significant role in ranking search results. Searchers can also view *who* is citing the work by clicking on the "Cited by" link.

Despite its utility, citation count as an indicator of relevance is imperfect. Inherent delays in reading and citing a particular work diminish the efficacy of citation count in detecting new articles that might become seminal.[1] Also, an article may be cited frequently because of the controversy—positive or negative—that it generates, rather than its relevance to standard of care.

Let's return to our scenario. We'll start our research into vasopressin, norepinephrine, and septic shock with a search of Google Scholar. Our intent is to quickly identify some key articles on the topic using the ranking algorithm.

Google Scholar Search Results: A seminal work by JA Russell on vasopressin and norepinephrine in septic shock is the first reference listed.

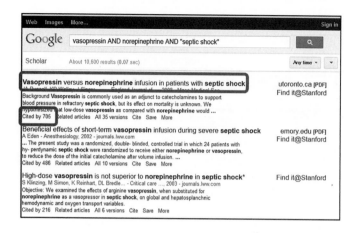

Google Scholar Search Tools and Techniques

- **Search Operators:** To exclude terms from a search, use the minus (–) symbol, for example, "skull base surgery" *–cadaver*. Use quotes to search an exact phrase, such as "postpartum hemorrhage."
- **Downloading:** Google Scholar has a "Settings" icon on the initial page that will allow you to activate an "Import to End-Note" link on your search results. Unfortunately, only one reference at a time can be imported from Scholar to EndNote. Zotero, a free citation management tool, provides an option for downloading *all* the results of a page with one click. Both of these reference management tools are discussed in more detail below.

Searching SCOPUS: *SCOPUS* is a subscription-based, multidisciplinary database covering topics ranging from astronomy to urology and virtually everything in between. In addition to supplying a huge database of article references, SCOPUS provides citation counts, researcher profiling tools (including H-Index scores), and metrics for evaluating an article's impact.

Now, let's search SCOPUS to locate any article on vasopressin and norepinephrine for treating septic shock and sort by citation count. For more information on the impact of the article, scan the SCOPUS "Metrics" report.

SCOPUS Search Results: The screenshot above shows the results of a title/abstract/keyword search of vasopressin AND

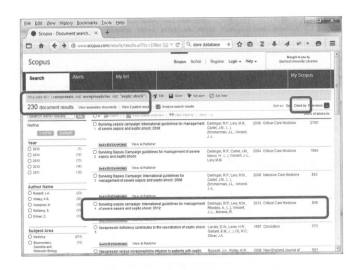

norepinephrine AND "septic shock" sorted by citation count (most to least cited). Click the title of citation 4 to retrieve the Metrics report on the Dellinger article.

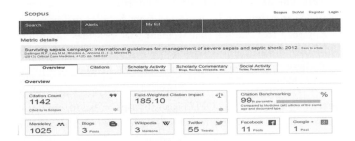

Note how Metrics tracks "the buzz" on an article via numerous social media tools and resources, such as Twitter, Facebook, Wikipedia, blogs, and Mendeley (a web tool for sharing research papers).

SCOPUS Search Tools and Techniques: SCOPUS uses the standard array of literature database search options:" Boolean operators AND, OR, and NOT; the asterisk * as a wild card; and double quotes for phrase searching. Searchers use pulldown menus to choose which fields within a reference to search.

Returning to the scenario, suppose that the intensivist wants to find out about any new articles that come up on this topic. There are multiple ways to stay current on the literature. Two of these strategies are BrowZine and Faculty of 1000.

Keeping Current with BrowZine: BrowZine is a service that allows you to browse and read articles from your favorite academic journals. If your institution subscribes to BrowZine, you can install the mobile application and use it to select and add specific journals to your own personalized digital library collection. Similar to an actual library reading room, BrowZine populates "shelves" with digital journals. New, unread articles are indicated by a number overlaying the image of the journal's cover. Alerts to new journal issues are sent as notifications to your device. BrowZine is currently available as an application for tablets and smartphones using either the Apple iOS or Android OS. BrowZine can also be used without subscription to access a much smaller collection of open-access journals.

The first screenshot of BrowZine shows surgery journal subcategories; the second screenshot shows final journal selection.

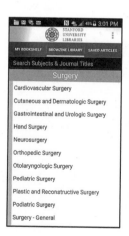
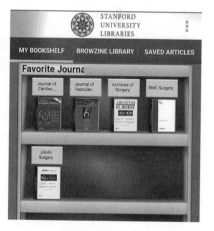

The third screenshot shows the table of contents for an issue of *Archives of Surgery*.

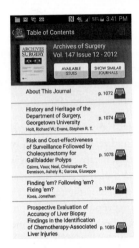

Keeping Current with Faculty of 1000 (F1000)—Prime: F1000 is a subscription-based service that provides article recommendations from thousands of world-renowned researchers in the clinical and life sciences. The topics and specialties in F1000 are often quite focused: pediatric anesthesiology, dermatologic and cosmetic surgery, and so on. In addition to providing options for creating auto-alerts, F1000 can also be searched as a standalone database.

Search for recommendations on articles relating to "septic shock" in the following screenshot:

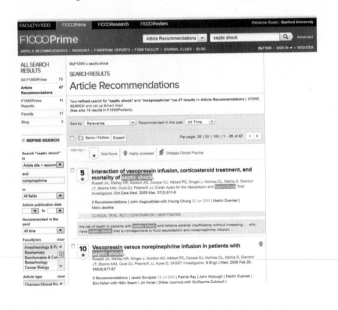

F1000 Search Results: Results include commentary and an overall "score" based on reviewer recommendations.

Additional Tools for Keeping up with the Latest Clinical Research: AutoAlerts, Recommendation Services, eTOCS, and More

Database Autoalerts: Most literature databases (eg, PubMed) and search engines provide utilities for building "autoalerts." Create an account in the database, run and save a search, and indicate how often alerts should be delivered.

Google Scholar Autoalerts: Access via http://scholar.google.com. Create a Google account. Run a search, then click on the "Create Alert" icon and follow the prompts.

Electronic Tables of Contents (eTOCS): A very popular method for receiving an email with the most recent issues of a journal, eTOCS are becoming increasingly available for most peer-reviewed journals. Signing up is usually a matter of visiting the journal's website, creating an account, locating an alert link (usually labeled "Alerts" or "eTOCS"), and activating the alert. The emails typically contain an attractively formatted list of articles from the latest issue of the journal, with embedded links to the full text.

READ (BY QXMD): READ is one of many customizable medical journal readers. Users select journals to follow, view article suggestions by specialty, or scan article collections created by other QxMD users. Available for Android and iOS and via a web browser. (Website: http://www.qxmd.com/apps/read-by-qxmd-app)

Scenario 2

Impressed by your ability to identify key articles on septic shock, norepinephrine, and vasopressin, the surgery attending asks you to give a presentation on the topic at next month's journal club. In preparation for the talk, you decide to design and run a well-constructed search on the topic in PubMed.

Searching PubMed: PubMed is a literature database of over 24 million references, primarily journal articles on biomedicine and the life sciences. Coverage extends to the mid-1940s. Over 5600 journals in 40 different languages are currently included in PubMed.

Step 1: Create a PubMed My NCBI account! Why? A My NCBI account allows you to save your searches, create auto-alerts, and color-highlight your search terms. After creating the account, click on "My NCBI," then "NCBI Site Preferences."

Click "Highlighting" and choose a color to highlight your search terms. Next, select "Abstract Supplemental Data" and click the "Open" checkbox: MeSH terms will now display automatically when viewing a full reference.

Step 2: Use the title tag [ti] to quickly locate relevant references with your search terms in the title. These initial references will form the basis of subsequent, more complex searches. What terms would likely occur in the title of a relevant article? How about *norepinephine, vasopressin,* and *septic shock?* Use the asterisk as a wildcard to capture any term that starts with *"vasopres."* The search should look like this:

- vasopres* [ti] AND norepinephrine [ti] AND "septic shock" [ti]

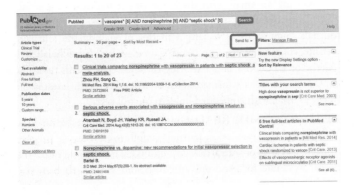

As you review the results, you can save relevant references to PubMed's Clipboard by clicking a reference's checkbox, then clicking "Send to," and then "Clipboard."

Step 3: Click the "Similar articles" link under a particularly useful reference to quickly locate other, related references.

Again, you can save what you find to the Clipboard by clicking "Send to" and then "Clipboard."

Step 4: Now it's time to use another powerful PubMed search tool: MeSH—Medical Subject Headings (see text below for more information on MeSH). MeSH can be extracted from any fully indexed reference; however, remember that not all references have been indexed (newer references are often, but not always, waiting "in queue" for indexers to add the MeSH terms).

Click the title of the MJ Daley article to view the MeSH terms (if you haven't selected "Abstract Supplemental Data" in your My NCBI preferences, you may have to click on the reference's "MeSH Terms" link).

Scan the terms, and note which seem most relevant. In this case, the MeSH terms are "Norepinephrine," "Vasopressins," and "Shock, Septic."

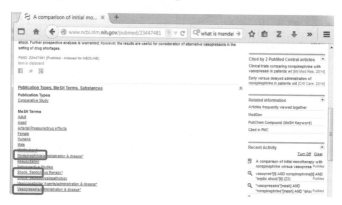

Now, simply plug the terms into the PubMed search box enclosed by double quotation marks, making sure to include the [mesh] tag. To keep things simple, use the MeSH terms, not the "subheadings" that follow the slash "/" (see below for more information on subheadings). The search should look like this:

- "vasopressins" [mesh] AND "norepinephrine" [mesh] AND "Shock, Septic" [mesh]

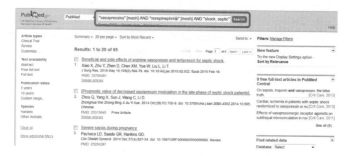

Step 5: Restrict the search to English-language articles published in the past 10 years using the filters to the left of the search results. Click on the last option, "Show

additional filters," and note the array of choices: age groups, subject categories, date range, etc. Check the box next to "Languages." Next, click "English," then restrict by date by clicking the "10 years" option under "Publication dates." Your results should look like this:

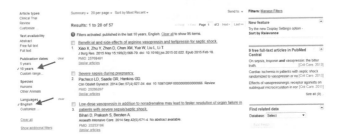

You can add the 57 results (or select from among the 57 using the checkboxes next to the references) to the Clipboard by clicking "Send to" and then "Clipboard." We'll discuss how to manage and store the references in more detail below.

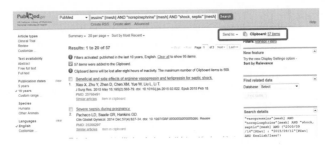

PubMed Autoalerts: Alerts enable you to automatically keep track of newly added PubMed references. To set up a PubMed alert, run a slightly different version of the initial title search from step 2. Why? Because the search will be run *only* against new PubMed references, so the search terms can be very broad without retrieving an unduly large set of references. One approach is to use the search tag [tw]. A [tw] search will look for terms in a number of fields within a reference, including titles, abstracts, author-supplied keyword(s), and MeSH. The search should look like this:

- vasopres* [tw] AND norepinephrine [tw] AND "septic shock" [tw] AND trial* [tw]

Apply the English-language filter, click "Save search," and then follow the prompts to activate monthly or weekly auto-alerts.

Medical Subject Headings (MeSH): Medical Subject Headings are the official, standardized terms or expressions used for a particular disease, drug, organism, study type, medical specialty, and so on, and as such are key components of well-constructed PubMed searches. Amazingly, human indexers (often topic experts with advanced degrees) actually scan or read most of the articles in PubMed (about 90% get indexed). Each reference is supplemented by approximately 5–25 MeSH terms.

Other terms added by indexers include type of publication (clinical trial, editorial, review, etc), age group (child, infant, aged, etc), and gender.

What is the main advantage of MeSH? Regardless of variants in terminology used by authors (eg, one author uses the term *kidney stones* while another uses *kidney calculi*), a properly indexed reference should include the official medical subject heading(s) that represents a concept; in this case, the medical subject heading is *kidney calculi*. Use it, and you should retrieve articles about kidney calculi regardless of variation in authors' terminology.

Additionally, MeSH terms are arranged hierarchically, and a search of one heading automatically includes headings "downstream." For example, a search of the MeSH heading "Respiration, Artificial" automatically searches narrower headings, including "High-Frequency Ventilation," "High-Frequency Jet Ventilation," "Liquid Ventilation," and "Positive-Pressure Respiration."

Subheadings: Terms that append some MeSH terms in a reference (separated by a slash) are known as *subheadings* or *qualifiers*. Subheadings focus on specific aspects of MeSH terms: for example, the subheading "etiology" is generally applied to a subject heading for a disease, such as "cystic fibrosis/etiology," while the subheading "adverse effects" or "administration & dosage" are applied to the subject heading for a drug or drug class, such as "vasopressins/administration & dosage." Knowing the correct usage of subheadings can be tricky, and a detailed description of how best to employ them is beyond the scope of this chapter. For more information, refer to one of the National Library of Medicine's[2] many online tutorials.

MEDLINE versus PubMed: Some confusion exists among searchers about the difference between PubMed and Medline. A simple way to think about it is to consider Medline the 90% of PubMed that contain indexing terms such as MeSH. The other 10% of PubMed does not include indexing terms such as MeSH.

The Default PubMed Search: A successful search of PubMed depends on avoiding the temptation to simply type words into the PubMed search box and click "Search." PubMed will often supplement searches with additional search terms or expand the number of fields (title, abstract, author affiliation, etc) searched within a reference, or both. The results can be perplexing. An extreme example might be a clinical instructor looking for new and innovative teaching tools and searching under "teaching aids." The search returns over 23,000 references, most of which are completely irrelevant. What happened? PubMed translated the term *aids* to the medical subject heading *acquired immunodeficiency syndrome*, dramatically increasing the number of references retrieved. To see what PubMed adds to a search, scroll down the right side of the results page and view "Search details."

To reduce the supplemental information PubMed adds, a searcher can design very specific searches that dictate *exactly* what terms should be searched and *precisely* what parts of the reference should be targeted. The following section provides guidance on how to accomplish this.

PubMed Search Tools and Techniques
- **Boolean Operators:** Combine and/or exclude search terms with the following three Boolean operators: AND, OR, and NOT. In PubMed, the operators *must* be in uppercase:
  - endoscopic **AND** skull base surgery
  - deep-brain stimulation **OR** dbs
  - skull base surgery **NOT** cadaver studies
- **Phrase Searching:** Quotation marks force PubMed to search for terms in a fixed sequence:
  - "laryngeal mask airways"
  - "laryngeal airways" OR "laryngeal mask airways"
- **Wild Cards:** Use the asterisk * to search for words beginning with the letters that precede it:
  - allerg* (retrieves allergy, allergic, allergens, etc)
  - microbio* (retrieves microbiota, microbiology, etc)
- **Tags:** Tags allow a searcher to dictate what parts of a PubMed reference (title, author, journal, etc) are searched. Enclosed in square brackets, tags are placed after the search terms. Some particularly useful tags include [ti] title, [tiab] title/abstract, [mesh] medical subject headings, [jour] journal, [pt] publication types, and [tw] title/abstract/medical subject headings/author-supplied keywords:
  - "carpal tunnel" [**ti**] AND "quality measures" [**tiab**]
  - ventilator [**ti**] AND wean* [**ti**] AND nejm [**jour**]

- organic* [**ti**] AND safe* [**ti**] AND stave c [**au**]
- "vasoconstrictor agents" [**mesh**] AND "shock, septic" [**mesh**] AND "clinical trial" [**pt**]

- **More on the Title Tag** [**ti**]: TITLE searching using the [ti] tag is a surprisingly simple but effective initial search strategy. Titles are often the purest distillation of the core meaning of an article, so if a thoughtfully selected set of search terms appear in the title, chances are that the reference will be relevant to the searcher. Retrieve a set of citations using the [ti] tag, and then build from the most relevant using either the "Related Citations" link or medical subject headings:

  - **Title Search:** weaning [**ti**] AND "mechanical ventilation" [**ti**]

Scenario 3

Having read through the relevant articles from the PubMed search, you begin to prepare your journal club presentation. Rather than building the presentation from scratch, you decide to check to see whether other presentations on the topic have already been given. Perhaps they can provide clues as to how to more effectively structure your talk.

Searching Google: Use Google to locate PowerPoint presentations on the topic of septic shock, norepinephrine, and vasopressin.

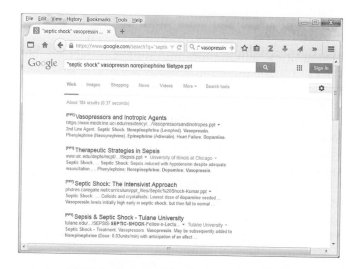

Obviously, attribution should be given, or permissions requested as appropriate.

Google Search Tools and Techniques
Filetype: Google's filetype allows searchers to target a variety of file types, not just PowerPoint slides, for example:

- procedural pain children filetype:**pdf**
- "total hip replacement" "united states" filetype:**docx**

Site: Frustrated by a website's seemingly underpowered search engine? Use "site" instead! After identifying the URL for the website, enter your search terms into Google followed by "site:" and the site's URL. For example:
- diabetes algorithm **site:**aace.com
- sepsis malnutrition **site:**who.int

Combining: To limit a search for PowerPoint slides to a particular website or domain, combine *site*, *filetype*, and search terms:
- surgical resident hours filetype:pdf site:acgme.org
- septic shock filetype:ppt site:who.int

Scenario 4

Having become somewhat of an expert on vasopressin, norepinephrine, and septic shock, you decide to write a review article on the topic. Excellent tools abound that can help you download, organize, and cite the literature accurately. You decide to use Zotero, a free reference manager with a simple interface and excellent collaboration tools.

Managing PDFs/References with Zotero: Zotero is a free, open-source application that works as a web browser plug-in or separate client. Terrific for grabbing items off the web (references, web pages, some PDFs), Zotero is available for Mac and PC operating systems. The references and PDFs maintained locally on a desktop or laptop computer can also be saved and synchronized in a web-based Zotero account. (Website: http://zotero.org.)

The following steps will showcase Zotero using the PubMed searches from Scenario 2:

Step 1: Go to http://www.zotero.org/download to download and install Zotero. A small black "Z" will appear in your browser. Click the "Z" to open the Zotero application, then click the 57 *items* link to view the 57 references you saved in Clipboard.

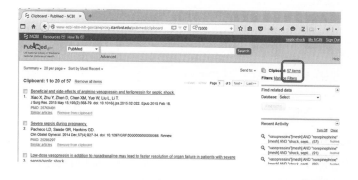

Step 2: Changing the page display limit from "20 per page" to "100 per page" will allow you to download all 57 citations in one step. Within the Zotero application, click on the "Collections" icon to create and name a folder for your references. Next, click on the small yellow folder next to the "Z" Zotero icon to pull up the reference download window.

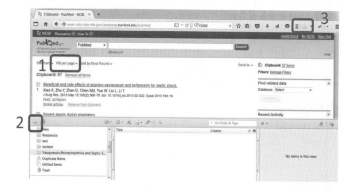

Step 3: After selecting items to save, click "OK" to save the results to the Zotero collection "Vasopressin/Norepinephrine" and "Septic Shock."

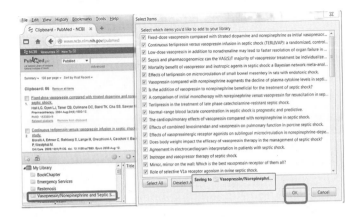

Step 4:   Locating articles. Use the small green arrow in the Zotero interface to activate the "Library Lookup" feature. Under "Actions/Preferences/Advanced" is a box for the address of your institution's journal link *resolver*. A link resolver is a utility that tries to connect the searcher with the full text of an article. If you add your institution's "link resolver," "Library Lookup" will try to locate the PDF of the article. Adobe Acrobat provides an option for saving the PDF directly into Zotero.

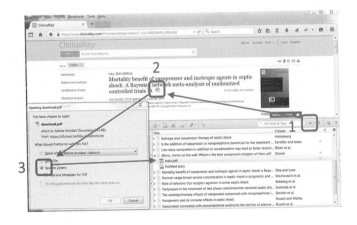

Step 5:   Searching and downloading results from Google Scholar to Zotero uses the same procedures as described above.

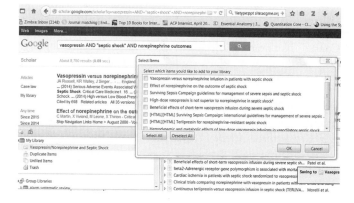

Step 6:   Creating bibliographies. An optional Zotero Word plug-in allows users to add references from Zotero "Collections" and "Groups" to a Word document. Zotero can then create bibliographies from these references in a variety of bibliographic styles. Additional styles (literally, thousands) are selectable via Zotero's "Actions/Preferences/Cite/Style" tab. For Zotero for Windows, the plug-in is located under the "ADD-INS" menu. The following screenshot shows a bibliography generated from the references added from Zotero:

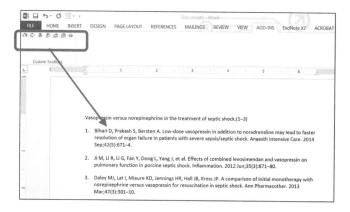

Cost: The application and the first 300 MB of storage space are free. Unlimited space is available for $120.00 per year.

Pros: The application Zotero is an excellent collaboration tool for sharing content with others. Create a "Group," load it into a Zotero account, and invite colleagues to share the content.

Cons: Not nearly as effective as EndNote for downloading large numbers of PDFs automatically. Current version lacks PDF text highlighters and sticky-note tools.

Managing PDFs/References with EndNote: EndNote is a popular and powerful commercial reference, PDF, and bibliography manager. Key features include (1) reference import from virtually any literature database; (2) depending on local subscriptions, automatic downloading of article PDFs; and (3) automatic bibliography generation in over 6000 different styles. (Website: http://endote.com.)

Cost: Price varies depending on site licenses and academic affiliation; however, a free, full version is available for a 30-day trial.

Pros: Terrific at downloading PDFs automatically. Powerful editing options for customizing bibliography styles.

Cons: Not as versatile as Zotero for sharing multiple collections of references/PDFs with collaborators. Not free.

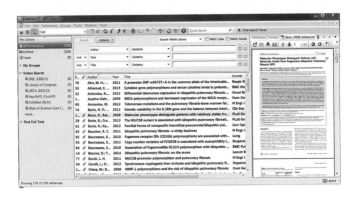

CONCLUSION

Clinicians are living in a veritable golden age of potent web-based search engines, extensive literature databases, powerful citation/PDF/bibliography managers, and tools for keeping current. The era of scanning print indexes and typing bibliographies by hand is clearly over (although some researchers may still not realize it). This chapter was intended to show how some very powerful tools and resources can be integrated logically and efficiently into a gradually unfolding clinical research scenario. Any clinician interested in getting more practical, hands-on experience with these topics should contact the obvious subject expert: the nearest biomedical librarian.

REFERENCES

1. Bae DHS, Hwang M, Kim SW, Faloutsos C. On constructing seminal paper genealogy. *IEEE Trans Cybernetics*. 2014;44(1):54–65.
2. National Library of Medicine. Applying subheadings and other features using the MeSH database (available from https://www.nlm.nih.gov/bsd/viewlet/mesh/subheadings/mesh3.html).

CHAPTER 3

How to Read a Journal Article

Laura Mazer • Kathryn Butler

This book intends to equip you with a foundational knowledge of landmark articles in general surgery. The introductory chapter, "Finding Answers," provides tools with which to conduct literature searches and identify high-impact articles. In this chapter, we describe a method for reading and interpreting journal articles in order to apply them to your clinical practice. Whether you are reading a landmark study within a field, running a literature search to answer a clinical question, or scanning an interesting abstract in the latest issue of a journal, assessment of the literature requires a logical and systematic approach to reading scientific manuscripts. The following discussion outlines key questions to consider when reading each section of a journal article.

1. **Title and abstract**

   Should I read this paper?

   Despite your new-found skills in literature searching, PubMed often produces lists of articles that vary in relevance to your clinical question. A good title and abstract should hint whether the study is worth your time to read.

   Abstracts are *insufficient*, however, to answer any clinical question, and should be used only to gauge whether to spend time reading the full article. Remember that the abstract is a 200–300-word advertisement for the paper. It is designed as much to hook the reader as to summarize the study. The abstract's conclusion section will provide one or two sentences that usually showcase the most impressive results, and most abstracts will avoid stating negative results.

For example, a study evaluating a new imaging test may reveal that the test has very poor sensitivity and specificity in the general population, but works well in a narrowly defined subset. The abstract's conclusion may state only the positive findings, ignoring the narrow range of applicability. The abstract will not reliably tell you whether the article's conclusions are generalizable, applicable to your patient population and practice, or conclusive. To answer such questions, you need to continue reading.

2. **Introduction**
   Why was this study done?

   The introduction section orients you to the study's topic with relevant citations to other important papers in the field. If you are not familiar with the field, the introduction is particularly helpful, and it serves as a good starting point in a search for landmark articles. Finally, the introduction provides insight into the authors' motivations for writing the article.

3. **Methods and results**

   The methods and results are the most important sections of the paper. These are the only sections that, taken alone, can answer a clinical question. If you want to read only two sections, after deciding a paper is relevant on the basis of its title and abstract, those sections should be the methods and results.

   Does this paper apply to my patient?

   Clinical studies generally present a description of the included patient population in "Table 1." This table provides the overall picture of the included population, and if the study has more than one group, it will indicate whether these groups have similar baseline characteristics (gender, age, comorbidities).

   In the text, the authors describe the inclusion and exclusion criteria used to choose the included population. These criteria can reveal the relevance of a study to your patient. For example, the study by Blakely et al[1] evaluating interval appendectomy for perforated appendicitis included only patients less than 18 years of age. If you are treating a 65-year-old man with multiple comorbidities who presents with perforated appendicitis, the Blakely study may not apply to your patient.

   Are these results generalizable to my practice?

   In addition to evaluating the study population, it is also important to evaluate the study method for generalizability. A study

TABLE 1: Description of study designs

Study Design	Description	Limitations
Descriptive		
Cross-sectional	Measures prevalence of risk factors and outcomes in a population at one time point	Cannot establish temporality
Case reports, case series	Tracks one or more subjects with a known exposure	No comparison group
Analytic: Observational		
Case–control	Selects participants based on outcome status (disease vs. no disease) and asks about past risk factors	Subject to recall bias
Prospective cohort	Ongoing observation of a group of people until they develop the outcome of interest	Loss to follow-up
Retrospective cohort	Often database studies, uses stored records to evaluate the association of risk factors and outcomes in a group	Only as good as the database, which was often created for another purpose
Analytic: Experimental		
Randomized controlled trial	Gold standard for establishing cause and effect: Participants are randomly assigned to interventions and followed prospectively	Expensive, potentially unethical to deny treatment to one group

evaluating a new treatment does so within the context of a larger clinical setting. If the larger setting does not reflect your practice, the results may not be generalizable. For example, Popadich et al[2] showed that patients have lower reoperation rates with no increase in complications with routine central lymph node dissection for cN0 papillary thyroid cancer. The included hospitals, however, were high-volume centers with specialized surgeons. If you are working at a community hospital without endocrine specialists, the results may not apply to your practice.

What is the study design?

The methods section should also allow you to describe the study's design. Understanding the study design is an important step toward understanding the study's level of evidence, potential limitations, and statistical outcomes. In general, studies fall into two major categories: descriptive and analytic. *Descriptive* studies do not try to quantify a relationship, but rather to describe the prevalence, incidence, or experience of an entire group. These studies provide a description of the problem, but do not attempt to provide a cause-and-effect analysis. *Analytic* studies attempt to quantify the relationship between two factors, usually between an exposure or intervention (for example, early goal-directed therapy) and an outcome (mortality). Analytic studies can be either *observational* or *experimental*. The major types of study designs within these categories are summarized in Table 1.[3,4]

4. **Discussion and conclusion**

What are the limitations to this study?

The methods and results should allow you to recognize the study's main limitations, especially as you identify the study design. The discussion should acknowledge these limitations explicitly, with the authors' comments. Every study faces a tension between generalizability and reliability. To be generalizable, a study needs to represent the real world; it needs to include patients with comorbidities and poor compliance in a variety of practice patterns. With all of those unknown variables, however, the study is at risk for confounders (see Box 1). To reduce confounders, authors try to make the population and study setting as restricted as possible. This makes it less likely that unknown confounders are impacting the outcome, but it also makes the study results less generalizable. These limitations are understandable and unavoidable, but they are important to identify when deciding if a study applies to your patients.

Confounder:
Some unmeasured factor that may confuse the true relationship you are interested in measuring.

Classic Example:
Smoking causes lung cancer. Smokers are more likely to drink. A study evaluating the association of alcohol with lung cancer could conclude that alcohol causes lung cancer. Smoking is the confounding variable that is confusing the relationship between alcohol and lung cancer. (Figure 1)

Where do the authors think the field is headed?

The discussion section will also help you understand the authors' views of the paper's relevance. They will usually explain how the results of the paper can change the field, and identify open questions that can drive further research. It is worth noting that the discussion section gives you only the author's opinions. Often, for a large clinical trial or particularly interesting paper, other researchers and clinicians will share their opinions as well. Many of the articles in this book sparked letters to the editor or even editorials within the same journal issue. When you access an article on a journal's website, "related articles" will almost always appear on the top or side margin. These related articles often include letters to the editor, editorials, or commentaries that can give you some understanding of how the study was received by other experts in the field. For example, the Rivers Trial on early goal-directed therapy for septic shock was published in the November 8, 2001 issue of the *New England Journal of Medicine* (*NEJM*). In that same issue, an editorial was published on hemodynamic and metabolic therapy in critically ill patients that provides significant context and critique of the Rivers Trial.[5]

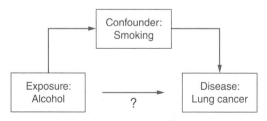

FIGURE 1. Impact of a confounder on the perceived relationship between exposure and disease.

Will this change my practice?

The final question to ask of any clinical study is whether the results of this study change or confirm your practice. All of the questions you ask yourself throughout the article culminate in this decision. As a result of this trial, will you prescribe (or stop prescribing) a drug? Will you change the way you perform a procedure? Will you continue to require a certain imaging test, or stop requiring an unnecessary test? This is the clinical judgment call every practicing surgeon makes: When reading a new study, how will you integrate the information into your existing knowledge base, and what choices will you make for your patients? This is our obligation as clinicians, and the fundamental reason why literature searches, journal articles, and evidence-based practice is so important.

REFERENCES

1. Blakely ML et al. Early vs interval appendectomy for children with perforated appendicitis. *Arch Surg.* 2011;146(6):660–665.

2. Popadich A et al. A multicenter cohort study of total thyroidectomy and routine central lymph node dissection for cN0 papillary thyroid cancer. *Surgery.* 2011;150(6):1048–1057.

3. Oxford Univ *Study Designs.* University of Oxford; 2016.

4. Sainani KL, Popat RA. Understanding study design. *Phys Med Rehab.* 2011;3(6):573–577 (PubMed PMID: 21665169).

5. Evans TW. Hemodynamic and metabolic therapy in critically ill patients. *NEJM.* 2001;345(19):1417–1418 (PubMed PMID: 11794176).

Essential Articles

Trauma Surgery

Amy Fiedler • Dante Yeh

Trauma is the oldest surgical subspecialty. Prehistoric evidence demonstrates early techniques for suturing lacerations, performing amputations, and setting fractures. Trephined skulls hint at early surgical attempts to relieve intracranial pressure after traumatic brain injury. The oldest known treatise on trauma care, the Edwin Smith Papyrus, dates back to 1600 BC and consists of 48 case descriptions of injuries. Such archaeological evidence reveals that ancient civilizations, from the Egyptians, to the Babylonyians, to the Mayans, treated wounds sustained from hand-to-hand and projectile-based combat.

Advancements in trauma care have closely paralleled technological advances on the battlefield. Ambulances were first introduced during the Siege of Malaga in 1487. Ambroise Paré first described the use of ligatures for hemostasis during his term as a military surgeon in 16th-century France. The practice of triage was developed during the Napoleonic Wars in the early 19th century, and the association of aggressive fluid resuscitation with pulmonary failure was described during the Vietnam Conflict. The Gulf Wars enhanced our understanding of massive transfusion ratios, management of traumatic brain injury, and tourniquet use. As weapons evolved with the invention of gunpowder and mechanized transportation, so evolved the understanding of blast injury and polysystem trauma.

In the civilian sector, research has historically consisted of expert opinion and single-center case series. High-quality studies on injured patients are extremely difficult to conduct, due to barriers to informed consent in the emergent setting, poor patient follow-up, and other methodological issues. However, in the past few decades, professional organizations such as the American Association for the Surgery of Trauma (AAST), the Eastern Association for the Surgery of Trauma (EAST), and the Western Trauma Association (WTA) have made great strides in organizing multicenter trials to enrich the quality of the trauma literature. This expanding evidence has steadily invalidated prior surgical dogma. In this chapter, we present several benchmark trials that have dramatically contributed to the trauma surgery literature. As the field of trauma surgery encompasses not only traumatology but also emergency surgery and surgical critical care, the importance of these trials spans multiple disciplines, and should influence the practices of trauma surgeons, general surgeons, and surgical intensivists alike.

a. NEXUS C-Spine Criteria

Validity of a set of clinical criteria to rule out injury to the cervical spine in patients with blunt trauma.

Hoffman JR, Mower WR, Wolfson AB, Todd KH, Zucker MI, National Emergency X-Radiography Utilization Study Group

NEJM 2000 Jul;343(2):94–99.

SYNOPSIS

Takeaway Point: A decision instrument based on a set of five clinical criteria can help identify a subset of patients who, after blunt trauma, are at extremely low risk for cervical injury and can safely forego cervical spine (c-spine) imaging.

Commentary: The authors present the results of a large, multicenter observational study on imaging of the cervical spine after blunt trauma. The decision instrument identifies five criteria that patients must meet following blunt trauma that, if met, identifies them as "low risk" for cervical spine injury. These five criteria are straightforward, and based on the results of this study, highly sensitive for diagnosing cervical spine injury. Utilizing this clinical decision instrument may significantly decrease costs and exposure to ionizing radiation by avoiding cervical spine imaging in low-risk blunt trauma patients. The Canadian c-spine rule[1] is another decision instrument that attempts to limit the amount of radiographs of the c-spine obtained after blunt trauma, which has a potentially lower sensitivity but higher specificity. American trauma centers tend to use the NEXUS criteria preferentially.

ANALYSIS

Introduction: Clinicians fear missing a cervical spine injury in a blunt trauma patient. For this reason, radiographs of the cervical spine are obtained for nearly every patient who presents after blunt trauma. A decision instrument based on five clinical criteria has been proposed to identify patients with a low probability of injury who therefore do not require radiographs of the cervical spine following blunt trauma. Sample size limitations have previously prevented widespread adoption of this decision instrument.

Objective: The National Emergency X-Radiography Utilization Study (NEXUS) was designed to validate this decision instrument and to test the hypothesis that patients with blunt trauma who meet all five criteria have a very low probability of clinically significant injury to the cervical spine.

Methods
Trial Design: Prospective observational study.
Participants
Inclusion Criteria: All patients with blunt trauma who underwent radiography of the cervical spine in the emergency department.

Exclusion Criteria: Patients with penetrating trauma and those who underwent cervical spine imaging for any reason unrelated to trauma, or patients without imaging.

Intervention: Observational study; a physician completed a data form to document presence or absence of the five clinical criteria: (1) absence of tenderness at the posterior midline of the cervical spine, (2) normal level of alertness, (3) no focal neurologic deficits, (4) no evidence of intoxication, and (5) no distracting injuries. Decision to proceed with radiography was made entirely at the discretion of the clinician.

Endpoints: To determine, within a confidence interval of 0.5%, the sensitivity of the decision instrument.

Sample Size: 34,069 patients were included in the study from 21 centers across the United States.

Statistical Analysis: Sample size calculation, sensitivity and specificity, negative and positive predictive value.

Results

Baseline Data: Patients ranged in age from <1 year to 101; 2.5% were under 8 years of age. Demographics were otherwise not reported.

Outcomes: 34,069 patients who sustained blunt trauma underwent cervical spine radiography. Of these patients, 818 (2.4%) had radiographically demonstrated cervical spine injury. The decision instrument yielded a false negative for 8 of the 818 patients with radiographically documented c-spine injury. 576 patients met predetermined criteria for a clinically significant c-spine injury, and of these two were cleared as "low risk" by the instrument. One patient who was judged low risk did require operative intervention for a laminal fracture. For all injuries, the sensitivity of the clinical criteria is 99% and negative predictive value (NPV) is 99.8%; for clinically significant injuries, the sensitivity is 99.6% and the NPV 99.9%. With the decision instrument criteria, 4309 patients (12.6%) could have been spared radiographic evaluation.

Discussion

Conclusion: This prospective, multicenter study confirms the validity and utility of a decision instrument based on five clinical criteria for identifying patients who, after blunt trauma, have a low probability of having sustained an injury to the cervical spine.

Limitations: This study included all patients with blunt trauma who were evaluated in the emergency department. Most of these patients were of low acuity and would not have triggered trauma activation. The documented rate of cervical spine injury is 2–3 times greater, or nearly 6%, in patients with higher acuity. Additionally, the study is observational, so it is possible that some patients who met the decision instrument criteria did not have cervical radiographs obtained and were therefore not included in the study. The study included all ages and did not control for any demographic information.

---

b. Penetrating Colon Injuries

Penetrating colon injuries requiring resection: Diversion or primary anastomosis? An AAST prospective multicenter study.

Demetriades D, Murray JA, Chan L, Ordoñez C, Bowley D, Nagy KK, Cornwell EE III, Velmahos GC, Muñoz N, Hatzitheofilou C, Rodriguez A, Cornejo C, Davis KA, Namias N, Wisner DH, Ivatury RR, Moore EE, Acosta JA, Maull KI, Thomason MH, Spain DA, Committee on Multicenter Clinical Trials

J Trauma. 2001 May;50(5):765–775.

SYNOPSIS

Takeaway Point: The surgical management of penetrating colon injury (primary anastomosis vs. diversion) does not affect the incidence of abdominal complications.

Commentary: The authors prospectively studied management and subsequent outcomes of patients with penetrating colon injury requiring resection from 19 trauma centers in an observational cohort. They compared patients who received primary anastomosis with those who were diverted, and identified risk factors for colon-related abdominal complications. They found that abdominal complications after penetrating colon injury are unrelated to surgical management (primary anastomosis vs. diversion). This is an observational trial, and the groups were not balanced; sicker patients were more likely to receive a diversion. Despite the authors' recommendations to attempt primary repair for all traumatic colon injuries, the conclusive data to support this recommendation are not yet available. This trial does provide compelling rationale for a potential randomized trial in the future.

ANALYSIS

Introduction: The optimal management of patients who have penetrating colonic injuries requiring resection is poorly defined because of the fairly small number of patients at any one center who require resection.

Objective: To evaluate the safety of primary anastomosis or diversion and identify independent risk factors for the development of colon related abdominal complications.

Methods

Trial Design: Observational multicenter prospective study.

Participants

Inclusion Criteria: Penetrating colon injuries requiring resection.

Exclusion Criteria: Patients with rectal injuries and all deaths occurring within 3 days of admission.

Intervention: Observational trial; surgical methods and antibiotic prophylaxis were surgeon's preference.

Endpoints: Colon-related mortality, colon-related abdominal complications (anastomotic leak, intra-abdominal abscess or peritonitis, fascial dehiscence, and colon obstruction or necrosis), ICU and hospital stay.

Sample Size: 297 patients from 19 institutions between December 1998 and July 2000.

Statistical Analysis: χ^2 test or two-tailed Fisher exact test, Wilcoxon rank sum test, Kruskal–Wallis test.

Results

Baseline Data: Mean age was 28.6 years, 93% of patients were men; 97% of injuries from gunshot wounds. Overall, 197 patients were managed with primary repair and anastomosis and 100 with diversion. There was a significantly higher incidence of delayed operation (>6 hours), shock at admission, left colon injury, small-bowel and liver injuries, blood transfusion requirements, and severe fecal contamination in the diversion group. The diversion group received significantly longer duration of antibiotics.

Outcomes: Overall colon-related mortality was 1.3% (four deaths), all in the diversion group. Overall incidence of abdominal complication was 22% after primary repair and 27% after diversion (p 0.37). Multivariate analysis identified three independent risk factors for abdominal complications: severe peritoneal contamination, >4 units of blood in the first 24 hours, and single-agent antibiotic prophylaxis. Average ICU stay was longer in the diversion group (3.7 days vs. 7.4 days) but this did not reach statistical significance (p 0.08), and overall hospital stay was similar (p 0.13).

Discussion

Conclusion: For penetrating colon injuries requiring resection, performing primary anastomosis versus diversion is not associated with the incidence of colon-related abdominal complications.

Limitations: As this is a prospective observational study with confounding variables, data presented are class II evidence and lack randomization. The clinical decision to perform a primary anastomosis versus diversion was likely related to patient factors, including the noted difference in baseline comorbidities between the two groups, with the diversion group being significantly sicker.

---

c. Management Guidelines for Penetrating Abdominal Trauma

Management of patients with anterior abdominal wall stab wounds: A Western Trauma Association multicenter trial.

Biffl WL, Kaups KL, Cothren CC, Brasel KJ, Dicker RA, Bullard MK, Haan JM, Jurkovich GJ, Harrison P, Moore FO, Schreiber M, Knudson MM, Moore EE

J Trauma. 2009 May; 66(5):1294–1301.

SYNOPSIS

Takeaway Point: Stable, asymptomatic patients with anterior abdominal stab wounds can be safely observed for symptoms of bleeding or hollow viscus injury, rather than proceeding to immediate exploratory laparotomy.

Commentary: The authors present a large, prospective observational study evaluating multiple techniques for assessing the hemodynamically stable patient with an anterior abdominal stab wound. They conclude that unless peritonitis, shock, or evisceration is present, an immediate exploratory laparotomy is *not* indicated. A number of additional studies and observation modalities are detailed in order to assist in the management of these patients to minimize resource utilization and the prevalence of nontherapeutic exploratory laparotomy. A large, prospective multicenter trial detailing the resource utilization of this approach is warranted.

ANALYSIS

Introduction: Patients with penetrating abdominal stab wounds who present with shock, peritonitis, or evisceration require exploratory laparotomy as a lifesaving surgical intervention. Other patients presenting with anterior abdominal stab wounds are hemodynamically stable and asymptomatic. The care of these patients is less well defined, and management remains controversial.

Objective: The purpose of this multicenter study was to evaluate the clinical course of patients managed by the various strategies, to determine whether there are differences in associated non-therapeutic laparotomy, emergency department discharge, or complication rates.

Methods

Trial Design: Observational multicenter prospective cohort study.

Participants

Inclusion Criteria: Age ≥ 16 with anterior abdominal stab wound, defined as that area bordered by the costal margin superiorly, the groin creases inferiorly, and the anterior axillary lines laterally.

Exclusion Criteria: Patients with back, flank, or presumed thoracoabdominal wounds, pregnancy, incarceration.

Intervention: No aspect of management was dictated by the study.

Endpoints: Hospital discharge, emergency department discharge.

Sample Size: 359 patients from 11 institutions between 2006 and 2007.

Statistical Analysis: Sensitivity, specificity, NPV, PPV.

Results

Baseline Data: 318 men and 41 women, mean age 33.4 years. 121 patients had two or more wounds.

Outcomes: 81 patients underwent immediate exploratory laparotomy, of which 68 (84%) were therapeutic. Of patients who were discharged from the emergency department, the decision was made by local wound exploration in 23%, CT scan in 21%, and diagnostic peritoneal lavage (DPL) in 18%. Exploratory laparotomy based on results from CT, local wound exploration, and DPL were nontherapeutic in 57%, 24%, and 31% of patients. 12% of patients who were admitted for serial clinical examinations underwent exploratory laparotomy, of which 33% were found to be nontherapeutic. There was no apparent morbidity due to delay in intervention. The authors compared CT scan, serial clinical assessments, focused assessment with sonography for trauma (FAST), DPL, and local wound exploration for predictive value. Local wound exploration and serial exams have 100% sensitivity, with 54% and 96% specificity, respectively. FAST has 21% sensitivity.

Discussion

Conclusion: Shock, evisceration, and peritonitis require immediate exploratory laparotomy after anterior abdominal stab wound. Patients without these findings may be safely observed for signs and symptoms of bleeding or hollow viscous injury.

Limitation: Morbidity following observation for asymptomatic patients is not clearly defined. No safety or cost-effectiveness data are provided. This is a purely observational study.

---

d. Prehospital RSI for TBI

Prehospital rapid sequence intubation improves functional outcome for patients with severe traumatic brain injury: A randomized controlled trial.

Bernard SA, Nguyen V, Cameron P, Masci K, Fitzgerald M, Cooper DJ, Walker T, Std BP, Myles P, Murray L, David T, Smith K, Patrick I, Edington J, Bacon A, Rosenfeld JV, Judson R

Ann Surg. 2010 Dec; 252(6):959–965.

SYNOPSIS

Takeaway Point: Prehospital rapid-sequence intubation (RSI) is associated with favorable neurological outcomes at 6 months post-trauma when compared to intubation on arrival at the hospital.

Commentary: Patients with severe traumatic brain injury (TBI) frequently require endotracheal intubation for airway protection to prevent hypoxia. Paramedics intubate many of these patients in the field. This randomized controlled trial evaluated the impact of prehospital intubation versus intubation in the hospital on neurologic outcomes at 6 months. Results demonstrate that in adults with severe TBI, RSI in the prehospital setting by paramedics increases the rate of favorable neurologic outcomes at 6 months compared with intubation in the hospital. While the trial design has sparked some controversy, including the question of whether neurologic recovery at 6 months was too far removed to reasonably link to timing of intubation, this trial has changed the standard of care and practice. Most paramedics are now confident in performing rapid sequence intubation with monitoring of end tidal carbon dioxide.

ANALYSIS

Introduction: There is a high morbidity and mortality associated with severe traumatic brain injury (TBI). In many areas, paramedics perform endotracheal intubation prior to hospital arrival without premedication. Observational studies have suggested that prehospital intubation may worsen outcomes.

Objective: To determine whether paramedic rapid-sequence intubation in patients with severe traumatic brain injury improves neurologic outcomes at 6 months compared with intubation in the hospital.

Methods
Trial Design: Prospective, randomized controlled trial.
Participants
Inclusion Criteria: Evidence of head trauma, Glasgow Coma Score (GCS) ≤9, age ≥15 years, and intact airway reflexes as documented by paramedic first responders.

Exclusion Criteria: Located within 10 minutes of a designated trauma hospital, no intravenous access, allergy to any of the rapid sequence intubation drugs, or transport by medical helicopter.

Intervention: Patients were randomized to either paramedic intubation (after preoxygenation and administration of fentanyl, midazolam, and succinylcholine), or hospital intubation (with high-flow supplemental oxygen by mask or assisted bag-mask ventilation if required).

Endpoints

Primary Endpoint: Median extended Glasgow Outcome Scale (GOS) at 6 months.

Secondary Endpoint: Favorable versus unfavorable outcome at 6 months, length of ICU and hospital stay, survival to hospital discharge.

Sample Size: 312 patients were randomized between April 2004 and January 2008 in four Australian cities, 160 to paramedic intubation and 152 to hospital intubation.

Statistical Analysis: Analysis of the principal outcome at 6 months was performed using a Mann Whitney U test. Additional results are expressed as risk ratios with 95% confidence intervals and compared using χ^2 test of independence.

Results

Baseline Data: Baseline characteristics were well distributed among the two groups, including age, mechanism of injury, initial GCS, and degree of intracranial injury on first CT scan.

Outcomes: A higher incidence of favorable neurologic outcome at 6 months was seen in the prehospital intubation patients compared with hospital intubation patients (51% vs. 39%, p 0.046). Median GOS, the primary outcome, was not different between the two groups (p 0.28). There was no difference in outcomes between the groups based on initial GCS 3–4 compared with initial GCS 5–9. There was no difference in survival.

Discussion

Conclusion: Patients with severe TBI should undergo prehospital intubation using a rapid-sequence approach in order to increase the likelihood of a favorable neurological outcome at 6 months.

Limitations: Study design did not allow for blinding of the paramedic personnel and hospital physicians for treatment allocation that may have affected management.

---

e. Blunt Traumatic Occult Pneumothorax: Is Observation Safe?

Blunt traumatic occult pneumothorax: Is observation safe?—Results of a prospective, AAST multicenter study.

Moore FO, Goslar PW, Coimbra R, Velmahos G, Brown CV, Coopwood TB Jr, Lottenberg L, Phelan HA, Bruns BR, Sherck JP, Norwood SH, Barnes SL, Matthews MR, Hoff WS, de Moya MA, Bansal V, Hu CK, Karmy-Jones RC, Vinces F, Pembaur K, Notrica DM, Haan JM

J Trauma. 2011 May;70(5):1019–1023.

SYNOPSIS

Takeaway Point: Most patients with occult pneumothorax can be managed with observation alone. Progression of pneumothorax and respiratory distress are independent risk factors associated with failure of observation.

Commentary: Rib fractures and pneumothoraces are the most common chest injuries in patients with blunt trauma. A significant number of pneumothoraces cannot be identified with chest radiograph alone; however, the identification of an occult pneumothorax on CT scan presents a diagnostic dilemma. Observation alone carries the risk of progression to symptomatic (and rarely, life-threatening) pneumothorax, while tube thoracostomy has a significant risk of iatrogenic injury and can prolong hospital stay. In this multicenter observational study, blunt trauma patients with occult pneumothorax managed with observation had a 6% failure rate, with no difference in mortality between the successful and unsuccessful observational cohorts. Importantly, the majority of "failures" were due to enlargement on serial x-rays without respiratory compromise. Future studies may consider higher thresholds for tube thoracostomy based on actual need rather than prophylaxis for perceived need.

ANALYSIS

Introduction: *Occult pneumothorax* (OPTX) is defined as a pneumothorax diagnosed on CT scan that was not identified on chest radiograph, and occurs in 2–15% of blunt trauma patients. The management of patients with occult pneumothorax remains poorly defined, and ranges from observation to tube thoracostomy.

Objective: The goal of this multicenter study was to assess the management strategies of OPTXs in level I and II trauma centers, and to determine which clinical factors predicted failure of observation.

Methods
Trial Design: Observational multicenter prospective study.
Participants
Inclusion Criteria: All patients of all ages with blunt trauma with an occult pneumothorax.
Exclusion Criteria: Pneumothorax identified on initial chest radiography.
Intervention: Observational study.

Endpoints: ICU length of stay, hospital length of stay (LOS), ventilator days, mortality, complications.

Sample Size: 569 patients at 16 trauma centers with 588 occult pneumothoraces.

Statistical Analysis: Student's t-test, Fisher's exact or χ^2 test, Mann–Whitney U test, multiple logistic regression analysis.

Results

Baseline Data: 121 patients were managed with immediate tube thoracostomy; 448 patients were observed.

Outcomes: Of 448 patients in the observation group, 27 patients failed and required tube thoracostomy for progression of pneumothorax, respiratory distress, or hemothorax. 14% failed observation while on positive-pressure ventilation. Patients who failed observation were significantly more likely to be on positive-pressure ventilation (37% vs. 16%, p 0.005), although positive-pressure ventilation was not an independent risk factor for failure in a multivariate analysis. There was no difference in injury severity score or number of rib fractures between the successful and unsuccessful observational cohorts. Mortality among successful and failed observation groups was similar, with the majority of deaths due to traumatic brain injury.

Discussion

Conclusion: Most blunt trauma patients with occult pneumothorax may be monitored closely without tube thoracostomy. Progression of pneumothorax and respiratory distress are independently associated with observation failure.

Limitations: This study is a prospective observational study, so clinical decisions introduce the possibility of selection bias. Very little data are presented on the patients treated with immediate tube thoracostomy, so risks and benefits of that option are not explored.

---

f. Management of Posttraumatic Retained Hemothorax

Management of post-traumatic retained hemothorax: A prospective, observational, multicenter AAST study.

DuBose J, Inaba K, Demetriades D, Scalea TM, O'Connor J, Menaker J, Morales C, Konstantinidis A, Shiflett A, Copwood B, AAST Retained Hemothorax Study Group

J Trauma Acute Care Surg. 2012 Jan;72(1):11–24.

SYNOPSIS

Takeaway Point: Retained hemothorax after trauma is associated with high rates of empyema and pneumonia. Video-assisted thoracoscopic surgery (VATS) has a high success rate for evacuation and clearance, although optimal timing and indications remain unclear.

Commentary: The authors of this large, multicenter prospective observational study enrolled trauma patients who had a tube thoracostomy performed within 24 hours after trauma admission with subsequent retained hemothorax. Patients were most likely to be observed successfully if the volume of retained hemothorax was <300 cm^3 as estimated on CT scan. VATS has a high success rate for preventing empyema; however, 25% of patients required more than one procedure and 20% required thoracotomy to effectively clear the retained hemothorax. This observational study provides several potential factors that can be used to predict success or failure of a conservative approach to retained hemothorax. Further research is needed before these data can be used to create a decision tool, which could be tested in a prospective fashion, in order to understand how these results can change practice.

ANALYSIS

Introduction: The natural history of retained hemothorax (RH) following trauma is unknown. Prior studies have identified RH as a risk factor for empyema, but recognition and treatment of this entity are still a matter of debate.

Objective: The objective of this study was twofold: to define practice patterns across trauma centers for the management of retained hemothorax following trauma, and to identify predictors of the need for thoracotomy.

Methods

Trial Design: Observational multicenter prospective study.

Participants

Inclusion Criteria: Posttraumatic retained hemothorax with tube thoracostomy within 24 hours of admission and a subsequent CT scan demonstrating retained hemothorax after initial placement.

Exclusion Criteria: Patients undergoing thoracotomy before tube thoracostomy.

Intervention: Observational study, all interventions at the discretion of the providers.

Endpoints

Primary Endpoint: Need for thoracotomy.

Secondary Endpoints: Successful utilization of less invasive management approaches for RH, correlation between CT scan estimation of RH volume, and results of operative evacuation.

Sample Size: 328 patients from 20 participating institutions in the United States, Canada, and South America between 2009 and 2011.

Statistical Analysis: χ^2 test with Yates correction, Fisher's exact test, Student's t-test, logistic regression model, Pearson–Moment correlation coefficient, and square correlation coefficient.

Results

Baseline Data: Mean age was 38.6, 86.6% of patients were male, and 33.8% of patients suffered critical injuries (ISS >25). The majority of initial thoracostomy tubes (65.5%) were placed in the emergency department.

Outcomes: VATS was the most commonly performed initial procedure in 110 of 328 patients. Thoracotomy was ultimately performed in 73 patients. 101 patients were initially managed with observation alone; of these, 18 required additional interventions. 120 patients required two or more procedures to either clear the retained hemothorax or a subsequently developed empyema. Patients who were successfully observed without further intervention were more likely to have RH ≤300 cm³ (80% vs. 54%, p <0.0001), rib fractures (64% vs. 51%, p 0.04), and to have been treated with a smaller (<34 french) thoracostomy tube size. RH volume <300 cm³ was the strongest independent predictor of successful observation (OR 3.7, p <0.001). Overall empyema and pneumonia rates for RH patients were 26.8% and 19.5%, respectively.

Discussion

Conclusion: Retained hemothorax following traumatic injuries carries a high rate of empyema and pneumonia. VATS has been demonstrated to be the initial procedure of choice for management; however, the optimal timing is not yet defined. RH volume ≤300 cm³ was the best predictor of successful management with tube thoracostomy alone.

Limitations: Practice style and ubiquity of CT scanning of the chest in centers may be selective for patients with quite small amounts of hemothorax that would have been missed on conventional chest radiography. Justification for CT scan in this setting is not clear. No data presented on duration of chest tubes.

g. Resuscitative Thoracotomy

Western Trauma Association critical decisions in trauma: Resuscitative thoracotomy.

Burlew CC, Moore EE, Moore FA, Coimbra R, McIntyre RC Jr, Davis JW, Sperry J, Biffl WL

J Trauma Acute Care Surg. 2012 Dec;73(6):1359–1363.

SYNOPSIS

Takeaway Point: Resuscitative thoracotomy has the highest success in patients who have sustained penetrating cardiac wounds, and outcome is extremely poor (1–2% survival) when performed for blunt-force trauma. Resuscitative thoracotomy should be reserved for blunt-force trauma patients who have less than 10 minutes of prehospital CPR and penetrating trauma patients with less than 15 minutes of prehospital CPR.

Commentary: Resuscitative thoracotomy has a long history of use in the trauma population. Over the course of the past three decades, there has been a paradigm shift toward a more selective use of resuscitative thoracotomy. It is unlikely that a prospective, randomized control trial will ever be performed in this patient population, so the Western Trauma Association (WTA) created the present algorithm for resuscitative thoracotomy in the trauma patient based on the best available observational and retrospective studies and expert opinions. They found that the use of resuscitative thoracotomy is most successful in trauma patients who have penetrating cardiac injury and quite poor in those patients who present in shock from blunt trauma.

ANALYSIS

Introduction: There has never been a published randomized clinical trial looking at the performance of resuscitative thoracotomy (RT). There has been a clinical shift away from the use of resuscitative thoracotomy in the trauma patient population over the past three decades, but no algorithm exists to guide clinical indications.

Objective: To create a bedside reference for clinicians to guide the use of RT in the trauma patient on the basis of the best available clinical evidence.

Methods
Trial Design: Literature query and expert opinion.
Participants: Not defined.

Intervention: Indications for resuscitative thoracotomy include the following: CPR with no signs of life (blunt-force trauma with <10 minutes of prehospital CPR, penetrating torso trauma patients with <15 minutes of CPR), or patients in profound, refractory shock.

Endpoints: Mortality.

Sample Size: Not applicable.

Statistical Analysis: Not applicable.

Results

Outcomes: Resuscitative thoracotomy was successful in 35% of patients with penetrating cardiac wounds, and 15% for all patients with penetrating wounds. Outcomes are poor for patients who undergo resuscitative thoracotomy after blunt trauma, with a 2% success rate for patients in shock and a 1% survival for patients with absent vital signs.

Discussion

Conclusion: Patients in profound refractory shock or who are undergoing CPR on arrival to the hospital should be stratified according to the algorithm presented based on transport time and injury to determine the utility of resuscitative thoracotomy.

Limitations: The algorithm presented is based on literature review and expert opinion. It is not level I evidence. There are a variety of provider, institutional, and situational factors that may confound the usefulness of the presented algorithm.

---

h. PROMMTT Study

The prospective, observational, multicenter, major trauma transfusion (PROMMTT) study: Comparative effectiveness of a time-varying treatment with competing risks.

Holcomb JB, del Junco DJ, Fox EE, Wade CE, Cohen MJ, Schreiber MA, Alarcon LH, Bai Y, Brasel KJ, Bulger EM, Cotton BA, Matijevic N, Muskat P, Myers JG, Phelan HA, White CE, Zhang J, Rahbar MH, PROMMTT Study Group

JAMA Surg. 2013 Feb;148(2):127–136.

SYNOPSIS

Takeaway Point: Higher plasma: RBC and platelet: RBC ratios early in resuscitation are associated with decreased mortality in adult trauma patients.

Commentary: This prospective cohort study documents the timing and component ratios of transfusions during active resuscitation for adult trauma patients. The authors attempted to correlate hospital mortality with early transfusion of either low, moderate, or high plasma: RBC and platelet: RBC ratios. They found that transfusion of a higher (≥1:1) platelets/plasma to RBC ratio early in resuscitation was associated with decreased 6-hour mortality. After 24 hours, plasma and platelet ratios were found to be unassociated with mortality. It is important to note that while this was an observational trial and the characteristics of the three groups were not balanced, PROMMTT represents an important step toward understanding the influence of transfusion ratio on outcomes in bleeding trauma patients. The debate regarding an ideal transfusion strategy is still ongoing, and was further addressed in the PROPPR trial in 2015 (see **j**, below).

ANALYSIS

Introduction: Hemorrhagic shock is a leading cause of potentially preventable death in the trauma population. *Damage control resuscitation* is a concept initially described by the military and entails early and aggressive transfusion of platelets, plasma, and RBC in a 1:1:1 ratio to reconstitute whole blood for hemorrhaging patients. Conflicting findings have been associated with this transfusion strategy, where observational studies are particularly at risk for survival bias.

Objective: To relate in-hospital mortality to early transfusion of plasma and/or platelets and to time-varying plasma:RBC and platelet:RBC ratios.

Methods
Trial Design: Multicenter prospective cohort study.
Participants
Inclusion Criteria: Age >16, requiring the highest level of trauma activation, and receiving a transfusion of *at least* 3 units of RBCs in the first hours after admission.

Exclusion Criteria: Transfer from other facilities, declared dead within 30 minutes of admission, have received more than five rounds of cardiopulmonary resuscitation prior to or within 30 minutes of admission, prisoners, burn injury of >20% total body surface area, inhalation injury as diagnosed on bronchoscopy, or pregnancy.

Intervention: Observational trial; cohort was divided into three groups based on plasma:RBC and platelet:RBC transfusion ratios (low, <1:2; moderate, 1:1–1:2; or high, >1:1)

Endpoints: In-hospital mortality.

Sample Size: 1245 trauma patients from 10 US level 1 trauma centers were evaluated; of these, 905 received a transfusion of ≥ 3 units of blood.

Statistical Analysis: Sample size calculations, Cox analysis, purposeful variable selection strategy.

Results

Baseline Data: Analyzed patients were 76% male, with median age of 37. Bleeding site was most commonly limbs (36.9%) or abdomen (35.4%). Baseline characteristics were not compared between transfusion groups.

Outcomes: There was significant variability in plasma: RBC and platelet: RBC ratios during the first 24 hours. Increased plasma: RBC and platelet: RBC ratios were independently associated with decreased 6-hour mortality. In the first 6 hours, patients were less likely to die if ratios were 1:1 or higher. Beyond the first 24-hour period, the ratio of plasma and platelets was not associated with mortality.

Discussion

Conclusion: Plasma and platelet to RBC ratios of 1:1 or higher early in the resuscitation of bleeding adult trauma patients requiring transfusion of at least 3 units of RBC is associated with decreased mortality in the first 6 hours. After 24 hours, the risk of death is not associated with plasma or platelet ratios.

Limitations: Most of the patients evaluated in the PROMMTT trial had blunt trauma and not penetrating trauma. Additionally, patients who died within 30 minutes of arrival were excluded from the analysis, which may indicate survivor bias. During the first 24 hours it should be noted that there was quite a bit of "catchup" with respect to transfusions, meaning that there was not a consistent transfusion ratio during the first 24 hours. Finally, this is an observational trial and no data are presented comparing baseline characteristics between the three observed groups. The impact of potential confounders cannot be assessed.

---

i. Surgical Management of Penetrating Liver Injury

A comprehensive five-step surgical management approach to penetrating liver injuries that require complex repair.

Ordoñez CA, Parra MW, Salamea JC, Puyana JC, Millán M, Badiel M, Sanjuán J, Pino LF, Scavo D, Botache W, Ferrada R

J Trauma Acute Care Surg. 2013 Aug;75(2):207–211.

SYNOPSIS

Takeaway Point: Patients who have sustained penetrating liver injury require emergent laparotomy for hemorrhage control, and when bleeding cannot be controlled with Pringle maneuver and packing, patients should undergo immediate intrahepatic exploration and direct vessel ligation.

Commentary: This single institution case series describes a five-step surgical approach for patients with penetrating liver injury. Over a period of eight years, 538 patients were operated on for thoracoabdominal trauma. Of these, 88 met American Association for the Surgery of Trauma-Organ Injury Scale (AAST-OIS) criteria for Grade III–V liver injury. These patients required complex techniques to achieve hemostasis such as the Pringle maneuver, perihepatic liver packing, and/or hepatotomy with selective vessel ligation. They found that patients who fail to respond to a Pringle maneuver and packing would benefit from immediate intraparenchymal exploration and selective vascular ligation. While this article presents only a single institution's experience without a comparison arm or long-term follow-up, it does provide an accessible and portable algorithm to assist in the management of these complex injuries.

ANALYSIS

Introduction: Patients with complex liver injuries following trauma have high mortality rates. The surgical management of these patients may be challenging even for the most experienced trauma surgeon. The surgical techniques employed to approach complex hepatic injuries have evolved through the years. On the basis of the authors' institutional experience, they propose a logical five-step approach to manage complicated hepatic injuries.

Objective: The objective of this study was to describe a comprehensive five-step surgical management approach for patients with penetrating liver trauma based on one institution's experience.

Methods
Trial Design: Single-institution case series.
Participants
Inclusion Criteria: All patients with penetrating trauma to the torso inferior to the nipple line and superior to the inguinal crease.
Exclusion Criteria: Patients who did not have penetrating liver trauma.

Endpoints: Overall mortality.

Sample Size: 538 patients presented with penetrating thoracoabdominal injuries between January 2003 and December 2011 requiring operative intervention. Of these, 146 had penetrating liver injuries that required surgical management; 88 of these patients had AAST-OIS Grade III–V injury requiring complex techniques to achieve hemostasis.

Statistical Analysis: Chi square (χ^2) or Fishers Exact Test.

Results:

Outcomes: A five-step surgical approach was created:

Step 1: Identify hemodynamically unstable patients with penetrating thoracoabdominal trauma requiring surgical intervention.

Step 2: Perform a midline exploratory laparotomy and pack all four abdominal quadrants.

Step 3: Remove anterior hepatic packs and inspect the liver. Assign an injury grade based on AAST-OIS.

Step 4: If a minor hepatic laceration is identified, achieve hemostasis with compression or topical agents. In major injuries, if packing fails to control bleeding, perform a Pringle maneuver. This is diagnostic and therapeutic. If bleeding continues with a clamp on the porta hepatis, there is back-bleeding from main hepatic veins and/or retrohepatic vena cava. This defines the anatomic injury.

Step 5: With Pringle maneuver in place, expose the bleeding through finger fracture or stapling devices. Directly control the bleeding and temporarily close the abdomen. Take the patient to the ICU for continued resuscitation.

Discussion

Conclusion: Patients who have sustained penetrating liver injury require emergent laparotomy for hemorrhage control. The authors present a five-step surgical approach wherein patients in whom bleeding cannot be controlled with Pringle maneuver and packing undergo immediate intra-hepatic exploration and direct selective vessel ligation for hemorrhage control.

Limitations: This is a single-institution case series of patients who required complex surgical management of penetrating liver injury. There is no comparison arm. A larger sample size would require multi-institutional collaboration. The use of angioembolization as an adjunct procedure has been demonstrated in various other trauma cohorts in patients with hepatic injury classified as AAST-OIS Grades IV and V; however, this was not an employed technique in this study.

j. PROPPR Study

Transfusion of plasma, platelets, and red blood cells in a 1:1:1 vs a 1:1:2 ratio and mortality in patients with severe trauma.

Holcomb JB, Tilley BC, Baraniuk S, Fox EE, Wade CE, Podbielski JM, del Junco DJ, Brasel KJ, Bulger EM, Callcut RA, Cohen MJ, Cotton BA, Fabian TC, Inaba K, Kerby JD, Muskat P, O'Keeffe T, Rizoli S, Robinson BRH, Scalea TM, Schreiber MA, Stein DM, Weinberg JA, Callum JL, Hess JR, Matijevic N, Miller CN, Pittet JF, Hoyt DB, Pearson GD, Leroux B, van Belle G, PROPPR Study Group

JAMA. 2015 Feb;313(5):471–482.

SYNOPSIS

Takeaway Point: For critically injured trauma patients, there is no difference in 24-hour or 30-day mortality with transfusion of plasma, platelets, and red blood cells in a 1:1:1 or 1:1:2 ratio.

Commentary: The majority of trials examining the ideal blood product ratio have been small, single-institution, and observational. The best available data comes from the PROMMTT study (see PROMMTT, above), a large, multicenter cohort study that demonstrated that most trauma patients actually receive blood products in a 1:1:1 or 1:1:2 transfusion ratio, with a potential survival advantage to higher proportion of plasma and platelets. The PROPPR study group sought to compare a 1:1:1 and 1:1:2 transfusion ratio for the first time in a large, randomized, controlled trial. The study demonstrated no significant difference in mortality between the two groups, although the 1:1:1 group had a higher rate of hemostasis and lower rate of death due to exsanguination. It is worth noting that the trial was designed to detect a 10% difference in mortality rate, and the observed 4.3% reduction in mortality rate in the 1:1:1 group could represent a type II error (failure to detect a true difference) due to small sample size. Additionally, the 1:1:2 group actually received blood products in an alternating 3:0:6 and 3:6:6 ratio, and the time delay in platelet transfusion may confound hemostasis. Despite these considerations, the PROPPR trial represents a major accomplishment in the ongoing search for the ideal transfusion strategy, and raises the bar in this field beyond observational studies.

ANALYSIS

Introduction: *Damage-control resuscitation* is the early adminis-tration of plasma, platelets, and red blood cells in a 1:1:1 ratio that approximates whole blood, along with rapid correction of coagulopathy. Damage-control resuscitation has become a stan-dard of care for trauma patients, despite the fact that no random-ized clinical trial has definitely established the ideal ratio of blood products.

Objectives: To determine the effectiveness and safety of transfus-ing patients with severe trauma and major bleeding using plasma, platelets, and red blood cells in a 1:1:1 ratio compared with a 1:1:2 ratio.

Methods
Trial Design: Multi-institution, pragmatic, phase 3, randomized clinical trial.

Participants

Inclusion Criteria: Severely injured patients meeting local crite-ria for highest-level trauma activation, at least 1 unit of any blood product transfused prior to arrival or within 1 hour of admission, age ≥15 or weight ≥50 kg if age unknown, received directly from the injury scene, and predicted to receive massive transfusion.

Exclusion Criteria: Received a lifesaving intervention from an outside hospital, devastating injuries with anticipated death within 1 hour of admission, direct admission from a correctional facility, thoracotomy prior to transfusion, known pregnancy, burns >20% TBSA, suspected inhalational injury, >5 minutes CPR, known do-not-resuscitate order, enrolled in another trial, or >3 units RBC given prior to randomization.

Intervention: Within each site, patients were randomized to a 1:1:1 or 1:1:2 ratio of blood products. The 1:1:1 group began with an initial container of 6 units each of platelets, plasma, and red blood cells. The 1:1:2 group began with an initial container of 3 units plasma, no platelets, and 6 units of red blood cells; subse-quent containers had either a 3:6:6 ratio or a 3:0:6 ratio.

Endpoints
Primary Endpoint: Mortality at 24 hours and 30 days.

Secondary Endpoints: Time to hemostasis, exsanguination within the first 24 hours, exsanguination within 30 days, number and type of blood products used from randomization until hemostasis achieved, number and type of blood products used after hemostasis, incidence of major surgical procedures, complication rates, functional status at discharge of 30 days, hospital-free days, ventilator-free days, and ICU-free days.

Sample Size: 680 patients were randomized between August 2012 and December 2013 from 12 level 1 trauma centers in North America; 338 to the 1:1:1 group and 342 to the 1:1:2 group.

Statistical Analysis: Sample size calculation required 680 patients to detect a 10% difference in 24-hour mortality with 95% power. Two-sided Mantel–Haenszel test for primary analysis, intention-to-treat analysis, Cox proportional hazards model.

Results:

Baseline Data: The two groups were balanced for baseline characteristics. Median Injury Severity Score overall was 26.

Outcomes: No significant difference was seen between the 1:1:1 and 1:1:2 groups in mortality at 24 hours (12.7% vs. 17%, p 0.12) or 30 days (22.4% vs. 26.1%, p 0.26). Rates of exsanguination were significantly lower in the 1:1:1 group (9.2% vs. 14.6%, p 0.03), and more patients in the 1:1:1 group achieved hemostasis (86% vs. 78%, p 0.006). No significant difference was seen in complication rates; functional status at discharge; or hospital-free, ventilator-free, or ICU-free days.

Discussion

Conclusion: There is no difference in mortality at 24 hours or 30 days between a 1:1:1 or 1:1:2 ratio of plasma, platelet, and red blood cell transfusion for critically injured trauma patients. The 1:1:1 ratio had a higher rate of hemostasis and lower rates of exsanguination.

Limitations: The trial was powered to detect a difference of 10%; to reach statistical significance for the observed effect (4.2% difference in 24-hour mortality) would have required a much larger sample size. The 1:1:2 group did not receive platelets until 9 units of other blood products were transfused, which may confound the response to the ratio of blood products.

REFERENCE

1. Steill IG, Wells GA, Vandemheen KL, Clement CM, Lesiuk H, DeMaio VJ, et al. The Canadian c-spine rule for radiography in alert and stable trauma patients. *JAMA*. 2001;286(15):1841–1848.

4

Surgical Critical Care

Laura Mazer • Kathryn L. Butler

Critical care medicine traces its origins to the Crimean War of the 1850s, when Florence Nightingale designated a separate treatment space for the most severely wounded soldiers.[1] At this point, the emphasis was on proximity to the nursing station and a higher level of nursing care. In 1923, Dr. Walter Dandy, a student of Harvey Cushing, created one of the first surgical intensive care units when he grouped his postoperative neurosurgical patients together in the same treatment area at Johns Hopkins.[2] The original emphasis on intensive nursing care continued into World War II, with the development of "shock units" for care of the severely wounded.[1]

As medicine evolved, so did critical care. With the advent of organ system support devices, intensive nursing units transitioned into intensive therapy units. In the 1940s, iron lung wards (supplemented, where necessary, by medical students providing round-the-clock manual ventilation) supported patients with respiratory paralysis from polio. In the 1950s, hantavirus became a major cause of renal failure in Korean War soldiers, leading to the development of the first hemodialysis units. Concurrently, electrical defibrillators and transvenous cardiac pacing allowed the creation of specialized cardiac care units.[1] In the 1960s, the creation of positive-pressure machines was a crucial step in the transition from iron lung wards to ventilatory care units.[3]

The isolated support of individual systems began to merge into true, multiorgan system support with the advent of improved vital sign monitoring, point-of-care analyzers, and STAT labs. This was supplemented by organizational restructuring, creating closed units and specialization for physicians and nurses.[2] With the structure in place, major advances in treatment became possible. In particular, with critical care units in hospitals throughout the world, multi-center clinical research groups developed. These groups allowed for larger sample sizes, higher statistical power, and more rigorous and generalizable studies.[4]

Many of these studies are described in detail in the following chapter. They include the ARDSNet group in the United States, who in the 1990s and early 2000s demonstrated the benefit of low-tidal-volume ventilation for ARDS.[5] In Canada, the Canadian Critical Care Trials Group demonstrated a mortality benefit to restrictive transfusion requirements that dramatically changed standard of care and resource utilization internationally.[6] When single-center studies called into question the standard of care, as with early goal-directed therapy in the Rivers Trial,[7] multicenter groups quickly formed to confirm or contest the results.[8]

Today, critical care units represent an increasing percentage of hospital beds, and that percentage is likely to continue to rise in the next few decades.[9] Although trauma and burn surgeons dedicate their practices to critical care, surgeons in all special-ties will be increasingly called on to care for patients with sep-tic shock, hemorrhagic shock, and multiorgan system failure. Surgeons must remain informed as critical care evolves; evidence may prove common practices in the multidisciplinary, highly monitored units of today to be as outdated as the iron lung wards of yesterday.

---

a. Yang–Tobin (RSBI) Trial

A prospective study of indexes predicting the outcome of trials of weaning from mechanical ventilation.

Yang KL, Tobin MJ

NEJM. 1991;324(21):1445–1450.

SYNOPSIS

Takeaway Point: The rapid shallow breathing index (RSBI), calculated as the ratio of respiratory frequency to tidal volume, predicts success of weaning from mechanical ventilation when < 105, and failure when > 105.

Commentary: The authors evaluate two new predictive indices of success at weaning from mechanical ventilation. Overall, the ratio of respiratory frequency to tidal volume, or *rapid shallow breathing index* (RSBI), was the best predictor of weaning success. The authors determined that a cutoff point of 105 yields the highest positive and negative predictive values. In a subsequent addendum, the authors calculated likelihood ratios for RSBI as a range, rather than an absolute cutoff. They concluded that RSBI < 80 is strongly predictive of weaning success, >100 is strongly predictive of failure, and 80–100 is a borderline group. The advantages of RSBI include ease of measurement and a simple calculation for use in the clinical setting.

ANALYSIS

Introduction: Predictive indices can assist in determining safe weaning from mechanical ventilation. Traditional parameters, including minute ventilation and vital capacity, have variable predictive value. The authors proposed two new indices: rapid shallow breathing index (RSBI), a ratio of respiratory frequency to tidal volume, and the CROP index, calculated from compliance, respiratory rate, oxygenation, and maximum inspiratory pressure.

Objectives: To evaluate the predictive power of two new indices to determine readiness to wean from a ventilator.

Methods
Trial Design: Single-center, prospective cohort study.
Participants
Inclusion Criteria: On ventilator support in the medical ICU and deemed appropriate for a weaning trial by their ICU physician.

Exclusion Criteria: Surgical patients.

Intervention: The first 36 patients enrolled constituted a "training set" to calculate a threshold value for each index that best differentiated patients who failed versus those who successfully weaned. The predictive power of the chosen threshold value was then tested prospectively in the next 64 patients enrolled.

Endpoints: The primary endpoint was successful weaning, defined as sustaining spontaneous breathing for >24 hours after extubation.

Sample Size: 100 patients at a single academic institution.

Statistical Analysis: Sensitivity and specificity, positive and negative predictive values, receiver-operating-characteristic (ROC) curves.

Results

Baseline Data: 100 patients were evaluated, 46 men and 54 women. Average length of ventilator support 8.2 ±1.1 days. 60 patients were successfully weaned. 40 patients required reintubation within 24 hours for either clinical or laboratory parameters.

Outcomes: The threshold values that best discriminated between successful and unsuccessful trails of weaning were calculated. For the RSBI, a ratio of ≤105 had a sensitivity of 0.97, specificity of 0.64, positive predictive value (PPV) of 0.78, and negative predictive value (NPV) of 0.95. Overall, RSBI performed better than the CROP index or isolated respiratory parameters. Area under the ROC curve for RSBI was 0.89, significantly higher than other predictors.

Discussion

Conclusion: The predictive powers of both proposed indices are better than traditional metrics. The RSBI has the highest predictive value and is easier to calculate.

Limitations: The trial included only medical patients. Definition of weaning failure included both clinical deterioration and abnormal lab values, and the difference was not explored. PPV and NPV depend on pretest probability, while likelihood ratios are independent of pretest probability and a better assessment of a predictive index. Additionally, a single cutoff point (105) has limited real-world applicability. After a letter to the editor from Jaeschke and Guyatt[10] making these points, the authors presented likelihood ratios for weaning success: for RSBI <80, LR 7.5; 80–100 LR 0.77; and >100 LR 0.04.

---

b. TRICC Trial

A multicenter, randomized, controlled clinical trial of transfusion requirements in critical care.

Hébert PC, Wells G, Blajchman MA, Marshall J, Martin C, Pagliarello G, Tweeddale M, Schweitzer I, Yetisir E, Transfusion Requirements in Critical Care Investigators for the Canadian Critical Care Trials Group

NEJM. 1999;340(6):409–417.

SYNOPSIS

Takeaway Point: In critically ill patients, transfusing for hemoglobin (Hgb) <7.0 is associated with improved survival compared with transfusing for hemoglobin <10.0.

Commentary: Prior to this trial, critically ill patients were routinely transfused to a goal Hgb of >10.0 g/dL (grams per deciliter). The authors performed a randomized parallel groups trial comparing liberal transfusion guidelines of Hgb>10 with a restrictive guideline recommending goal Hgb of 7.0–9.0. The restrictive group had a trend toward improved 30-day mortality, although the difference was not significant. The restrictive group had a 54% decrease in blood product utilization. The authors demonstrate that a restrictive transfusion guideline with a goal Hgb of 7.0–9.0 is at least equivalent, and possibly superior, to the liberal transfusion strategy. Although these results have been widely applied to many patient populations, it is worth remembering that the study population included only critically ill patients, and excluded cardiac patients.

ANALYSIS

Introduction: Critically ill patients are at increased risk for the immunosuppressive and microcirculatory complications of blood transfusions. Because of the risks associated with anemia and decreased oxygen delivery, transfusion guidelines in the ICU often have a goal Hgb of >10.0 g/dL.

Objectives: To compare a red cell transfusion protocol for goal Hgb 7.0–9.0 g/dL to a strategy of 10.0–12.0 g/dL in euvolemic, critically ill patients.

Methods
Trial Design: Randomized, nonblinded, parallel group controlled trial.
Participants
Inclusion Criteria: Anticipated ICU stay >24 hours, Hgb <9.0 within 72 hours of admission to the ICU, euvolemic after initial treatment.

Exclusion criteria: Age <16 years, inability to receive blood products, active/ongoing blood loss, chronic anemia, brain death, admission after routine cardiac surgery.

Intervention: Restrictive transfusion guideline, with transfusions given when Hgb fell below 7.0 as opposed to below 10.0.

Endpoints
Primary Endpoint: 30-day all-cause mortality.
Secondary Endpoints: 60-day all-cause mortality, ICU and hospital stay mortality, 30-day survival time, organ failure scores, composite outcomes of death and organ dysfunction.

Sample Size: 838 patients enrolled (6451 screened) from 22 tertiary care centers and three community hospitals in Canada. 420 randomized to liberal group, 418 to restrictive group.

Statistical Analysis: Intention-to-treat analysis, Tukey's honestly-significant-difference test for pairwise comparisons, Fisher's exact test, logistic regression, Kaplan–Meier curves, χ^2 test, Wilcoxon rank sum test.

Results
Baseline Data: Baseline characteristics were balanced between the two groups. Most common reasons for ICU admission were respiratory and cardiac disease. Over 80% required intubation. 26.5% were admitted with infection.

Outcomes: Average daily Hgb in the liberal group was 10.7, with an average of 5.6 units transfused per patient. The restrictive group had an average daily Hgb of 8.5 and an average of 2.6 units transfused per patient (54% decrease in transfusions). 33% of restrictive patients received no transfusions; all patients in the liberal group received transfusions. The 30-day mortality for the restrictive group was 18.7%, compared with 23.3% in the liberal group (p 0.11). In-hospital mortality, ICU mortality, and 60-day mortality were lower in the restrictive group, although not significantly. Rates of cardiac complications were significantly lower in the restrictive group (13.2% vs. 21%, $p < 0.01$).

Discussion
Conclusion: The use of a restrictive threshold for red cell transfusion, with a goal Hgb of 7.0–9.0, is equivalent or superior to a more liberal goal of 10.0–12.0 g/dL.

Limitations: The study did not include cardiac surgery patients, and study results cannot be generalized to that population. Overall enrollment was significantly lower than expected, and only 13% of patients screened were enrolled in the study, raising concerns for external validity.

---

c. ARDSNet Trial

Ventilation with lower tidal volumes as compared with traditional tidal volumes for acute lung injury and the acute respiratory distress syndrome.

Brower RG, Matthay MA, Morris A, Schoenfeld D, Thompson BT, Wheeler A, for the Acute Respiratory Distress Syndrome Network

NEJM. 2000;342(18):1301–1308.

SYNOPSIS

Takeaway Point: In critically ill patients with acute respiratory distress syndrome (ARDS), a ventilation strategy using tidal volumes of 6 cm^3/kg is associated with lower mortality and greater number of ventilator-free days when compared with 12 cm^3/kg tidal volumes.

Commentary: The authors presented a large, multi-institution randomized controlled trial comparing traditional tidal volumes of 12 cm^3/kg with a low tidal volume of 6 cm^3/kg for patients with ARDS. The trial was stopped early when an interim analysis showed a clear mortality benefit in the lower tidal volume group. The trial has been criticized for using 12 cm^3/kg as a standard tidal volume, when many centers at that time used an intermediate goal of 10 cm^3/kg. Additionally, the lower tidal volume group had higher average positive end-expiratory pressure (PEEP) than did the control group, raising questions of whether PEEP or tidal volume contributed most to the beneficial effects. Overall, however, this trial demonstrated a significant benefit to lower tidal volume ventilation for patients with ARDS. Their findings have been validated by a Cochrane review in 2013, and have been incorporated into the Surviving Sepsis Campaign 2012 guidelines.

ANALYSIS

Introduction: ARDS is associated with atelectasis, edema, and fibrosis, and has traditionally been treated with high-tidal-volume ventilation to counteract respiratory acidosis and hypoxia. Animal trials, however, suggested worsening inflammation and barotrauma with this strategy.

Objectives: The present trial was conducted to determine whether the use of a lower tidal volume with mechanical ventilation would improve important clinical outcomes.

Methods

Trial Design: Multicenter randomized controlled trial.

Participants

Inclusion Criteria: Intubated on mechanical ventilation, diagnosis of ARDS [ratio of partial pressure of O_2 to fraction of inspired oxygen <300, bilateral pulmonary infiltrates; no clinical evidence of left atrial (LA) hypertension, or pulmonary capillary wedge pressure (PCWP) <18].

Exclusion Criteria: >36 hours since meeting ARDS criteria, age <18 years, pregnant, increased intracranial pressure (ICP), neuromuscular disease, sickle cell disease, severe chronic respiratory disease, morbid obesity, burns >30% of body surface area (BSA), estimated 6-month mortality >50%, bone marrow or lung transplant, Child–Pugh class C liver disease.

Intervention

Lower-Tidal-Volume Group: Tidal volume 6 cm^3/kg predicted body weight, reduced by 1 cm^3/kg to maintain plateau pressure <30, minimal tidal volume of 4 cm^3/kg.

Control Group: Tidal volume 12 cm^3/kg predicted body weight, decreased by 1 cm^3/kg if necessary to maintain plateau pressure <50; minimum tidal volume 4 cm^3/kg predicted body weight.

Endpoints

Primary Endpoint: Death prior to discharge home off the ventilator.

Secondary Endpoints: Ventilator-free days, organ system failure, time until barotrauma.

Sample Size: 861 patients were randomized, 432 to lower tidal volumes and 429 to traditional, at 10 university centers from 1996 to 1999.

Statistical Analysis: Student's *t*-test or Fisher's exact, analysis of covariance, Wilcoxon's test, χ^2; planned interim analyses.

Results:

Baseline Data: Baseline characteristics were overall balanced between the two groups.

Outcomes

Primary: The lower-tidal-volume group had significantly lower tidal volumes and plateau pressures. Mortality at 180 days was 39.8% in the traditional tidal volume group, compared with 31% in the lower tidal volume group (*p* 0.007). The difference was sufficiently significant that the trial was stopped early.

Secondary: The lower-tidal-volume group had a significantly higher number of ventilator-free days (12 vs. 10, *p* 0.007), and organ-failure-free days. Incidence of barotrauma was similar in the two groups.

Discussion

Conclusion: In patients with ARDS, ventilation with lower tidal volumes of 6 cm^3/kg are associated with lower mortality at 180 days when compared with 12 cm^3/kg tidal volumes.

Limitations: The two comparison groups may both have represented a departure from standard practice. Volumes of 12 cm^3/kg are higher than standard, and the standardized PEEP strategy used in the trial resulted in higher average PEEP in the lower-tidal-volume group. Additionally, the majority of analyses in the trial were univariate comparisons of mean values. Causes of death were not reported. The trial was cited by OHRP for providing insignificant informed consent to participants.

---

d. Rivers Trial

Early goal-directed therapy in the treatment of severe sepsis and septic shock.

Rivers E, Nguyen B, Havstad S, Ressler J, Muzzin A, Knoblich B, Peterson E, Tomlanovich M, for the Early Goal-Directed Therapy Collaborative Group

NEJM. 2001;345(19):1368–1377.

SYNOPSIS

Takeaway Point: Early goal-directed therapy for sepsis or septic shock reduces in-hospital, 30- and 60-day mortality.

Commentary: Goal-directed therapy for septic shock involves treatment targeted to cardiac preload, afterload, and contractility to balance oxygen delivery and oxygen demand. The authors targeted these goals within the "golden hours" between presentation with systemic inflammatory response syndrome (SIRS) and development of global tissue hypoxia. Prior studies enrolled patients within 72 hours of ICU admission; this trial targeted the first 6 hours after presentation to the emergency department. Of note, some components of early goal-directed therapy (EGDT) have come under controversy: specifically, transfusion goal hematocrit (Hct) of 30 contradicts the previously published TRICC Trial (see **b**, above), and use of CVP as surrogate for blood volume is not well established.[11] The overall results of the trial, however, are compelling, with a 16% reduction to in-hospital mortality. These results were replicated in other centers[12,13] but had not been evaluated in a multi-institution trial until 2014 (see **j**, below).

ANALYSIS

Introduction: Goal-directed therapy for sepsis involves manipulation of cardiac preload, afterload, and contractility to balance oxygen delivery with oxygen demand. Studies of goal-directed interventions have rarely shown a benefit, and have enrolled patients up to 72 hours after admission to the ICU.

Objectives: To determine whether early goal-directed therapy before admission to the intensive care unit effectively reduces the incidence of multiorgan dysfunction, mortality, and the use of health care resources among patients with severe sepsis or septic shock.

Methods

Trial Design: Prospective, randomized nonblinded trial.

Participants

Inclusion Criteria: Adult patients presenting to the emergency department (ED) meeting SIRS criteria, plus systolic blood pressure <90 or lactate >4 after fluid bolus.

Exclusion Criteria: Age <18 years, pregnancy, acute cerebrovascular accident, acute coronary syndrome, acute pulmonary edema, status asthmaticus, cardiac dysrhythmias as primary diagnosis, active GI bleed, seizure, drug overdose, burn, trauma, need for surgery, on chemotherapy, immunosuppression, do-not-resuscitate (DNR) status.

Intervention: Early goal-directed therapy (EGDT) in the emergency department prior to ICU admission, defined as placement of a central venous catheter and use of fluid resuscitation, blood, and vasoactive agents to keep central venous pressure (CVP) 8–12, mean arterial pressure (MAP) >65, and central venous oxygen saturation (Scv O$_2$) >70%. Resuscitation endpoints and clinical parameters were the same in both groups.

Endpoints

Primary Endpoint: In-hospital mortality.

Secondary Endpoints: Resuscitation endpoints (oxygen saturation, lactate, base deficit, pH), organ dysfunction scores, coagulation-related variables, healthcare costs.

Sample Size: 263 patients between 1997 and 2000 at a single tertiary care hospital, 130 randomized to early goal-directed therapy, and 133 to standard emergency room treatment.

Statistical Analysis: Intention-to-treat analysis, Kaplan–Meier curves, mixed models, alpha spending function.

Results

Baseline Data: Treatment groups were balanced in terms of baseline characteristics. 92% of standard therapy patients were given antibiotics in the first 6 hours, compared with 86% of treatment group; this difference was not significant. The most common admitting diagnoses were pneumonia and urosepsis.

Outcomes: In-hospital mortality rates were higher in the standard therapy group (46% vs. 30%, *p* 0.009), as was mortality at 28 days (61% vs. 40%, *p* 0.01) and 60 days (70% vs. 50%, *p* 0.03). In the first 6 hours, the EGDT group received more fluid, more RBC transfusions, and more inotropic support; from 7 to 72 hours, the standard therapy arm received more of all three interventions. From 7 to 72 hours, standard therapy patients also had significantly higher APACHE II, MODS, and SAPS II scores (*p* <0.0001 for all). Of patients who survived until discharge, the standard therapy arm had a significantly longer length of stay (18.4 vs. 14.6 days, *p* 0.04).

Discussion

Conclusion: Early goal-directed therapy for sepsis is associated with lower in-hospital, 30- and 60-day mortality and shorter hospital stays.

Limitations: The exclusion criteria make the population more homogeneous, but may limit general applicability. The study was not blinded. The protocol tested contained multiple interventions, and it is not clear which component is responsible for the observed benefit.

---

e. SAFE Trial

A comparison of albumin and saline for fluid resuscitation in the intensive care unit.

Finfer S, Bellomo R, Boyce N, French J, Myburgh J, Norton R, SAFE Study Investigators

NEJM. 2004;350(22):2247–2256.

SYNOPSIS

Takeaway Point: ICU patients resuscitated with either albumin or saline have similar outcomes at 28 days.

Commentary: This trial addresses the uncertain choice of ideal resuscitative fluid in critically ill patients. Prior data from two meta-analyses disagreed on the impact of albumin resuscitation on risk of mortality, and no adequately powered trial had addressed this question. The authors enrolled 7000 patients, in accordance with power calculations intended to detect a 3% difference in absolute mortality rates with 90% power. No significant differences were seen in primary or secondary outcomes. The authors did attempt subgroup analyses, and although there was a significantly higher risk of death in patients with traumatic brain injury who received albumin, the trial was not adequately powered for this analysis.

ANALYSIS

Introduction: Fluid resuscitation for critically ill patients can involve crystalloid or colloid solutions. Prior meta-analyses have disagreed on the relative benefit of these options.

Objectives: To compare 4% albumin with 0.9% sodium chloride for intravascular fluid resuscitation in patients in the ICU.

Methods
Trial Design: Stratified, double-blinded, randomized parallel-group trial.

Participants
Inclusion Criteria: Patients >18 years, admitted to the ICU, requiring fluid resuscitation.

Exclusion Criteria: Cardiac surgery, liver transplant, and burn patients.

Intervention: Patients were randomized to receive either 4% albumin or 0.9% normal saline for resuscitation fluid. Treating physicians determined the amount and rate of fluid administration, but were blinded to the type of fluid. Study treatment was used until discharge from ICU, death, or 28 days after randomization. Maintenance fluids were at the discretion of the physician.

Endpoints
Primary Endpoint: All-cause mortality within 28 days.

Secondary Endpoints: Survival time during the first 28 days, proportion of patients with new organ failure, duration of mechanical ventilation, duration of renal replacement therapy, length of ICU and hospital stay.

Sample Size: 6997 patients were enrolled from 16 ICUs in Australia and New Zealand between 2001 and 2003. 3497 patients were randomized to the albumin group, and 3500 to the saline group.

Statistical Analysis: Intention-to-treat analysis, χ^2 or Fisher's exact test, unpaired t-test, relative risks, Kaplan–Meier curves, subgroup analysis of all-cause mortality.

Results

Baseline Data: Baseline data were similar in both groups. 17% of patients were admitted for trauma, 18% for sepsis, and 1–2% for ARDS. 43% were surgical admissions, 57% medical.

Outcomes: All-cause mortality during the first 28 days was similar, 20.9% in the albumin group versus 21.1% in the saline group (p 0.87). Survival times did not significantly differ. Rates of organ failure were also similar (p 0.85), as were ICU and hospital length of stay. Patients randomized to albumin received significantly less fluid in the first 3 days; after day 4, there was no difference in volume of study fluids.

Discussion

Conclusion: 4% albumin or 0.9% saline solution for fluid resuscitation in the ICU result in equivalent all-cause mortality in 28 days.

Limitations: Exclusion criteria (no cardiac surgery, burn, or transplant patients) limits applicability. Relative risk of mortality differed in the subgroup analysis (in trauma patients, the saline group did better; in sepsis patients, albumin was better), but the trial was not adequately powered to investigate this difference. The trial compared 4% albumin but did not assess potential utility of concentrated (25%) albumin.

---

f. VASST Trial

Vasopressin versus norepinephrine infusion in patients with septic shock.

Russell JA, Walley KR, Singer J, Gordon AC, Hébert PC, Cooper DJ, Holmes CL, Mehta S, Granton JT, Storms MM, Cook DJ, Presneill JJ, Ayers D, VASST Investigators

NEJM. 2008;358(9):877–887.

SYNOPSIS

Takeaway Point: Among patients with septic shock requiring vasopressors, all-cause mortality at 28 days does not differ with the addition of vasopressin compared to norepinephrine alone.

Commentary: Vasopressin promotes vascular tone via smooth muscle vasoconstriction, elevating blood pressure. Prior studies have demonstrated relative vasopressin deficiency in septic shock, suggesting a possible role for vasopressin to restore vascular tone in these patients.[14] To investigate this hypothesis, the VASST trial sought to determine whether vasopressin could improve survival in septic shock. Patients were enrolled within 12 hours of diagnosis, and randomized to receive either exclusively norepinephrine at escalating doses, or combined vasopressin and norepinephrine infusions in a blinded fashion. No difference was detected in mortality or rates of organ failure between the two cohorts. The trial has been criticized for enrolling patients up to 12 hours after diagnosis, which contradicts the potential benefits associated with early goal-directed therapy (see **d**, above). Additionally, since the majority of patients were enrolled with mean arterial pressure (MAP) >65 while on low dose norepinephrine, vasopressin served as a catecholamine-sparing drug, rather than as an adjunct for refractory shock. These results may not be generalizable to patients with more severe shock.

ANALYSIS

Introduction: Studies suggest that patients in septic shock may have a relative vasopressin deficiency, and exogenous vasopressin is often used as an adjunct to catecholamines to restore vascular tone and blood pressure. Potential risks of use include decreased blood flow to the heart, kidneys, and intestine.

Objectives: To determine whether the addition of vasopressin compared with norepinephrine alone decreased 28-day mortality in patients with septic shock.

Methods

Trial Design: Multicenter, stratified, randomized, parallel-group, double-blind trial. Patients were stratified according to baseline norepinephrine dose.

Participants

Inclusion Criteria: Septic shock resistant to fluids and requiring low-dose norepinephrine.

Exclusion Criteria: Age <16 years, unstable coronary syndrome, >24 hours since patient met entry criteria, use of vasopressin for blood pressure support prior to enrollment, anticipated 6-month mortality >50% due to other conditions, acute mesenteric ischemia, chronic heart disease New York Heart Association (NYHA) class III or IV, severe hyponatremia, traumatic brain injury, pregnancy.

Intervention: Patients were randomized to either vasopressin plus norepinephrine infusions or norepinephrine infusion alone, titrated to maintain a target mean arterial pressure (determined by attending ICU physician). Other vasopressors were added if the target MAP could not be obtained by the study drugs.

Endpoints

Primary Endpoint: All-cause mortality at 28 days.

Secondary Endpoints: 90-day mortality, time to death, days free from mechanical ventilation or renal replacement therapy, length of ICU and hospital stay.

Sample Size: 802 patients from 27 centers in three countries, from 2001 to 2006; 778 were analyzed, 396 in the vasopressin group and 382 in the norepinephrine group.

Statistical Analysis: Sample size analysis to detect 10% difference in mortality, O'Brien–Fleming stopping rules, χ^2 test, Kaplan–Meier curves, logistic regression.

Results

Baseline Data: Baseline characteristics were well balanced. The included population was 84% Caucasian. The most common source of infection was lung (43% in control group, 40% for vasopressin); the second most common was abdomen. The majority of patients in both groups (>70%) were also treated with corticosteroids.

Outcomes: Rates of death at 28 days were not significantly different for the vasopressin versus norepinephrine group (35% vs. 39%, p 0.26). Mortality at 90 days was also similar. Among patients with less severe septic shock (defined as lower initial norepinephrine requirements), there was a nonsignificant trend toward lower mortality at 28 and 90 days.

Discussion

Conclusion: No significant difference in mortality or secondary outcomes was seen with the addition of vasopressin to norepinephrine for septic shock.

Limitations: Analysis was not intention-to-treat. Vasopressin levels were not measured. Baseline MAPs averaged >65, meaning that vasopressin was acting primarily as a catecholamine-sparing drug rather than adjunctive therapy for catecholamine-resistant shock. Power calculation was based on expected mortality of 60%, which was much higher than the observed mortality, making the trial underpowered.

---

g. CORTICUS Trial

Hydrocortisone therapy for patients with septic shock.

Sprung CL, Annane D, Keh D, Moreno R, Singer M, Freivogel K, Weiss YG, Benbenishty J, Kalenka A, Forst H, Laterre PF, Reinhart K, Cuthbertson BH, Payen D, Briegel J, CORTICUS Study Group

NEJM. 2008;358(2):111–124.

SYNOPSIS

Takeaway Point: Low-dose hydrocortisone hastens reversal of septic shock, but is not associated with any mortality benefit.

Commentary: Prior studies suggested a survival benefit of hydrocortisone and fludrocortisone administered to patients with septic shock, particularly in those with documented adrenal insufficiency.[15,16] Corticosteroids became standard of care for septic shock, despite the failure of subsequent trials to duplicate these results. To address this contradiction, the CORTICUS group administered low-dose hydrocortisone to 500 patients with septic shock, regardless of response to corticotropin test. No survival benefit was demonstrated in either responders or nonresponders. The hydrocortisone group did have a more rapid reversal of shock, but the overall percentage of patients with shock reversal did not change.

The role of corticosteroids in septic shock remains controversial. The most recent Surviving Sepsis Guidelines recommend hydrocortisone only in the setting of shock refractory to resuscitation with fluids, pressors, and inotropes. The corticotropin stimulation test is no longer recommended as a diagnostic or prognostic indicator in septic shock.

ANALYSIS

Introduction: The use of corticosteroids in septic shock has been controversial for decades. Hydrocortisone has been trialed at both high and low doses, and results have been mixed. Studies suggested that patients with adrenal insufficiency suggested by a corticotropin stimulation test have the greatest benefit from steroid treatment.

Objectives: To evaluate the efficacy and safety of low-dose hydrocortisone therapy in a broad population of patients with septic shock and specifically in patients who had had a response to a corticotropin test.

Methods
Trial Design: Multicenter, randomized, double-blind, placebo-controlled trial.
Participants
Inclusion Criteria: Clinical evidence of infection within the previous 72 hours, evidence of systemic response, evidence of shock.

Exclusion Criteria: Age <18 years, pregnancy, underlying disease with expected survival <3 months, cardiopulmonary resuscitation (CPR) within 72 hours, drug-induced immunosuppression, chronic corticosteroids, HIV, DNR status, acute MI or PE (myocardial infarction or pulmonary embolism), likely to die within 24 hours.

Intervention: Hydrocortisone administered as 50 mg IV bolus every 6 hours for 5 days, then tapered to 50 mg IV every 12 hours on days 6–8, then 50 mg daily for days 9–11, then stopped.

Endpoints

Primary Endpoint: Rate of death at 28 days in patients who did not have a response to corticotropin.

Secondary Endpoints: Rate of death at 28 days for all patients, rate of death at 28 days for patients who had a response to corticotropin, rates of death in ICU and in-hospital death at 1 year, reversal of shock, duration of ICU and hospital stay.

Sample Size: From 2002 to 2005, 500 patients from 52 ICUs in nine countries were randomized, 252 to hydrocortisone and 248 to placebo.

Statistical Analysis: Sample size calculation to detect 10% decrease in mortality, intention-to-treat analysis, Fisher's exact test, Kaplan–Meier curves.

Results

Baseline Data: 46.7% of patients had no response to corticotropin, 125 of the treatment arm and 108 of the placebo arm. Baseline characteristics were well balanced.

Outcomes: There was no significant difference in rate of death at 28 days among patients who did not respond to corticotropin; there was also no significant difference among the responders. No mortality difference was seen at any other timepoint. The time until reversal of shock was significantly shorter for all patients receiving hydrocortisone ($p<0.001$, 3.3 days vs. 5.8 days).

Discussion

Conclusion: Low-dose hydrocortisone had no significant effect on rate of death regardless of patients' adrenal responsiveness to corticotropin. The rate of reversal of shock was similar, but the time until shock reversal was significantly faster in patients receiving hydrocortisone.

Limitations: The study was not adequately powered (sample size calculations projected 800 patients needed, only 500 were enrolled).

h. NICE–SUGAR Trial

Intensive versus conventional glucose control in critically ill patients.

Finfer S, Chittock DR, Yu-Shuo DR, Su SY, Blair D, Foster D, Dhingra V, Bellomo R, Cook D, Dodek P, Henderson WR, Hébert PC, Heritier S, Heyland DK, McArthur C, McDonald E, Mitchell I, Myburgh JA, Norton R, Potter J, Robinson BG, Ronco JJ, NICE-SUGAR Study Investigators

NEJM. 2009;360(13):1283–1297.

SYNOPSIS

Takeaway Point: A blood glucose target of less than 180 is associated with lower mortality at 90 days than a target of 81–108.

Commentary: Hyperglycemia is common in critical illness. The Leuven Surgical Trial[17] demonstrated a mortality benefit to intensive glycemic control (blood glucose 80–110 for surgical ICU patients). This was not replicated in subsequent trials, leading the NICE–Sugar group to pursue a large, multi-institution parallel- group trial comparing conventional control (blood glucose <180) with intensive control (goal 81–108). Unlike the Leuven Trial, they demonstrated a higher 90-day mortality in patients with intensive control. The NICE–Sugar trial had a much higher percentage of patients receiving enteral nutrition, compared with the higher frequency of TPN in older trials. Additionally, this trial, with over 6000 patients, has greater statistical power than prior studies. On the basis of this study, the 2012 Surviving Sepsis Campaign recommends blood glucose target of <180 in critically ill patients as grade 1A evidence.

ANALYSIS

Introduction: Hyperglycemia is common in critical illness, and is associated with increased morbidity and mortality. Tight glucose control carries its own risks, including potential hypoglycemia and increased resource utilization.

Objectives: To test the hypothesis that intensive glucose control reduces mortality at 90 days.

Methods
Trial Design: Parallel-group, randomized controlled trial.

Participants
Inclusion Criteria: Medical and surgical patients admitted to the ICU, anticipated ICU stay ≥ 3 days, arterial line in place.

Exclusion Criteria: Age < 18 years, death expected within 24 hours or DNR, admission for diabetic ketoacidosis (DKA), expected to be eating within 3 days, prior episodes of hypoglycemia without full neurologic recovery, abnormally high risk of hypoglycemia (eg, insulin-secreting tumor).

Intervention: Comparison of glucose control with one of two target ranges: intensive/tight control group with target 81–108 mg/dL, or conventional control target of ≤180 mg. Glucose control was achieved with IV insulin.

Endpoints

Primary Endpoint: All-cause mortality within 90 days.

Secondary Endpoints: Survival time within 90 days, cause-specific death, durations of mechanical ventilation and renal replacement therapy, ICU and hospital length of stay.

Sample Size: 6104 patients from 42 hospitals (38 tertiary care, 4 community) in Australia and New Zealand 2004–2008; 3054 randomized to intensive therapy, and 3050 to conventional glucose control.

Statistical Analysis: Sample size calculation to detect 3.8% difference between groups, intention-to-treat analysis, χ^2 test, logistic regression, Welch's test, Wilcoxon rank sum, odds ratios, Kaplan–Meier curves and Cox models, subgroup analysis.

Results

Baseline Data: Baseline characteristics were balanced between the two groups.

Outcomes: Intensive control patients were significantly more likely to receive insulin (97% vs. 69%, $p < 0.001$), and blood glucose remained significantly lower in the intensive-control group. Mortality at 28 days was not significantly different between the groups. At 90 days, 27.5% of the intensive control group had died, compared with 24.9% of the conventional control group [OR 1.14 (1.02–1.28; p 0.02)]. Median survival time was also lower in the intensive control group. Length of ICU and hospital stay were similar between the two groups. In the intensive control group, 206 patients (6.8%) had severe hypoglycemia, versus 15 (0.5%) in the conventional approach.

Discussion

Conclusion: Intensive glucose control, defined as goal blood glucose of 81–108, is associated with increased mortality at 90 days when compared with a blood glucose target of < 180.

Limitations: Not blinded, primary endpoint was a univariate analysis. Although a mortality difference was seen at 90 days, the authors do not explain why mortality was equivalent at day 28.

i. CRASH-2 Trial

Effects of tranexamic acid on death, vascular occlusive events, and blood transfusion in trauma patients with significant haemorrhage (CRASH-2): A randomised, placebo-controlled trial.

CRASH-2 trial collaborators, Shakur H, Roberts I, Bautista R, Caballero J, Coats T, Dewan Y, El-Sayed H, Gogichaishvili T, Gupta S, Herrera J, Hunt B, Iribhogbe P, Izurieta M, Khamis H, Komalafe E, Marrero MA, Mejía-Mantilla J, Miranda J, Morales C, Olaomi O, Olldashi F, Perel P, Peto R, Ramana PV, Ravi RR, Yutthakasemsunt S

Lancet. 2010;376(9734):23–32.

SYNOPSIS

Takeaway Point: Administration of tranexamic acid reduces the risk of all-cause mortality in bleeding trauma patients if given within 3 hours of injury.

Commentary: This trial is an extension of previous observations that tranexamic acid—a fibrinolysis inhibitor—reduces blood transfusion requirements in elective surgical patients. The authors demonstrate a mortality benefit in bleeding trauma patients as well. As the majority of deaths due to bleeding occur on the day of injury, early administration of tranexamic acid is crucial. The dose selected in this study, of 1 g over 10 minutes as the loading dose followed by a second 1 g dose over 8 hours, had been shown in prior studies to be safe for patients <50 kg while still effective in patients >100 kg. A single-dose protocol is a more practical intervention in an emergency setting than previously suggested weight-based regimens. Tranexamic acid presents an easy to administer intervention with the possibility of decreased mortality in a large and vulnerable population. A subgroup analysis of the CRASH-2 trial suggested improved mortality when given within 3 hours of injury, but potentially increased rate of death from bleeding if given thereafter.

ANALYSIS

Introduction: Tranexamic acid (TXA), a synthetic derivative of lysine, inhibits fibrinolysis by blocking lysine binding sites on plasminogen. It has been shown to significantly decrease the need for blood transfusion in patients undergoing elective surgery. The coagulation abnormalities seen after surgery and major trauma are similar.

Objectives: To assess the effects of early administration of a short course of tranexamic acid on death, vascular occlusive events, and the receipt of blood transfusion in trauma patients with or at risk of significant hemorrhage.

Methods

Trial Design: Prospective, block-randomized, double-blinded trial.

Participants

Inclusion Criteria: Adult (age >16) trauma patients with significant ongoing hemorrhage as evidenced by hypotension and/or tachycardia, or who are considered at risk for significant hemorrhage, presenting within 8 hours of injury.

Exclusion Criteria: Patients for whom there is a clear contraindication to or obvious benefit from antifibrinolytic therapy; treating physicians should be "uncertain" regarding the potential benefit of the proposed treatment.

Intervention: Loading dose of 1 g TXA over 10 minutes, followed by infusion of 1 g over 8 hours, with matching placebo doses of 0.9% saline.

Endpoints

Primary Endpoint: Death in hospital within 4 weeks of injury.

Secondary Endpoints: Vascular occlusive events, surgical intervention, receipt of blood products and units transfused.

Sample Size: 20,211 patients randomized from 274 hospitals in 40 countries: 10,096 to tranexamic acid and 10,115 to placebo.

Statistical Analysis: Intention-to-treat analysis, χ^2 test, risk ratios with 95% confidence intervals.

Results

Baseline Data: A total of 3076 patients (15.3%) died, of whom 1086 died on the day of randomization. There were 1063 deaths due to bleeding, of which 637 (59.9%) were on the day of randomization. Treatment groups were balanced with respect to baseline characteristics.

Outcomes: All-cause mortality was significantly reduced in the TXA group [14.5% vs. 16.0%, RR 0.91 (0.85–0.97), p 0.0035]. Risk of death due to bleeding was also significantly reduced [4.9% vs. 5.7%, RR 0.85 (0.76–0.96), p 0.0077]. The risk of vascular occlusive event (1.7% vs. 2.0%, p 0.084) or of death from vascular occlusive event (0.3% vs. 0.5%, p 0.096) was not significantly increased with TXA. The rates of multiorgan failure, head injury, and death from other causes did not differ significantly between the groups. There was no significant difference in other secondary outcomes, including need for blood products, median units of blood transfused, or surgical intervention.

Discussion

Conclusion: All-cause mortality is significantly reduced in bleeding trauma patients with early administration of tranexamic acid. There is no observed increased risk of vascular occlusive events.

Limitations: All inclusion criteria and outcome measures are clinical parameters; while this increases feasibility, it may decrease specificity of results. In particular, defining a patient "at risk" for significant hemorrhage is nonspecific. Exclusion criteria (nonequipoise on the part of treating physicians) are vague.

---

j. ProCESS Trial

A randomized trial of protocol-based care for early septic shock.

Yealy DM, Kellum JA, Huang DT, Barnato AE, Weissfeld LA, Pike F, Terndrup T, Wang HE, Hou PC, LoVecchio F, Filbin MR, Shapiro NI, Angus DC, ProCESS Investigators

NEJM. 2014;370(18):1683–1693.

SYNOPSIS

Takeaway Point: Among patients with early septic shock, there is no difference in all-cause mortality with management driven by (1) early goal-directed therapy, (2) a less invasive protocol-based therapy, or (3) usual care at the discretion of treating physicians.

Commentary: This trial is a direct response to the Rivers Trial (see **d**, above), which demonstrated a significant reduction in mortality with early goal-directed therapy (EGDT) for septic shock. The Rivers protocol included central venous oxygen saturation monitoring by central venous catheter, and aggressive transfusion requirements (goal Hct >30). It was not clear which elements of that strategy accounted for the mortality benefit. The ProCESS investigators sought to compare the Rivers EGDT protocol to a less invasive protocol, which did not require central monitoring and had lower transfusion requirements, and a third group receiving "usual care" at the discretion of their providers. They found that mortality rates at 60 days, 90 days, and one year were similar between all three groups. Since EGDT had already become standard of care for patients with sepsis, it is likely that all three groups were heavily influenced by the Rivers Trial. Although none of the protocols tested carried a mortality benefit, all of the enrolled patients necessarily had early identification and treatment of sepsis, which may have influenced the equivalent outcomes.

ANALYSIS

Introduction: The Rivers Trial of EGDT for septic shock proposed a specific protocol to guide treatment of sepsis in the emergency department, rather than delaying treatment until arrival in the ICU. The protocol includes measuring central venous pressure (CVP) and central venous oxygenation saturation (Scv O_2) to guide treatment. Following the Rivers Trial, the standard of care for septic shock became early goal-directed therapy.

Objectives: To determine whether all elements of the sepsis protocol proposed by Rivers et al in 2001 are necessary to achieve the survival benefits associated with EGDT.

Methods

Trial Design: Multicenter, randomized trial.

Participants

Inclusion Criteria: Patients presenting to the Emergency Department with sepsis, meeting at least two SIRS criteria, with refractory hypotension or lactate >4.

Exclusion Criteria: Age <18 years; development of shock >2 hours prior to enrollment; presenting diagnosis of cerebrovascular accident (CVA), acute coronary syndrome (ACS), acute pulmonary edema, status asthmaticus, GI bleed, drug overdose, trauma, or need for immediate surgery; pregnancy; CD4 count <50; contraindication to central venous line (CVL).

Intervention: Patients were randomly assigned to one of three groups: protocol-based EGDT, protocol-based standard therapy, or usual care. Protocol-based EGDT mimics the Rivers Trial, with CVL and Scv O_2 monitoring determining vasopressor use. The protocol-based standard therapy was less aggressive, requiring only peripheral access and setting goals for systolic blood pressure and shock index. The transfusion goals were lower than EGDT (goal Hgb > 7.5 vs. Hct >30). For the usual-care arm, the study did not dictate any specific interventions; patients were treated by providers without interference.

Endpoints

Primary Endpoint: In-hospital death at 60 days.

Secondary Endpoints: All-cause mortality at 90 days and one year, duration of need for vasopressors, acute respiratory or renal failure, duration of ICU and hospital stay, discharge disposition.

Sample Size: 1341 patients at 31 academic hospitals in the United States, from 2008 to 2013; 439 in the protocol-based EGDT group, 446 in the protocol-based standard therapy group, and 456 in the usual-care group.

Statistical Analysis: Intention-to-treat analysis, sample size calculation to detect 6–7% decrease in mortality, Fisher's exact, Kaplan–Meier, log-rank test, Breslow–Day test.

Results

Baseline Data: Baseline characteristics were well matched. For all groups, the most common source of sepsis was pneumonia, followed by UTI and then intraabdominal sources.

Outcomes: In the first 6 hours, the protocol-based standard therapy group received significantly more fluid (3.3 L vs. 2.8 L in EGDT and 2.3 L in usual-care arm). Both protocol groups received more vasopressors than did the usual-care group. The EGDT group received significantly more blood cell transfusions (14.4% vs. 8.3% for standard therapy protocol and 7.5% for usual care, p 0.001). At 60 days, mortality did not significantly differ between the groups, with 21% of EGDT patients dead, 18.2% of standard therapy patients, and 18.9% of usual-care patients. 90-day mortality and time to death were also similar between the groups.

Discussion

Conclusion: Adherence to either an invasive early goal-directed therapy protocol or a more relaxed protocol based on noninvasive blood pressure and heart rate measurements did not significantly alter mortality compared with nonprotocol sepsis management.

Limitations: The usual-care arm was not well defined; patients likely had less severe sepsis than in the Rivers Trial. In all arms, sepsis was diagnosed and antibiotics administered early, which may have influenced the equivalent mortality rates.

REFERENCES

1. Weil MH, Tang W. From intensive care to critical care medicine: A historical perspective. *Am J Respir Crit Care Med.* 2011;183(11): 1451–1453.

2. Vincent JL. Critical care—where have we been and where are we going? *Crit Care*. 2013;17(Suppl 1):S2.

3. Marini JJ. Mechanical ventilation: Past lessons and the near future. *Crit Care*. 2013;17(Suppl 1):51–61.

4. Cook D, et al. Multicenter clinical research in adult critical care. *Crit Care Med*. 2002;30(7):1636–1643.

5. Brower RG, Matthay MA, Morris A, Schoenfeld D, Thompson BT, Wheeler A, for the Acute Respiratory Distress Syndrome Network. Ventilation with lower tidal volumes as compared with traditional tidal volumes for acute lung injury and the acute respiratory distress syndrome. *NEJM* 2000;342(18):1301–1308.

6. Hebert PC, et al. A multicenter, randomized, controlled clinical trial of transfusion requirements in critical care. Transfusion Requirements in Critical Care Investigators, Canadian Critical Care Trials Group. *NEJM*. 1999;340(6):409–417.

7. Rivers E, et al. Early goal-directed therapy in the treatment of severe sepsis and septic shock. *NEJM*. 2001;345(19):1368–1377.

8. Pro CI, et al. A randomized trial of protocol-based care for early septic shock. *NEJM*., 2014;370(18):1683–1693.

9. Halpern NA, Pastores SM, Greenstein RJ. Critical care medicine in the United States 1985-2000: An analysis of bed numbers, use, and costs. *Crit Care Med*. 2004;32(6):1254–1259.

10. Yang K, Tobin MJ. Indexes predictive of weaning from mechanical ventilation. *NEJM*. Nov. 1991;325:1442–1444.

11. Evans TW. Hemodynamic and metabolic therapy in critically ill patients [editorial]. *NEJM*. Nov. 2001;345(19):1417–1418.

12. Sivayoham N. Outcomes from implementing early goal-directed therapy for severe sepsis and septic shock: A 4-year observational cohort study. *Eur J Emerg Med*. 2012;19(4):235–240.

13. Natanson C, Danner RL, et al. Resuscitation and stabilization of the critically ill child. *Chest*. 2006;129(2):225–232.

14. Sharshar T, Blanchard A, Paillard M, et al. Circulating vasopressin levels in septic shock. *Crit Care Med*. 2003;31:1752–1758.

15. Schumer W. Steroids in the treatment of clinical septic shock. *Ann Surg*. 1976;184(3):333–341.

16. Annane D, Sebille V, Charpentier C, et al. Effect of treatment with low doses of hydrocortisone and fludrocortisone on mortality in patients with septic shock. *JAMA*. 2002;288(7):862–871.

17. Van den Berghe G, Wouters P, Verwaest C, et al. Intensive insulin therapy in critically ill patients. *NEJM*. 2001;345:1359–1367.

5

Breast Surgery

Andrea Merrill • Upahvan Rai • Michelle Specht

While breast cancer has been recognized as a disease process since the Egyptians described it in 3000 BC,[1] treatment is generally thought to have originated with Dr. William Halsted. In 1894 with his publication "The Results of Operations for the Cure of Cancer of the Breast,"[2] radical mastectomy (removal of the breast, muscle, and lymph nodes) was introduced as the mainstay of treatment for breast cancer. Halsted wrote, "I was led to adopt this procedure because, on microscopical examination, I repeatedly found when I had not expected it that the fascia was already carcinomatous, whereas the muscle was certainly not involved." He then went on to say, "There are undoubtedly many surgeons still in active practice who have never cured a cancer of the breast."

Fortunately, with improved understanding of the biology of cancer, specifically the hormonal aspect of breast cancer, along with the advent of mammography, treatment has evolved significantly since Halsted's initial description of the morbid and disfiguring radical mastectomy. Breast cancer has paved the way in cancer research and treatment, and the majority of patients today can be cured. Advances in chemotherapy and radiation therapy have allowed for more limited surgery, creating the modern systemic, multidisciplinary approaches.

The first major change in therapy came in 1971 with initiation of the National Surgical Adjuvant Breast and Bowel Project (NSABP) B04 Trial, which established total mastectomy (removal of only the breast) as equally effective for early breast cancer with the benefit of lower morbidity than radical mastectomy.[3] This led to the NSABP B06 trial for invasive cancer and the NSABP B17 trial for DCIS, which demonstrated that lumpectomy plus radiation, today's breast conservation therapy (BCT), is equivalent to more radical surgery.[4,5] Breast surgery continued to scale down with the NSABP B32 trial establishing the role of the sentinel lymph node biopsy[6] and the Z0011 trial eliminating need for axillary node dissection in women with early-stage breast cancer and one or two positive nodes.[7]

Advancements were also achieved in the area of systemic therapy. The NSABP B18 trial established the role of neoadjuvant therapy in breast cancer treatment,[8] while the NSABP P1 and NSABP P2 trials introduced the use of hormonal therapy, namely, tamoxifen and raloxifene.[9,10] Additional trials have led to improvements in chemotherapy and use of more targeted agents. Breast cancer therapy today would be unrecognizable to Dr. Halsted, and research continues to look for ways to provide individualized targeted treatment while minimizing morbidity and improving outcomes.

Breast cancer therapy has benefited from large, multinational trials with extended follow-up, made possible in large part by the NSABP consortium. Many of the trials described in this chapter began in the 1970s, and interval follow-up has now been published in several manuscripts. We present the long-term results when they are available, as 25-year data can build on, and occasionally contradict, results from shorter follow-up periods. Since many of these trials build on the hypotheses and early results of prior studies, the articles presented in this chapter are presented chronologically by recruitment dates, rather than by date of publication.

---

a. NSABP B-04 25-Year Follow-Up

Twenty-five-year follow-up of a randomized trial comparing radical mastectomy, total mastectomy, and total mastectomy followed by irradiation.

Fisher B, Jeong J-H, Anderson S, Bryant J, Fisher ER, Wolmark N

NEJM. 2002;347(8):567–575.

SYNOPSIS

Takeaway Point: After 25 years of follow-up, this large randomized trial fails to demonstrate any survival advantage to radical mastectomy for women with invasive cancer and clinically positive or negative axillary nodes. It also fails to demonstrate a survival benefit to total mastectomy plus postoperative radiation compared to total mastectomy alone in patients with clinically negative nodes.

Commentary: The National Surgical Adjuvant Breast and Bowel Project (NSABP) is a clinical trial cooperative group established in 1958 to conduct large-scale clinical trials in breast and colorectal surgery. Its research has significantly shaped the current treatment of breast cancer with multiple important clinical trials. The NSABP B04 trial was the first landmark trial in breast cancer, initiated in 1971, and was the basis for moving away from Halsted's radical mastectomy and toward less extensive surgery. This specific publication is an update to the original trial with 25 years of follow-up and maintains the original conclusion that there is no survival advantage to radical mastectomy (breast, chest wall muscles, and axillary lymph nodes) over total mastectomy (removal of breast and skin only) in breast cancer.

ANALYSIS

Introduction: Previously, the Halsted radical mastectomy was the standard of care for all stages of breast cancer. High morbidity and anecdotal reports of less extensive surgery led the NSABP to initiate the B04 study in 1971 to explore other operative approaches to treating breast cancer. Initial analysis of this cohort demonstrated differences in local control of disease, but no survival difference. This study presents the 25-year follow-up data.

Objectives: The aims of the study were to determine whether patients with either clinically negative or clinically positive axillary nodes who received local or regional treatments other than radical mastectomy would have outcomes similar to those achieved with radical mastectomy.

Methods
Trial Design: Multicenter randomized controlled trial.
Participants
Inclusion Criteria: Women with operable breast cancer with either clinically positive or negative nodes.
Exclusion Criteria: Secondary or metastatic disease.
Intervention: Randomized to either total mastectomy alone, total mastectomy plus irradiation, or radical mastectomy. Node-positive subjects received an additional boost as compared with node-negative subjects undergoing radiation therapy. No adjuvant systemic therapy was administered.
Endpoints
Primary Endpoint: First local regional or distant recurrence of tumor, contralateral breast cancer or a second primary tumor other than a tumor of the breast, and death without evidence of cancer.

Secondary Endpoints: Death due to breast or other cancer.

Sample Size: 1765 women were enrolled between July 1971 and September 1974. For those with clinically negative axillary nodes, one-third underwent radical mastectomy, one-third total mastectomy with regional radiation, and one-third total mastectomy alone. For the women with clinically positive nodes, half underwent radical mastectomy and the other half underwent total mastectomy and regional radiation.

Statistical Analysis: Kaplan–Meier survival curves for disease-free survival (DFS), distant disease-free survival (DDFS), relapse-free survival (RFS), and overall survival. Cox proportional hazards models. Nonparametric models, Gray's K-sample test statistic.

Results
Baseline Data: The three groups were well matched for baseline characteristics. Approximately 70% of women in each group were over 50 years of age at time of enrollment. Mean tumor diameter was 3.3 cm for patients with negative nodes and 3.7 cm for patients with positive nodes.

Outcomes
Node-Negative Disease: No significant difference is DFS, RFS, DDFS, or overall survival was observed among the three node-negative groups. The lowest cumulative incidence of local or regional recurrence was for women treated with mastectomy and radiation (p 0.002), although there was no significant difference between groups in cumulative incidence of distant recurrence. Overall, approximately 40% of women with clinically negative nodes who underwent radical mastectomy had tumor-positive nodes on pathology.

Node-Positive Disease: No significant different in DFS, RFS, DDFS, or overall survival between the two node-positive treatment groups. 81.7% of women with clinically positive nodes had breast cancer–related events within the first 5 years of follow-up.

Regardless of nodal status, most first events were related to distant recurrences of tumor and to deaths that were unrelated to breast cancer.

Discussion
Conclusion: After 25 years of follow-up, there is no survival advantage from radical mastectomy over total mastectomy in the treatment of node-negative or node-positive breast cancer. Additionally, there is no advantage to postmastectomy radiation in patients with node-negative breast cancer. Finally, leaving occult positive nodes behind does not significantly increase the rate of distant recurrence or breast cancer–related mortality.

Limitations: Lymph nodes were sometimes found in specimens removed during operations designated as total mastectomy alone, which may skew results. Also, whereas the study was relatively large, subgroups were small, which may have limited the ability to detect significant differences with the addition of radiation therapy to total mastectomy.

---

b. NSABP B-06 20-year Follow-Up

Twenty-year follow-up of a randomized trial comparing total mastectomy, lumpectomy, and lumpectomy plus irradiation for the treatment of invasive breast cancer.

Fisher B, Anderson S, Bryant J, Margolese RG, Deutsch M, Fisher ER, Jeong J-H, Wolmark N

NEJM. 2002;347(16):1233–1241.

SYNOPSIS

Takeaway Point: After 20 years of follow-up, breast-conserving therapy with lumpectomy plus radiation continues to be adequate treatment for invasive breast cancer.

Commentary: The NSABP initiated the B04 trial (see **a**, above) in 1971 to resolve controversy over the surgical management of breast cancer. The 25-year findings showed no significant difference in survival between women treated with the Halsted radical mastectomy and those treated with the less extensive total mastectomy. The B06 trial, which began in 1973, sought to evaluate the efficacy of breast-conserving therapy in women with stage 1 or 2 tumors. Although no significant difference in survival was noted among the three groups (mastectomy, lumpectomy, lumpectomy plus irradiation), lumpectomy plus irradiation resulted in significantly lower ipsilateral breast tumor recurrence (IBTR) as compared to lumpectomy without breast irradiation regardless of nodal status. NSABP B06 continues to be the basis for recommending breast-conserving therapy today. Of note, a substantial proportion of events in the study occurred after 5 years of follow-up, emphasizing the need for long-term follow-up and outcomes.

ANALYSIS

Introduction: This study reports on the B06 trial, initiated in 1973 to evaluate the efficacy of breast-conserving surgery (lumpectomy with or without radiation) compared with total mastectomy in women with stages 1 and 2 breast tumors measuring 4 cm or less. Initial analyses had demonstrated no significant survival difference, but a decrease in ipsilateral recurrence associated with radiation was observed. The present study reports the 20-year follow-up data.

Objectives: To determine whether lumpectomy with or without radiation is as effective as total mastectomy for the treatment of stage 1 and 2 invasive breast cancer.

Methods

Trial Design: Multicenter randomized controlled trial.

Participants

Inclusion Criteria: Invasive breast tumors ≤4 cm in diameter with negative or positive nodes.

Exclusion Criteria: Stage 3 or 4 cancer.

Intervention: Women were randomly assigned to lumpectomy with or without 50 Gy (grey unit) radiation, or mastectomy. If tumor-free margins were unattainable, mastectomy was performed even if randomized to lumpectomy initially. Level I and II axillary nodes were removed with lumpectomy, and complete axillary dissection was performed with mastectomy.

Endpoints

Primary Endpoint: Disease-free survival (DFS), distant disease-free survival (DDFS), and overall survival.

Secondary Endpoints: Local, regional, and distant recurrences in the ipsilateral breast. Diagnosis of a second cancer. Distant metastases after a local or regional recurrence. Tumors in the contralateral breast. Death without evidence of cancer.

Sample Size: 2163 women were enrolled between August 1976 and January 1984. 1852 (86%) had follow-up data available at 20 years. Women were randomized independent of nodal status to lumpectomy ($n = 634$), lumpectomy plus irradiation ($n = 628$), and total mastectomy ($n = 589$).

Statistical Analysis: Kaplan–Meier curves; log-rank tests, log-rank statistic, and log-rank subtraction; tests for heterogeneity, Cox proportional-hazards models, and Gray's K-sample test statistic to determine significance.

Results

Baseline Data: The three groups were similar in age, tumor size, and nodal status.

Outcomes: Incidence of recurrence in the ipsilateral breast 20 years after surgery was 14.3% for lumpectomy plus irradiation group and 39.2% for lumpectomy without irradiation ($p < 0.0001$); this difference was significant for women with positive and negative nodes. There were no significant differences in DFS ($P=0.26$), DDFS ($P=0.034$), or overall survival ($P=0.57$) among the three treatment groups. There was no significant difference in DDFS between the women in the two lumpectomy groups who had specimens with tumor-free margins.

Discussion
Conclusion: After 20 years, mastectomy compared with lumpectomy plus or minus radiation results in no significant difference in DFS, DDFS, and overall survival. The addition of irradiation to lumpectomy significantly decreases the rate of ipsilateral breast recurrence.

Limitations: In this study, only women with positive nodes received chemotherapy and the regimen used at the time was older and less effective. For this reason, the incidence of recurrence in this study is higher than more current studies. All women also underwent some form of axillary dissection at time of surgery, whereas sentinel lymph node biopsy is the current standard of care for clinically node-negative disease.

---

c. NSABP B-17 Trial for the Treatment of Intraductal Cancer

Lumpectomy compared with lumpectomy and radiation therapy for the treatment of intraductal breast cancer.

Fisher B, Constantino J, Redmond C, Fisher E, Margolese R, Dimitrov N, Wolmark N, Wickerham DL, Deutsch M, Ore L, Mamounas E, Poller W, Kavanah M

NEJM. 1993;328(22):1581–1586.

SYNOPSIS

Takeaway Point: Lumpectomy plus breast irradiation significantly reduced the rate of second ipsilateral breast tumors (both invasive and noninvasive) compared to lumpectomy alone for localized ductal carcinoma in situ.

Commentary: In the 1980s, utilization of mammography lead to increased diagnosis of ductal carcinoma in situ (DCIS). Prior to this study, mastectomy was still the standard of care for DCIS. After results from the NSABP B06 trial shifted treatment for invasive cancer to lumpectomy, there was a push to test the outcome of breast conserving therapy in DCIS. This is the first large, multicenter trial to compare lumpectomy alone to lumpectomy plus radiation therapy in DCIS. The B17 trial showed significantly decreased rates of recurrence with the addition of radiation therapy and is the basis for including radiation therapy in DCIS treatment today, although this continues to be a subject of debate.

ANALYSIS

Introduction: Ductal carcinoma in situ is being diagnosed more frequently at a clinically undetectable stage with the advent of mammography. Previous studies on the incidence of recurrence after local excision are based on women with palpable tumors. Appropriate treatment for tumors that are not clinically detectable is uncertain.

Objectives: "To test the hypothesis that in women with localized ductal carcinoma in situ thought to have been completely removed, lumpectomy (or more accurately, local excision, since most women did not have a palpable mass) plus breast irradiation is more effective than local excision alone in preventing a second cancer in the ipsilateral breast."

Methods
Trial Design: Multicenter randomized controlled trial.
Participants
Inclusion Criteria: Women receiving lumpectomy for noninvasive cancer identified either clinically or mammographically; tumors with both DCIS and lobular carcinoma in situ (LCIS) and multiple lesions were also included.

Exclusion Criteria: Clinically positive axillary nodes, positive nodes after axillary dissection, previous cancer (other than cervical or skin cancer), tumor-embedded microcalcifications on final pathology.

Intervention: After lumpectomy, women were randomly assigned to either ipsilateral breast irradiation (50 Gy at 10 Gy per week) or no radiation therapy. Randomization was stratified according to age (<49 or >49), axillary dissection (performed or not performed), tumor type (DCIS or DCIS+LCIS), and method of detection (clinically, mammographically, or both). The cohort of women randomly assigned to breast irradiation received therapy within 2 months postoperatively.

Endpoints

Primary Endpoint: Event-free survival as defined by the presence of no new ipsilateral or contralateral breast cancers, regional or distant metastases, or other cancers.

Secondary Endpoints: Death.

Sample Size: 818 subjects enrolled between October 1, 1985 and December 31, 1990; 790 were included in the final analysis with 391 receiving lumpectomy alone and 399 receiving lumpectomy plus radiation therapy.

Statistical Analysis: Women having no event occurring had percentages computed by the actuarial method with a life table estimate. A two-sided summary χ^2 (log-rank) test was used to compare time before the occurrence of a first event. Multivariate proportional-hazards analysis was used to test for specific interactions.

Results

Baseline Data: Baseline characteristics were balanced between the two groups.

Outcomes: Women treated with lumpectomy alone had significantly worse event-free survival at 5 years compared with lumpectomy plus radiation (73.8% vs. 84.4%, p 0.001). Radiation therapy reduced the incidence of ipsilateral breast cancer by 58.8% ($p < 0.001$). Ipsilateral invasive cancer incidence was 10.5% in lumpectomy patients as compared to 2.9% in those treated with lumpectomy and radiation therapy ($p < 0.001$).

Discussion

Conclusion: Radiation therapy after lumpectomy improves overall event-free survival as compared with lumpectomy alone in women with DCIS.

Limitations: Pathology analysis may differ between centers because of difficulty in differentiating between benign breast lesions and DCIS, between DCIS and LCIS, and between DCIS and invasive cancer associated with DCIS. Sampling error accounted for some of the limitations due to discordance in diagnosis.

d. NSABP B-17 and B-24 15-year Follow-Up

Long-term outcomes of invasive breast tumor recurrences after lumpectomy in NSABP B-17 and B-24 randomized clinical trials for DCIS.

Wapnir IL, Dignam JJ, Fisher B, Mamounas EP, Anderson SJ, Julian TB, Land SR, Margolese RG, Swain SM, Costantino JP, Wolmark N

J Natl Cancer Inst. 2011;103(6):478–488.

SYNOPSIS

Takeaway Point: Radiation and tamoxifen in addition to breast-conserving surgery for treatment of DCIS reduce the rate of invasive breast tumor recurrence.

Commentary: Diagnosis of DCIS has increased dramatically over the past two decades because of the increased usage and improved resolution of mammographic techniques. The initial report of the NSABP B17 trial in 1993 showed similar overall 5-year survival for patients with DCIS when comparing mastectomy to lumpectomy alone (LO) or lumpectomy with radiation (LRT), although the addition of radiation decreased the rate of ipsilateral breast tumor recurrence (IBTR). This trial represents an update of the B17 trial after 15 years of follow-up, and the B24 trial, which randomized patients with DCIS undergoing lumpectomy plus radiation (LRT) to tamoxifen (TAM) or no tamoxifen. This update specifically focuses on the occurrence of invasive IBTR (I-IBTR) and its effect on survival in patients in both the NSABP B17 and B24 trials. An important key finding in this study was that half of all IBTR were invasive, which was associated with an increased mortality risk. It is this finding that has emphasized the need for local control of DCIS to prevent invasive recurrences. The study also found that radiation and tamoxifen in addition to lumpectomy significantly reduced the rate of I-IBTR. Overall, survival remained high for all treatment groups with DCIS.

ANALYSIS

Introduction: Ipsilateral breast tumor recurrence (IBTR) is the most common failure event after lumpectomy for DCIS. This study evaluated invasive IBTR (I-IBTR) and its influence on survival among participants in two NSABP randomized trials for DCIS. The NSABP B7 trial demonstrated a 60% lower risk of IBTR with lumpectomy followed by radiation compared with lumpectomy alone at 5 years. The B24 trial investigated the addition of tamoxifen to lumpectomy and radiation, and demonstrated an additional risk reduction. This study presents an update on those cohorts after 15 years of follow-up.

Objectives: To investigate the impact of I-IBTR on the long-term mortality of patients receiving breast-conserving treatments for DCIS.

Methods

Trial Design: Two multicenter randomized controlled trials.

Participants

Inclusion Criteria: Women with DCIS undergoing lumpectomy with clear margins in the B17 cohort with follow-up information available. B24 also allowed women with DCIS at the tumor margins.

Exclusion Criteria: Patients undergoing mastectomy or having primary invasive tumor.

Intervention: In the B17 trial, patients were randomized to lumpectomy plus radiation (LRT) or lumpectomy alone (LO). In the B24 trial, patients were randomized to LRT with either placebo or tamoxifen (TAM) for 5 years.

Endpoints

Primary Endpoint: I-IBTR.

Secondary Endpoints: DCIS-IBTR, contralateral breast cancers (CBC), second primary cancer, all-cause mortality, and breast-cancer-specific mortality.

Sample Size: B17 trial enrolled 818 patients between 1985 and 1990, 495 randomized to LO and 413 to LRT. B24 enrolled 1804 patients between 1991 and 1994, with 902 randomized to placebo and 902 to tamoxifen.

Statistical Analysis: Cause-specific hazard ratios using the Cox proportional-hazards model. Proportional-hazards assumption evaluated using Schoenfeld residual plots. Indicator variables in conjunction with a time-varying covariate were used in the hazard regression model.

Results

Baseline Data: Patient and disease characteristics were similar between all groups. In B24, 25% of patients were reported as positive margins.

Outcomes: 46.3% of all IBTR events were noninvasive; 53.7% were invasive. Rate of contralateral breast cancer was similar in the LO and LRT groups but lower in the LRT + TAM group. Rate of second primary cancers was similar among treatment groups. LRT group showed 52% reduction in risk of I-IBTR compared with the LO group ($p < 0.001$). Tamoxifen in combination with radiation therapy (LRT + TAM) showed 32% reduction in risk for I-IBTR compared with LRT + placebo (p 0.025). Radiation therapy reduced incidence of I-IBTR at 15 years from 19.4% in LO to 8.9% in B17 LRT, and to 10% in the B5 LRT + placebo group. There was a twofold increase in risk of endometrial cancers in LRT + TAM group compared with the LRT + placebo group.

Positive margin status in B24 trial carried a twofold increased risk of I-IBTR.

No statistically significant differences in the hazard of local, regional, or distant disease between LRT and LO groups.

Discussion

Conclusion: 50% of all IBTR after treatment for DCIS is invasive cancer, which is associated with an increased risk of mortality. Radiation therapy and tamoxifen both decrease the rate of invasive breast tumor recurrences in women with DCIS.

Limitations: Study designed more than 20 years ago, and imaging quality is now far superior. The effect of surgical margins particularly in the B24 trial introduces heterogeneity to the study as B17 and B24 had differing margin exclusion criteria. Finally, tumor hormone receptor status was unknown and not commented on in this report.

---

e. NSABP B-18 Preoperative Therapy Effects

(1) Effect of preoperative chemotherapy on local–regional disease in women with operable breast cancer: Findings from National Surgical Adjuvant Breast and Bowel Project B-18.

Fisher B, Brown A, Mamounas E, Wieand S, Robidoux A, Margolese RG, Cruz AB Jr, Fisher ER, Wickerham DL, Wolmark N, DeCillis A, Hoehn JL, Lees AW, Dimitrov NV

J Clin Oncol. July 1997;15:2483–2493.

(2) Effect of preoperative chemotherapy on the outcome of women with operable breast cancer.

Fisher B, Bryant J, Wolmark N, Mamounas E, Brown A, Fisher ER, Wickerham DL, Begovic M, DeCillis A, Robidoux A, Margolese RG, Cruz AB Jr, Hoehn JL, Lees AW, Dimitrov NV, Bear HV

J Clin Oncol. 1998;16(8):2672–2685.

SYNOPSIS

Takeaway Point: Preoperative chemotherapy in women with primary operable (stage 1 and 2) breast tumors does not impact DFS, DDFS, or overall survival compared with postoperative chemotherapy, but does: reduce the size of most tumors; increase the likelihood of lumpectomy; and decrease the number of positive nodes.

Commentary: Prior to this study a few small studies had demonstrated potential benefit of preoperative (neoadjuvant) chemotherapy in the treatment of operable (stage 1 and 2) breast cancer. However, a large randomized controlled trial (RCT) had yet to be conducted. NSABP B18 is the first large RCT analyzing the outcomes of preoperative chemotherapy in patients with operable breast cancer. The first study, published in 1997, looked specifically at the effects of preoperative chemotherapy on tumor size reduction, clinical and pathological response, decrease in node positivity, and increase in likelihood of lumpectomy. This finding led to the current use of neoadjuvant therapy to downsize large breast tumors initially found to be too large for lumpectomy. The second publication in 1998 compared outcomes of those who received postoperative chemotherapy to those who received preoperative chemotherapy and also assessed outcomes according to local response to preoperative chemotherapy. They concluded that preoperative chemotherapy should be considered in stage 1 or 2 breast cancer patients who would otherwise be eligible for postoperative chemotherapy, as it increases the likelihood of breast-conserving therapy.

ANALYSIS

Introduction: Since the 1950s, postoperative chemotherapy for breast cancer has aimed at controlling local, regional, and micrometastatic disease. More recently, preoperative neoadjuvant (or induction) chemotherapy has demonstrated a decrease in the size of primary breast cancers and an increase in breast-conserving therapy in operable (stage 1 or 2) breast cancer, although these benefits have not been demonstrated in a large randomized trial.

Objectives: The aim of the manuscript published in 1997 was "to determine whether preoperative doxorubicin and cyclophosphamide (AC) permits more lumpectomies to be performed and decreases the incidence of positive nodes in women with primary breast cancer." The 1998 manuscript compares outcomes of patients who received preoperative versus postoperative chemotherapy in the treatment of stage 1 and 2 breast cancer.

Methods
Trial Design: Multicenter randomized controlled trial.
Participants
Inclusion Criteria: Women with primary palpable, operable (T13, N01, M0) breast cancer receiving either pre- or postoperative

chemotherapy, with tumors confined to breast and axilla and life expectancy at or above 10 years.

Exclusion Criteria: Tumors immobile in relation to the underlying chest wall; fixed axillary nodes; ulceration, erythema, skin fixation, peau d'orange, satellite breast nodules, or parasternal nodules.

Intervention: Subjects were randomized to either pre- or postoperative systemic chemotherapy. Randomization was stratified according to age, clinical tumor size, and clinical nodal status. Degree of surgery (lumpectomy vs. mastectomy) was at the discretion of the surgeon. In all patients undergoing preoperative chemotherapy, surgeons were asked to declare whether they would perform lumpectomy or mastectomy at initial staging. All lumpectomy patients also received postoperative radiation.

Endpoints

Primary Endpoint: 1997—tumor response to preoperative therapy (size, clinical and pathological response). 1998—disease-free survival (DFS), distant disease-free survival (DDSF), and survival.

Secondary Endpoints: 1997—nodal response to preoperative chemotherapy, increase in number of lumpectomies. 1998—correlation between tumor response to preoperative therapy and outcome.

Sample Size: 1523 women at participating NSABP institutions in the United States and Canada enrolled between October 1988 and April 1993. 763 women were randomized to the postoperative therapy arm, and 760 women were randomized to the preoperative therapy arm.

Statistical Analysis: Multivariate modeling using logistic regression. Kaplan-Meier method. Log-rank test. Cox proportional-hazards model. 95% intervals. Wald tests for significance. Mantel–Haenszel approach.

Results

Baseline Data: The two groups were well balanced for baseline characteristics. Approximately 50% of the cohort were under 50 years of age; 26% were clinically node-positive; 28% had tumors ≤ 2 cm.

Outcomes: 80% of patients had reduction in tumor size after preoperative therapy. Patient age failed to predict outcome, but positive nodal status (p 0.003) and smaller tumor size (p <0.0001) were significant predictors of complete response. 36% had a complete clinical response to preoperative chemotherapy. Preoperative chemotherapy also decreased the number of clinically and pathologically positive nodes and increased the likelihood of lumpectomy surgery, especially in those with tumors >5.1 cm.

There was no different in DFS, DDSF, or overall survival between pre- and postoperative therapy. Women who had a complete pathologic response to preoperative chemotherapy had better overall outcomes.

Discussion

Conclusion: In women with primary operable breast tumors, preoperative chemotherapy decreases the tumor size and node positivity and should be considered in patients with tumors initially too large for lumpectomy. Additionally, preoperative chemotherapy has outcomes similar to those for postoperative chemotherapy in eligible patients and can help predict tumor response and biology.

Limitations: Physician bias may be present in recommendations for degree of surgery with respect to age, potentially confounding the relationship between age and outcome. The negative nodes cohort consisted of both patients who had negative nodes before therapy, and those that were downstaged as a result of preoperative therapy. There is also the concern that some women underwent therapy unnecessarily due to a false-positive fine-needle aspiration (FNA), or that some did not start therapy because of an absence of invasive cancer on the FNA.

---

f. EBCTCG: Effect of Radiotherapy

Effect of radiotherapy after breast-conserving surgery on 10-year recurrence and 15-year breast cancer death: Meta-analysis of individual patient data for 10,801 women in 17 randomised trials.

Early Breast Cancer Trialists' Collaborative Group (EBCTCG), Darby S, McGale P, Correa C, Taylor C, Arriagada R, Clarke M, Cutter D, Davies C, Ewertz M, Godwin J, Gray R, Pierce L, Whelan T, Wang Y, Peto R

Lancet. 2011;378(9804):1707–1716.

SYNOPSIS

Takeaway Point: Radiotherapy after breast-conserving surgery (BCS) significantly reduces the risk of recurrence and has a moderate effect on reducing the risk of ultimate death from breast cancer.

Commentary: This meta-analysis evaluated 17 randomized clinical trials of node-positive (pN+) and node-negative (pN0) women allocated to BCS plus radiotherapy or BCS alone. Follow-up at 10 years and 15 years showed a significant reduction in first recurrence as well as death from breast cancer. For node-positive women, radiotherapy significantly reduced the 10-year recurrence risk and the 15-year risk of death due to breast cancer. For node-negative patients, the absolute recurrence risk reduction with radiotherapy varied by age, grade, ER status, tamoxifen use, and extent of surgery. These patient factors were then used in a model to predict absolute reductions in both recurrences and death from breast cancer. This was one of the first studies to note that specific patient/tumor characteristics can predict response to radiotherapy.

ANALYSIS

Introduction: Breast-conserving surgery is a well-accepted treatment for women with early-stage breast cancer. However, recurrence of distant metastases can result from macroscopic tumor foci left in the conserved breast. This EBCTCG meta-analysis evaluated 17 randomized controlled trials, focusing primarily on women with known nodal status.

Objectives: To assess the extent to which the radiotherapy-related absolute reduction in 10-year risk of first recurrence at any site (locoregional or distant) varies for women with different prognostic and other factors. It then relates the absolute reduction in the 15-year risk of breast cancer death to the absolute reduction in the 10-year risk of recurrence.

Methods
Trial Design: Meta-analysis of 17 randomized trials.
Participants
Inclusion Criteria: Eligible trials began before 2000, evaluating adjuvant radiotherapy versus no radiotherapy after breast-conserving surgery for invasive cancer.
Exclusion Criteria: Subjects for which follow-up data of at least 10 years was unavailable.
Intervention: Meta-analysis of trials of breast conserving surgery with or without radiotherapy.
Endpoints
Primary Endpoint: Locoregional or distant recurrences, contralateral breast cancer.
Secondary Endpoints: Metastases, death.
Sample Size: 10,801 women from 17 randomized trials with 8337 of known nodal status assigned to either lumpectomy alone or lumpectomy and radiotherapy. Included trials from 1976 to 1999.
Statistical Analysis: Log-rank analyses are stratified by trial, individual follow-up year, and nodal status. Poisson regression fitted by

maximum likelihood. Confidence intervals and p values based on two-sided tests.

Results

Baseline Data: 13 trials evaluated radiotherapy after lumpectomy; 4 were of radiotherapy after quadrentectomy. Median follow-up was 9.5 years. Overall, 7287 women had negative nodes and 1050 had positive nodes (2464 unknown node status).

Outcomes: The 10-year risk of any first recurrence was 19.3% in women allocated to radiotherapy and 35.0% in women allocated to breast-conserving surgery only, corresponding to an absolute risk reduction of 15.7% ($p < 0.00001$). Radiotherapy also reduced breast cancer death: 15-year absolute risk reduction was 3.8% (p 0.00005). Allocation to radiotherapy halved the average annual rate of any first recurrence and reduced the annual breast cancer death rate by one-sixth. In node-negative subjects receiving radiotherapy, the 10-year risk of any first recurrence was reduced from 31.0% to 15.6% with an absolute risk reduction of 15.4% ($p < 0.00001$). In node-positive subjects receiving radiotherapy, the one-year recurrence risk was reduced from 26% to 5.1%. In both pN0 and pN+ disease, first recurrence was more often locoregional for women who did not receive radiotherapy.

Discussion

Conclusion: This meta-analysis shows that radiotherapy after BCS not only substantially reduces the risk of recurrence but also moderately reduces the risk of death from breast cancer.

Limitations: Since only 1050 women had pN+ disease in these trials, the relevance of prognostic factors and other characteristics could not be explored reliably. Beyond year 10, information about recurrence in this period was incomplete as number of events was small. Nodal status was not known for all patients, but was known in a majority.

---

g. SSO/ASTRO Margin Consensus Guideline

Society of Surgical Oncology–American Society for Radiation Oncology consensus guideline on margins for breast-conserving surgery with whole-breast irradiation in stages I and II invasive breast cancer.

Moran MS, Schnitt SJ, Giuliano AE, Harris JR, Khan SA, Horton J, Klimberg S, Chavez-MacGregor M, Freedman G, Houssami N, Johnson PL, Morrow M

Ann Surg Oncol. 2014;21:704–716.

SYNOPSIS

Takeaway Point: New guidelines state that a margin of "no tumor on ink" (ie, with no tumor cells touching the margin inked by the pathologist) is an adequate clear margin for stage 1 and 2 invasive breast cancer.

Commentary: Prior to this meta-analysis by the Society for Surgical Oncology (SSO) and the American Society for Radiation Oncology, there was no consensus as to what constituted a negative or clear margin for lumpectomy in invasive breast cancer. As a result, rates of positive margins and subsequent reexcisions were high. The SSO and ASTRO therefore conducted this meta-analysis to determine the acceptable negative margin standard. "No tumor on ink" is now the current margin standard for lumpectomy surgery, and this more lenient standard has the potential to reduce the frequency of reexcision.

ANALYSIS

Introduction: Previously there was no consensus as to what constitutes a negative margin for lumpectomy surgery in invasive cancer. With conflicting standards, rates of positive margins and reexcisions were high.

Objectives: To determine what margin width minimizes the risk of ipsilateral breast tumor recurrence (IBTR) and, additionally, whether other factors affect this margin width.

Methods
Trial Design: Meta-analysis.
Participants
Inclusion Criteria: Studies published from 1965 to 2013 that allowed for calculation of IBTR in relation to margin width. Patients in the studies were required to have early-stage (stage 1 or 2) invasive breast cancer and to have undergone breast-conserving therapy with whole-breast irradiation. Age and microscopic margins had to be reported and a minimum follow-up time of 4 years was required.
Exclusion Criteria: Pure DCIS. Patients receiving neoadjuvant chemotherapy.
Intervention: None.
Endpoints
Primary Endpoint: Relationship of margin width to IBTR.

Secondary Endpoints: Effect of other factors on margin width and IBTR, such as tumor histology, patient age, use of systemic therapy, and technique of radiation delivery.

Sample Size: 33 studies were included with 28,162 patients.

Statistical Analysis: A study-level analysis was conducted, adjusted for study-specific median follow-up time as well as covariates.

Results

Baseline Data: The majority of included studies were retrospective, and lacked patient-level data. The studies had a median of 701 patients each and a median follow-up time of 79.2 months.

Outcomes: Risk of IBTR was doubled with positive margins (defined as tumor touching ink) during lumpectomy surgery regardless of biology, radiation boost, or endocrine therapy. Margins wider than no tumor on ink did not confer a recurrence benefit. This remained true even when looking at higher risk factors such as young age, tumors with unfavorable biology, lobular cancer, or cancer with an extensive intraductal component.

Discussion

Conclusion: No tumor on ink is an adequate margin standard for breast-conserving surgery in early invasive breast cancer. Wider margins do not decrease the risk of recurrence even in the presence of other known high risk factors.

Limitations: This study is a meta-analysis and not an RCT. It pools data from a wide timeframe (dating back to 1965) when mammography, radiation, and adjuvant therapy were inferior to what we have today; this may render the included studies more heterogeneous and more difficult to compare in a meta-analysis. Additionally, all patients were required to undergo whole-breast radiation, which is not generalizable to patients who opt out of radiation or those who undergo partial breast irradiation.

---

h. Update of NSABP P-1

Tamoxifen for prevention of breast cancer: Current status of the National Surgical Adjuvant Breast and Bowel Project P-1 study.

Fisher B, Costantino JP, Wickerham DL, Cecchini RS, Cronin WM, Robidoux A, Bevers TB, Kavanah MT, Atkins JN, Margolese RG, Runowicz CD, James JM, Ford LG, Wolmark N

J Natl Cancer Inst. 2005;97(22):1652–1662.

SYNOPSIS

Takeaway Point: Tamoxifen is effective in the prevention of non-invasive and estrogen receptor (ER)-positive invasive breast cancer in high-risk women, although it carries an increased risk of uterine cancer, thromboembolism, and cataracts.

Commentary: This is an update on the initial NSABP P1 study that investigated the benefits and risks of using tamoxifen for prevention of noninvasive and invasive breast cancer in high-risk women. The extended follow-up after unblinding the study in 1998 confirms the initial findings that tamoxifen reduces the risk of non-invasive and invasive cancer but increases the risk of uterine cancer, thromboembolism, and cataracts. At the time of this publication, it was estimated that approximately 2.5 million women at high risk for breast cancer could derive a net benefit from the drug. Before this study, we had nothing to offer these high-risk patients (strong family history, LCIS, ADH, etc.) aside from close imaging follow-up or prophylactic mastectomy. This study allows clinicians to discuss the potential risks and benefits of using tamoxifen in those patients at high risk for breast cancer, which has become commonplace today.

ANALYSIS

Introduction: In 1992, the NSABP P1 trial randomized women with high risk of breast cancer to 5 years of placebo or tamoxifen as a preventive agent in breast cancer. Initial results showed a significant risk reduction in noninvasive and invasive breast cancer, as well as a reduction in osteoporotic fractures. However, administration of tamoxifen resulted in an increased risk of endometrial cancer and thromboembolism. The current publication provides an extended follow-up on that cohort.

Objectives: To give updated results after 7 years of follow-up on the preventive effect of tamoxifen on noninvasive and invasive breast cancer in high-risk women and on side effects including endometrial cancer and thromboembolism.

Methods
Trial Design: Double-blinded, randomized placebo-controlled trial.
Participants
Inclusion Criteria: Women over 60, or between 35 and 59 with a 5-year predicted risk for breast cancer of at least 1.66%, or history of ADH or LCIS.

Exclusion Criteria: Taking estrogen/progesterone, oral contraceptive therapy, or androgens within 3 months of randomization, history of deep-vein thrombosis/pulmonary embolism (DVT/PE).

Intervention: Initially double-blinded; participants randomized to 5 years of placebo or tamoxifen. After trial results were announced in 1998, the study was unblinded and those taking the placebo were allowed to receive a 5-year course of tamoxifen or enter the STAR trial (tamoxifen vs. raloxifene; see **k**, below).

Endpoints

Primary Endpoint: Reduction in invasive and noninvasive cancer.

Secondary Endpoints: Rates of osteoporotic fractures, ischemic heart disease, uterine cancer, thromboembolic events, cataracts, and other cancers.

Sample Size: 13,388 women randomized between June 1992 and September 1997, with 6707 to placebo and 6681 to tamoxifen. After unblinding in 1998, 32% of women in the placebo group elected to either receive tamoxifen or enroll in the STAR trial. Seven-year follow-up was available for 4379 from placebo group and 4931 for tamoxifen group.

Statistical Analysis: Incidence rates with two-sided p values determined by exact method, risk ratios with 95% confidence interval (CI), cumulative incidence rates.

Results

Baseline Data: Baseline characteristics were similar between the two groups.

Outcomes: Updated estimates of risk ratios (RRs) for all beneficial and undesirable outcomes of tamoxifen are similar to those in the initial report. Rates of invasive cancer and noninvasive cancer were reduced in the tamoxifen group, RR = 0.57 (95% CI 0.46–0.70) and 0.63 (95% CI 0.45–0.89), respectively. For women who developed cancer, those on tamoxifen were more likely to develop ER-negative breast cancer than were those taking placebo (38.6% vs. 16.8%). Tamoxifen was protective against osteoporotic fractures, RR = 0.68 (95% CI 0.51–0.92). There was an increased risk of endometrial cancer in those taking tamoxifen, RR = 3.28 (95% CI 1.87–6.03). There was a trend toward an increased risk of stroke and DVT in those taking tamoxifen, but this was not statistically significant. Risk of PE was increased in those taking tamoxifen, as was risk of cataracts. There was no significant increase in risk of other cancers. Death rates were similar between both groups.

Discussion

Conclusion: This updated study confirms the reduction in risk of noninvasive and invasive breast cancer seen in those taking tamoxifen in the P1 trial. It also confirms the increased risk of endometrial cancer, thromboembolism (significant only for PE), and cataracts.

Limitations: Trial was not designed to look at reduction in mortality. Trial was unblinded after 1998, and women were allowed to switch to tamoxifen, which resulted in less follow-up data for those in the placebo group, creating potential bias and confounding.

---

i. NSABP B-32

(1) Sentinel-lymph-node resection compared with conventional axillary-lymph-node dissection in clinically node-negative patients with breast cancer: Overall survival findings from the NSABP B-32 randomized phase 3 trial.

Krag DN, Anderson SJ, Julian TB, Brown AM, Harlow SP, Costantino JP, Ashikaga T, Weaver DL, Mamounas EP, Jalovec LM, Frazier TG, Noyes RD, Robidoux A, Scarth HM, Wolmark N

Lancet Oncol. 2010;11(1):927–933.

(2) Morbidity results from the NSABP B-32 trial comparing sentinel lymph node dissection versus axillary dissection.

Ashikaga T, Krag DN, Land SR, Julian TB, Anderson SJ, Brown AM, Skelly JM, Harlow SP, Weaver DL, Mamounas EP, Costantino JP, Wolmark N, National Surgical Adjuvant Breast and Bowel Project

J Surg Oncol. 2010;102(2):111–118.

SYNOPSIS

Takeaway Point: Sentinel lymph node dissection (SLND) in breast cancer patients with negative SLN is a safe alternative to axillary lymph node dissection (ALND) with similar overall survival, disease-free survival, and rates of local recurrence, and lower associated morbidity.

Commentary: This is a pivotal trial in breast cancer surgery and why we are able to perform SLN biopsy without ALND in patients with negative SLN today. ALND carries high morbidity, and SLND is a potential alternative to reduce morbidity while still hopefully achieving the same staging, survival, and recurrence results. This randomized controlled trial was designed to assess overall survival, disease-free survival, rates of local recurrence, and associated morbidity in SLN-negative patients who underwent SLN resection only versus ALND. Outcomes were very similar in both groups with a slight, although nonsignificant, survival advantage in patients who underwent ALND. With regard to morbidity (arm abduction deficits, lymphedema, and subjective numbness and tingling), while patients undergoing SLND did have significant morbidity, all measures and follow-up points favored SLND over ALND. On the basis of this pivotal trial, current practice for patients with invasive breast cancer and clinically negative axillary lymph nodes is to perform SLN resection initially and completion ALND only if the SLN is positive.[11]

ANALYSIS

Introduction: Axillary lymph node dissection (ALND) is important for regional control, survival, and prognosis in breast cancer but is associated with many side effects. Sentinel lymph node (SLN) resection has fewer side effects, but it is unknown whether it achieves the same outcomes as ALND and to what degree the associated morbidity is reduced on a long-term basis.

Objectives: To establish whether SLN resection in patients with SLN-negative breast cancer achieves the same survival and regional control as ALND and to compare 3-year morbidity between SLND and ALND treatment groups in patients with pathologically negative nodes.

Methods

Trial Design: Multicenter randomized controlled trial.

Participants

Inclusion Criteria: Women with invasive breast cancer and clinically negative nodes.

Exclusion Criteria: Clinically positive nodes.

Intervention: Group 1–SLND plus immediate ALND; group 2–SLND alone and ALND only if SLNs are positive. The analysis included only those with negative SLN.

Endpoints

Primary Endpoint: Overall survival in patients with negative SLNs. Morbidity defined as shoulder abduction deficits, arm volume differences (measured by water displacement), and self-reports of numbness and tingling.

Secondary Endpoints: Overall disease-free survival, and regional control in patients with negative SLNs. The study on morbidity used incidence of residual morbidity (ie, incidence of residual shoulder abduction deficits at follow-up).

Sample Size: 3983 SLN-negative patients from 80 institutions in the United States and Canada from May 1, 1999 to February 29, 2004, with 1975 patients randomized to group 1 (ALND) and 2008 to group 2 (SLN)

Statistical Analysis: Intention-to-treat analysis, Fisher's exact test, Kruskal–Wallis rank sum test, odds ratio, simple log-rank tests and Cox proportional-hazards models, Kaplan–Meier curves, cumulative incidence curves.

Results

Baseline Data: The two groups were similar in age, tumor size, and surgical treatment plan. The SLND group had a slightly higher rate of the dominant arm affected (52% vs. 48%, p 0.037) and a lower rate of supraclavicular radiation therapy (XRT) (0.8% vs. 1.6%, p 0.012).

Outcomes: Overall survival between the two groups was not significantly different using log-rank comparisons or Cox proportional-hazards analyses. The 5- and 8-year Kaplan–Meier estimates for overall survival were similar, 96.4% versus 95%, and 91.8% versus 90.3%, respectively. The 5- and 8-year Kaplan–Meier estimates for disease-free survival were also similar, 89% versus 88.6%, and 82.4% versus 81.5%, respectively. Local recurrence rates were not significantly different.

Prevalence of shoulder abduction deficits $\geq 10\%$ were higher in ALND group versus SLND starting at 1 week (75% vs. 41%, p <0.001) and continued until the end of follow-up at 6 months (9% vs. 6% p <0.001). Arm volume differences were lower in the SLND group (7–9%) versus ALND (13–14%) at 6–36-month follow-up (p <0.001 at all timepoints). At 36 months, SLND patients had an odds ratio (OR) of 0.52 (0.41–0.67) for tingling and 0.19 (0.16–0.24) for numbness. Incidence rates of residual shoulder abduction deficits at 6 months, residual arm volume differences at 36 months, and residual arm numbness/tingling at 36 months were lower in the SLND group (p <0.001). Logistic regression showed that XRT and chemotherapy affected residual shoulder abduction morbidity; age, treatment of the dominant side, and receipt of XRT affected residual arm volume morbidity; and age and tumor size affected residual numbness.

Discussion

Conclusion: Overall survival, disease-free survival, and regional control are all statistically equivalent in SLN-negative patients who had an ALND or SLN surgery alone. While patients undergoing SLND still suffer significant morbidity, measurements of arm abduction, arm volume and self-reported numbness and tingling favor SLND over ALND at all follow-up points.

Limitations: Group 1 included 75 patients with negative SLN but a positive nonsentinel node; 95% of this subset received adjuvant therapy compared to 84% in group 2. This difference in adjuvant therapy may have falsely, although nonsignificantly, increased the hazard ratio for survival in favor of group 1. Non–breast cancer deaths were also randomly in favor of group 1 and may have contributed to survival differences. Some of the morbidity measurements were subjective in nature.

---

j. Z0011

(1) Locoregional recurrence after sentinel lymph node dissection with or without axillary dissection in patients with sentinel lymph node metastases: The American College of Surgeons Oncology Group Z0011 randomized trial.

Giuliano AE, McCall L, Beitsch P, Whitworth PW, Blumencranz P, Leitch AM, Saha S, Hunt KK, Morrow M, Ballman K

Ann Surg. 2010;252(3):426–432; discussion 432–433.

(2) Axillary dissection vs. no axillary dissection in women with invasive breast cancer and sentinel node metastasis: A randomized clinical trial.

Giuliano AE, Hunt KK, Ballman KV, Beitsch PD, Whitworth PW, Blumencranz PW, Leitch AM, Saha S, McCall LM, Morrow M

JAMA. 2011;305(6):569–575.

SYNOPSIS

Takeaway Point: In women with clinical T1–T2, N0, M0 breast cancer undergoing breast conservation therapy (lumpectomy, whole breast irradiation and systemic therapy) with one or two positive SLNs, ALND does not demonstrate any advantage in locoregional control or survival over SLND.

Commentary: Before the Z0011 trial, the standard of care for patients with positive SLNs was to undergo ALND. Unfortunately, ALND carries high morbidity, including postoperative paresthesias, wound infections, and lymphedema. Additionally, there was no clear evidence that ALND had any impact on rates of local recurrence or overall survival, especially given advances in surgery, radiation, and systemic therapy. The Z0011 trial was designed to look at whether ALND in women with positive SLNs offers any locoregional or survival benefit in a specific subset: women with T1–T2 invasive breast cancer undergoing lumpectomy, whole breast irradiation, and systemic therapy. The results found no additional locoregional control or survival benefit of ALND for this subset of women. It is important to note that these findings do not apply to women undergoing mastectomy or those with clinically detectable axillary disease. The Z0011 study is widely cited today and has helped avoid much surgical morbidity in many women who would have otherwise undergone unnecessary ALND.

ANALYSIS

Introduction: SLND alone has replaced ALND in clinically node-negative women with pathologically negative SLN. However, ALND is still recommended for women with positive SLN, although some initial small studies suggest that selected patients may be managed without completion ALND.

Objectives: The Z0011 RCT was initiated to compare the overall survival and locoregional control in women with clinical T1–T2, N0, M0 breast cancer with a positive SLN undergoing ALND versus SLND alone.

Trial Design: Multicenter randomized phase 3 controlled trial.

Participants
Inclusion Criteria: Adult women with clinical T1–T2 invasive breast cancer <5 cm, no palpable adenopathy, and one or two SLNs containing metastatic breast cancer documented by frozen section, touch preparation, or hematoxylin + eosin (H + E) staining. All underwent lumpectomy (to negative margins) and tangential whole-breast irradiation. Adjuvant systemic therapy was determined by the treating physician.

Exclusion Criteria: Patients with metastases identified initially or solely with immunohistochemical staining. Three or more positive SLNs, matted nodes, gross extranodal disease, or neoadjuvant hormonal therapy or chemotherapy. Pregnant or lactating patients. Bilateral breast cancer. History of ipsilateral axillary surgery.

Intervention: Before randomization, all women underwent SLND and were stratified by age, estrogen receptor status, and tumor size. Eligible women were then randomized to axillary lymph node dissection (10 or more nodes) or no further axillary treatment.

Endpoints

Primary Endpoint: Disease recurrence (local, regional, distant) and overall survival.

Secondary Endpoints: Time to recurrence and disease-free survival.

Sample Size: 891 patients from 115 sites, 445 randomized to ALND, and 446 to SLND alone. Enrollment from May 1999 to December 2004.

Statistical Analysis: χ^2 test, two-sample t-test, Cox proportional-hazards model, Cox regression model, Kaplan–Meier survival curves, log-rank test, Fisher exact test, intention-to-treat analysis, and treatment-received analysis.

Results

Baseline Data: Patient characteristics were similar between the two groups, including rates of adjuvant therapy and radiation.

Outcomes: 40.8% of the ALND group had two or more positive nodes compared to 21.9% in SLND group. 27.3% of the ALND group had additional metastatic disease in the ALND sample. After median of 6.3 years' follow-up, locoregional recurrence was 3.4% in the entire cohort. There was no significant difference in local or regional recurrences in either group. The median time of local recurrence-free survival was not reached in either group and did not differ. 5-year overall survival rates were 92.5% in SLND-only group and 91.8% in ALND group. Disease-free survival did not differ significantly: 5-year disease-free survival was 83.9% for SLND-only group and 82.2% for ALND group. Surgical morbidities (paresthesias, infecton, lymphedema) were significantly higher in the ALND group.

Discussion

Conclusion: In women with low to moderate axillary tumor burden undergoing breast conservation therapy, ALND does not show any advantage in locoregional control or overall survival compared to SLND alone.

Limitations: Most patients had low axillary tumor burden; if the surgeon felt that there was extensive axillary disease during dissection, the patient was excluded from the study. Patients with three or more positive SLNs were not eligible for randomization (although a few were randomized before SLND and therefore included). Study was not stratified for volume of disease, and those SNs detected by immunohistochemistry (usually micrometastases or isolated tumor cells) were excluded. Initial sample size calculations estimated 1900 patients were needed for a hazard ratio for overall survival of 1.3 with 90% power; trial was closed early with only 891 patients enrolled because of lower than anticipated accrual rates. Possible randomization imbalance favoring SLND-alone group. Does not include patients undergoing mastectomy or those undergoing lumpectomy treated without XRT, or with partial XRT.

---

k. STAR P-2

Update on the National Surgical Adjuvant Breast and Bowel Study of Tamoxifen and Raloxifene (STAR) P-2 Trial: Preventing breast cancer.

Vogel VG, Costantino JP, Wickerham DL, Cronin WM, Cecchini RS, Atkins JN, Bevers TB, Fehrenbacher L, Pajon ER, Wade JL 3rd, Robidoux A, Margolese RG, James J, Runowicz CD, Ganz PA, Reis SE, McCaskill-Stevens W, Ford LG, Jordan VC, Wolmark N, National Surgical Adjuvant Breast and Bowel Project

Cancer Prev Res. 2010;3(6):696–706.

SYNOPSIS

Takeaway Point: After prolonged follow-up, raloxifene remains effective in preventing invasive and noninvasive breast cancer in postmenopausal patients. Raloxifene is less effective than tamoxifen but carries a reduced risk of side effects, including endometrial cancer and thromboembolic events.

Commentary: This study is an update to the original STAR study comparing the effectiveness of raloxifene and tamoxifen in preventing breast cancer. The original study followed patients for 47 months and showed similar outcomes for invasive cancer and a slight advantage for tamoxifen for noninvasive cancer (although not statistically significant). While raloxifene had an overall better side effect profile, there was no significant difference in rates of endometrial cancer. This study represents an extended follow-up of 81 months and shows more pronounced differences between the two drugs over time. Tamoxifen is more effective in preventing invasive and noninvasive breast cancer than raloxifene, but we are now seeing a significant increase in endometrial cancer in patients taking tamoxifen compared to raloxifene. On the basis of this study, both drugs are effective in prevention of primary breast cancer but because of their side effect profiles, should be tailored to fit individual risk (ie, may favor tamoxifen in a high-risk patient who has undergone hysterectomy).

ANALYSIS

Introduction: Tamoxifen has been proven to prevent breast cancer but carries an increased risk of endometrial cancer and thromboembolic events. Raloxifene, a selective estrogen receptor modulator initially studied in the prevention of osteoporotic fractures, has also proved effective for preventing breast cancer but with fewer side effects. This study is an update to the original STAR study, which showed equal risk reduction but decreased side effects for raloxifene compared with tamoxifen.

Objectives: To compare the efficacy and side effect profiles of tamoxifen and raloxifene in preventing breast cancer after prolonged follow-up.

Methods
Trial Design: Two-arm, randomized, double-blinded trial.
Participants
Inclusion Criteria: Postmenopausal women, at least 35 years old, with a 5-year predicted breast cancer risk of at least 1.66% (based on the Gail model).

Exclusion Criteria: Taking tamoxifen, raloxifene, hormonal therapy, oral contraceptives, or androgens in the 3 months prior to randomization. Taking warfarin or cholestyramine. History of stroke, transient ischemic attack (TIA), PE, DVT, atrial fibrillation, uncontrolled diabetes mellitus or hypertension, or a psychiatric condition that would interfere with compliance. Poor performance status. History of prior malignancy aside from skin, carcinoma in situ of cervix, and LCIS of the breast.

Intervention: Initially double-blinded; randomly assigned to tamoxifen or raloxifene. Unblinded in April 2006.
Endpoints
Primary Endpoint: Incidence of invasive breast cancer.
Secondary Endpoints: Incidence of noninvasive cancer, endometrial cancer, other cancers, and vascular-related events.

Sample Size: 19,747 women initially enrolled from July 1999 to November 2004, with 257 women lost to follow up. Remaining 19,490 analyzed (9736 tamoxifen and 9754 raloxifene). At time of unblinding and at time of the original report (April 2006), participants were given option to switch to raloxifene, which 879 women did.

Statistical Analysis: Intention-to-treat analysis, risk ratios, cumulative incidence, log-rank test.

Results

Baseline Data: Similar baseline characteristics. Followed for median of 81 months (60 months of treatment).

Outcomes: Invasive breast cancer RR (raloxifene:tamoxifen) is 1.24 (95% CI 1.05–1.47) and 1.22 (95% CI 0.95–1.59) for noninvasive breast cancer. Raloxifene is about 76% as effective as tamoxifen in reducing invasive breast cancer risk and 78% as effective for reducing noninvasive cancer risk. Compared to a theoretical placebo (using the Breast Cancer Prevention Trial and the Gail model of risk prediction), raloxifene reduces risk of invasive cancer by 38% versus 50% for tamoxifen and for noninvasive cancer by 39% versus 50% for tamoxifen. RR of uterine cancer for raloxifene:tamoxifen was 0.55 (p 0.003) and for uterine hyperplasia was 0.19. Twice the number of hysterectomies was performed in the tamoxifen group. No significant differences were seen for other cancers. RR of thromboembolic events for raloxifene:tamoxifen was 0.75 (95% CI 0.60–0.93). Incidence of cataracts was increased in the tamoxifen group. There were no significant differences in mortality.

Discussion

Conclusion: After prolonged follow-up (median 81 months), raloxifene was found to be 76% as effective as tamoxifen in preventing invasive breast cancer and 76% as effective in preventing noninvasive breast cancer. However, tamoxifen continues to carry a higher risk of endometrial cancer, hysterectomies for benign disease, cataracts, and thromboembolic events.

Limitations: Allowed crossover when study was unblinded, which may have affected results. Non-adherence may affect raloxifene more than tamoxifen, due to bioavailability.

I. ACOSOG Z1071 (Alliance) Trial

Sentinel lymph node surgery after neoadjuvant chemotherapy in patients with node-positive breast cancer: The ACOSOG Z1071 (Alliance) Clinical Trial.

Boughey JC, Suman VJ, Mittendorf EA, Ahrendt GM, Wilke LG, Taback B, Leitch AM, Kuerer HM, Bowling M, Flippo-Morton TS, Byrd DR, Ollila DW, Julian TB, McLaughlin SA, McCall L, Symmans WF, Le-Petross HT, Haffty BG, Buchholz TA, Nelson H, Hunt KK, Alliance for Clinical Trials in Oncology

JAMA. 2013;310(14):1455–1461.

SYNOPSIS

Takeaway Point: The false-negative rate for sentinel lymph node surgery in patients with patients with clinically positive lymph nodes (cN1) following neoadjuvant chemotherapy is 12.6%, higher than the accepted rate of 10%.

Commentary: This study investigated whether SLND is an acceptable alternative to complete axillary lymph node dissection (ALND) for accurately determining lymph node status in women with cN1 disease after neoadjuvant chemotherapy. All patients underwent SLND of at least two lymph nodes aided by radiolabeled colloid and/or blue dye, followed by ALND. The false-negative rate (FNR) of SLN surgery was calculated and compared to the FNR for SLND in patients with clinically node-negative disease (cN0). The FNR was found to be 12.6%, higher than the acceptable rate of 10% (the rate expected for SLND in women who initially present with clinically negative axillary lymph nodes). The FNR decreased with dual mapping techniques and SLND of at least three lymph nodes. The switch to SLND from ALND has the potential to reduce the surgical morbidity in cN1 patients receiving neoadjuvant therapy. However, more data and perhaps improved patient selection are needed before supporting the use of SLN surgery as an alternative to ALND in this patient population.

ANALYSIS

Introduction: 50–60% of women presenting with clinically node-positive disease (cN1) have residual axillary nodal disease after neoadjuvant therapy. Although accurate determination of axillary lymph node status is important in guiding treatment, ALND carries a high risk of morbidity. Sentinel lymph node biopsies have lower morbidity; however, current limited data show false-negative rates as high as 25%.

Objectives: To determine the FNR for SLND following chemotherapy in women initially presenting with biopsy-proven cN1 breast cancer.

Methods

Trial Design: Prospective cohort study.

Participants

Inclusion Criteria: Women ≥18 years with histologically proven clinical stage T0–T4, N1–N2 (by FNA or core needle biopsy), and M0 primary invasive breast cancer undergoing neoadjuvant chemotherapy.

Exclusion Criteria: History of prior ipsilateral axillary surgery.

Intervention: SLND (at least two nodes identified with radiolabeled colloid and/or blue dye) followed by complete ALND after neoadjuvant chemotherapy.

Endpoints

Primary Endpoint: FNR of SLND after chemotherapy when at least two SLNs were excised in women who presented with cN1 disease.

Secondary Endpoints: The pathologic complete nodal response (pCR) rate.

Sample Size: 701 women from 136 institutions from July 2009 to June 2011, of which 663 had cN1 disease and 38 had cN2 disease.

Statistical Analysis: Bayesian clinical trial design, Fisher exact test, multivariable logistic regression, likelihood ratio tests.

Results

Baseline Data: 74.6% of chemotherapy regimens included anthracycline and taxane. After completion of chemotherapy, clinical examination of the axilla revealed no palpable lymphadenopathy in 83%, palpable nodes in 12%, and fixed/matted nodes in 0.6%.

Outcomes: Among the 525 patients with cN1 disease who had at least two SLNs excised, 108 patients had residual disease confined to the SLN (20.6%), 39 patients had disease confined to the nodes removed on ALND (7.4%), 163 patients had disease in both SLN and ALND (31.1%), and 215 patients had no residual disease, yielding a pCR rate of 41%. 39 of the 310 patients with residual disease had a false-negative SLN, yielding a FNR of 12.6% (90% BCI 9.85–16.05%). Likelihood of a false-negative SLN finding was significantly reduced when both blue dye and radiolabeled colloid were used and when at least three SLNs were examined. In multivariable logistic modeling, only the number of SLNs examined was significant. For women with cN2 disease, the pCR rate was 46.1% and FNR was 0% (95% CI, 0–23.2%).

Discussion

Conclusion: The FNR for SLN surgery (at least two nodes) after neoadjuvant chemotherapy in women with cN1 disease is 12.6%, higher than the accepted threshold of 10% for women with cN0 disease. The FNR may be reduced by using a dual-mapping technique and examining at least three SLNs. Changes in approach and patient selection would be necessary to support use of SLN surgery as alternative to ALND in this patient population.

Limitations: There were no exclusion criteria for type or length of chemotherapy, reason for discontinuing chemotherapy, or nodal response after chemotherapy. This does not allow for selection of patients with the highest likelihood of nodal response and/or lowest likelihood of residual disease.

REFERENCES

1. Rayter Z, Mansi J. *Medical Therapy of Breast Cancer*. St George's Hospital Medical School, University of London; 2008.

2. Halsted W. The results of operations for the cure of cancer of the breast performed at the Johns Hopkins Hospital from June 1889 to January 1894. *Ann Surg*. 1894;20(5):497–555.

3. Fisher B, Jeong J-H, Anderson S, Bryant J, Fisher ER, Wolmark N. Twenty-five year follow-up of a randomized trial comparing radical mastectomy, total mastectomy, and total mastectomy followed by irradiation. *NEJM*. 2002;347(8):567–575.

4. Fisher B, Anderson S, Bryant J, Margolese RJ, Deutsch M, Fisher ER, Jeong J-H, Wolmark N. Twenty-year follow-up of a randomized trial comparing total mastectomy, lumpectomy, and lumpectomy plus irradiation for the treatment of invasive breast cancer *NEJM*. 347(16):1233–1241.

5. Fisher B, Constantino J, Redmond C, Fisher E, Margolese R, Dimitrov N, Wolmark N, Wickerham DL, Deutsch M, Ore L, Mamounas E, Poller W, Kavanah M. Lumpectomy compared with lumpectomy and radiation therapy for the treatment of intraductal breast cancer. *NEJM*. 328:1581–1586.

6. Ashikaga T, Krag DN, Land SR, Julian TB, Anderson SJ, Brown AM, Skelly JM, Harlow SP, Weaver DL, Mamounas EP, Costantino JP, Wolmark N. Sentinel-lymph-node resection compared with conventional axillary-lymph-node dissection in clinically node-negative patients with breast cancer: Overall survival findings from the NSABP B-32 randomised phase 3 trial. *Lancet Oncol*. 2010;11(10):927–933.

7. Giuliano AE1, McCall L, Beitsch P, Whitworth PW, Blumencranz P, Leitch AM, Saha S, Hunt KK, Morrow M, Ballman K. Axillary dissection vs no axillary dissection in women with invasive breast cancer and sentinel node metastasis: A randomized clinical trial. *JAMA*. 2011;305(6):569–575.

8. Fisher B, Bryant J, Wolmark N, Mamounas E, Brown A, Fisher ER, Wickher DL, Begovic M, Deilisz A, Robidoux A, Margolese RG, Cruz AB Jr, Hoeh JL, Lees AW, Dimitrov NV, Bear HD. Effect of preoperative chemotherapy on local-regional disease in women with operable breast cancer: Findings from National Surgical Adjuvant Breast and Bowel Project B-18. *J Clin Oncol.* 1997;15:2483–2493.

9. Fisher B, Costantino J, Wickerham DL, Cecchini RS, Cronin WM, Robidoux A, Bevers TB, Kavanah M, Atkins J, Margolese R, Runowicz CD, James J, Ford L, Wolmark N. Tamoxifen for the prevention of breast cancer: Current status of the National Surgical Adjuvant Breast and Bowel Project P-1 Study. *J Natl Cancer Inst.* 2005;97(22):1652–1662.

10. Vogel VG, Costantino JP, Wickerham DL, Cronin WM, Cecchini RS, Atkins JN, Bevers TB, Fehrenbacher L, Pajon ER, Wade JL 3rd, Robidoux A, Margolese RG, James J, Runowicz CD, Ganz PA, Reis SE, McCaskill-Stevens W, Ford LG, Jordan VC, Wolmark N. Update of the National Surgical Adjuvant Breast and Bowel Project Study of Tamoxifen and Raloxifene (STAR) P-2 Trial: Preventing breast cancer. *Cancer Prev Res.* 2010;3(6):696–706.

11. Lyman GH, Temin S, Edge SB, et al. Sentinel lymph node biopsy for patients with early-stage breast cancer: American Society of Clinical Oncology Clinical Practice Guideline update. *J Clin Oncol.* 2014; 32:1365–1383.

6

Endocrine Surgery

Hadiza Kazure • Dana Lin

Prior to the late 1800's, the function of endocrine glands was unknown. Surgeons excised the thyroid gland for severe goiters, but operative mortality was over 40% due to massive hemorrhage.[1] Outcomes for patients who survived the operation were ambiguous, but as neither antisepsis nor the existence of parathyroid glands was recognized, it was unclear whether postoperative mortality reflected infection or organ failure.[2]

Major advances in the mid-19th century, namely, the advent of effective anesthesia, adoption of aseptic technique, and the invention of hemostatic forceps, enabled significant strides in thyroid surgery. Swiss surgeon Theodor Kocher (1841–1917) refined the operation over the course of his 40-year career and approximately 5000 thyroidectomies, reducing mortality rates to 0.5%.[3] Crucially, Kocher also characterized the vital role of the thyroid gland in metabolism and organ function. At the behest of a referring physician, Kocher reexamined a girl he had previously performed a total thyroidectomy on 9 years earlier, and found her to be cretinoid. This prompted him to initiate follow-up on 102 of his postthyroidectomy patients (the largest reported single-surgeon series at the time) and review an additional 134 cases collected from 15 colleagues in Germany and Switzerland. He catalogued in detail the clinical features and outcome of each patient, and coined the term *cachexia strumipriva* (decay resulting from lack of goiter).[2] His work represents a milestone in surgery, as a classic example of a surgical audit and investigation into the long-term effects of a procedure. For his groundbreaking work on the physiology, pathology, and surgery of the thyroid gland, Kocher was awarded the Nobel Prize in 1909, and is considered the father of endocrine surgery.

Thyroid and parathyroid surgery today boasts very low complication rates in experienced hands. The more common disease entities requiring surgical interventions, such as well-differentiated thyroid cancer and primary hyperparathyroidism, have excellent long-term survival and cure rates.[4,5] A comparison of different treatment approaches in a prospective randomized controlled fashion would, therefore, require a prohibitively high number of subjects, as demonstrated by Carling et al in a feasibility study concerning prophylactic central lymph node dissection for papillary thyroid cancer.[6] Given these considerations, as well as the rarity of many endocrine disorders, the majority of published reports in the field of endocrine surgery are retrospective in nature. Without good randomized clinical trials, surgeons rely on clinical practice guidelines developed and endorsed by reputable professional societies such as the American Thyroid Association, American Association of Endocrine Surgeons, and American Association of Clinical Endocrinologists. We will review several of these guidelines in this chapter.

The modern age of clinical practice guidelines began in 1992 with an Institute of Medicine report advocating for "systematically developed statements to assist practitioner and patient decisions about appropriate health care for specific circumstances."[7] Clinical practice guidelines aim to create consistent practice patterns based on the best available evidence. Guidelines are formulated according to a structured process. A panel of "expert" stakeholders convenes to vet and summarize the total weight of evidence on a specific subject area or clinical question, taking into consideration the quality and strength of the data. The summarized evidence is then categorized according to its susceptibility to bias. When conclusive evidence is absent, expert opinion is relied on to interpret or extrapolate the evidence and derive recommendations. This subjectivity is an inherent weakness of practice guidelines. Recommendations are typically graded in terms of strength, indicating the panel's level of confidence that the guidelines will produce the desired outcome. In general, recommendation grades are a reflection of research methodology ranging from strong (randomized controlled trials), to weak (cross-sectional studies, case reports), to anecdotal (opinion, consensus, or review). After critical review of the quality of evidence, various subjective factors are incorporated, such as risk–benefit analysis, cost-effectiveness, clinical relevance, and dissenting opinions. A final recommendation grade is then established, with grade A and B representing strong recommendations, grade C weaker recommendations, and grade D expert opinion.[8]

The guidelines then undergo external review to ensure content validity, clarity, and applicability.[9] Thus, while tremendously practical and informative, it is wise when reading guidelines to keep in mind that they are (1) derived only in part from randomized trials, (2) reliant on the expertise and judgment of the appointed task force, and (3) meant to be customized to the individual patient rather than prescriptively applied.

Some of the greatest surgeon scientists of all time have been endocrine surgeons: Theodor Kocher, Theodor Billroth, William Stewart Halsted, and Charles Mayo, to name only a few. Their contributions and impact far transcend the subspecialty of endocrine surgery. In their relentless pursuit of technical excellence, optimal surgical outcomes, and scientific progress, they revolutionized the world of surgery in their day. Their legacy has served as an inspiration and model for countless young surgeons through the generations to this day.

a. Management Guidelines for Thyroid Nodules and Differentiated Thyroid Cancer

Revised American Thyroid Association management guidelines for patients with thyroid nodules and differentiated thyroid cancer.

American Thyroid Association (ATA) Guidelines Taskforce, Cooper DS, Doherty GM, Haugen BR, Kloos RT, Lee SL, Mandel SJ, Mazzaferri EL, McIver B, Pacini F, Schlumberger M, Sherman SI, Steward DL, Tuttle RM

Thyroid. 2009;19(11):1167–1214.

SYNOPSIS

Takeaway Point: In contrast to guidelines published by American Thyroid Association (ATA) in 2006, the revised 2009 guidelines advise total or near-total thyroidectomy for differentiated thyroid carcinoma (DTC) > 1 cm, and central lymph node dissection (CLND) for any cN1 disease. The glaring paucity of level I studies to guide the surgical management of thyroid cancer remains apparent in these guidelines.

Commentary: In 2006, the ATA issued an updated set of management guidelines for thyroid nodules and DTC, advising "routine central compartment (level VI) neck dissection for patients with papillary thyroid carcinoma and suspected Hurthle cell carcinoma."

This sparked heated controversy due to its susceptibility to varying interpretations and the absence of strong supporting data. Proponents of prophylactic central lymph node dissection (pCLND) cite the high incidence of cervical lymph node metastasis[10] and possible attendant increase in recurrence and decrease in survival.[11–13] Preoperative ultrasound and intraoperative assessment have low sensitivity for microscopic lymph node involvement.[14,15] In addition, central neck dissection during the initial surgery affords valuable staging information to determine the need for and dosing of adjuvant radioactive iodine.[16] Arguments against pCLND focus on the unproven benefit[17,18] and concern for increased surgical morbidity. Neck dissection carries a low complication rate in experienced hands;[19] however, studies have shown that the majority of thyroid surgeries in the United States are performed by low-volume surgeons—a group that has been associated with higher complication rates.[20,21]

In light of the limited and conflicting data regarding the initial management of the central compartment lymph nodes in clinically node-negative papillary thyroid cancer, the ATA revised and clarified their stance in 2009, as detailed in the following summary. Prophylactic CLND may be considered, especially for advanced primary tumors, but with the acknowledgment that this approach can be associated with increased morbidity, especially among low-volume surgeons. Following publication of the 2009 guidelines, several large-volume trials were conducted to further investigate the role of central compartment neck dissection in DTC, two of which are discussed later in this chapter (see **b** and **c**, below).

Although it has been shown that care in accordance with guidelines for DTC is associated with improved patient outcomes, a wide variability in the degree of adherence to the revised ATA recommendations has been noted among practitioners.[22]

ANALYSIS

Introduction: Differentiated thyroid cancer (DTC), which includes papillary and follicular cancer, occurs in 5–10% of thyroid nodules, and represents 90% of all thyroid cancers. Incidence is increasing, and surgery is essential for management. In 1996, the American Thyroid Association (ATA) published its first treatment guidelines for patients with thyroid nodules and DTC. These guidelines were updated in 2006, and a surge of high-quality studies led to another update in 2009.

Methods

A task force of 13 experts on short- and long-term medical and surgical management of thyroid nodules and thyroid cancer reviewed the previously published ATA guidelines from 2006 in light of new data and produced updated *consensus* guidelines. Given the paucity of randomized controlled trials in the treatment of DTC, the panel relied on all available published evidence. When evidence was judged to be insufficient, the task force members relied on their personal experience and judgment.

Results

In keeping with the previous version, the revised guidelines cover the management of thyroid nodules and DTC, including diagnostic approach and algorithms for initial and long-term medical and surgical management. Of particular interest to surgeons, the updated guidelines address controversial topics, including extent of thyroidectomy based on tumor size, and prophylactic central neck dissection:

Extent of surgery for differentiated thyroid cancer (lobectomy vs. thyroidectomy). **The guidelines previously recommended total or near-total thyroidectomy for documented thyroid cancers greater than 1–1.5 cm. The 2009 guidelines reduced the size criteria to >1 cm (recommendation rating A). This was based in part on a retrospective study of more than 50,000 patients that demonstrated significantly improved recurrence and survival rates after thyroidectomy as opposed to lobectomy for tumors larger than 1 cm.[23] Lobectomy for management of DTC should be restricted to subcentimeter, unifocal lesions.**

Central lymph node dissection. **The 2006 guidelines proposed that "routine central node dissection should be *considered* for patients with papillary or suspected Hurthle cell carcinoma." The revised guidelines are more explicit in the distinction between prophylactic neck dissection (for patients clinically and radiologically N0) and therapeutic neck dissection (for patients cN1) and their respective indications. For patients with clinically involved central or lateral neck lymph nodes, central compartment neck dissection *should* accompany total thyroidectomy (recommendation rating B). For patients with clinically uninvolved central neck lymph nodes, prophylactic central compartment neck dissection *may* be performed, especially for advanced primary (T3 or T4) tumors (recommendation rating C). Accompanying the recommendation is** the caveat that it should be interpreted in light of available surgical expertise. The benefit of decreased locoregional recurrence must be weighed against possible increased surgical morbidity.

Discussion

Conclusion: Total or near-total thyroidectomy should be performed for DTC > 1 cm. Patients with cN1 disease should undergo therapeutic CLND. Prophylactic CLND may be considered in patients with cN0 disease, especially for advanced primary tumors.

Limitations: The majority of data informing the guidelines are derived from retrospective, single-institution studies. In addition, the recommendations may reflect the bias of the experts on the task force.

---

b. Routine Central Lymph Node Dissection for cN0 Papillary Thyroid Cancer

A multicenter cohort study of total thyroidectomy and routine central lymph node dissection for cN0 papillary thyroid cancer.

Popadich A, Levin O, Lee JC, Smooke-Praw S, Ro K, Fazel M, Arora A, Tolley NS, Palazzo F, Learoyd D, Sidhu S, Delbridge L, Sywak M, Yeh MW

Surgery. 2011;150(6):1048–1057.

SYNOPSIS

Takeaway Point: Routine central lymph node dissection (CLND) in papillary thyroid carcinoma (PTC) is associated with lower postoperative thyroglobulin levels and reduces the need for reoperation in the central compartment.

Commentary: The authors evaluated the impact of routine CLND after total thyroidectomy in the management of patients with cN0 PTC in three international endocrine surgery centers over a 14-year period. The authors demonstrated that patients who underwent CLND with thyroidectomy had statistically lower postoperative thyroglobulin (Tg) levels (prior to radioiodine ablation) and lower reoperation rates compared with thyroidectomy alone. In addition, there was no significant difference in complication rates between those who underwent CLND versus those who did not. While this study indicates that routine prophylactic CLND is associated with positive outcomes without an increase in morbidity, it is limited by its retrospective nature and the use of data from high-volume centers, which restricts generalizability.

ANALYSIS

Introduction: The role of routine, or prophylactic, central lymph node dissection (CLND) for papillary thyroid cancer (PTC) remains controversial.

Objectives: The aim of this study was to evaluate the impact of routine CLND after total thyroidectomy (TTx) in the management of patients with PTC who were clinically node negative at presentation with emphasis on stimulated thyroglobulin (Tg) levels and reoperation rates.

Methods
Trial Design: Retrospective, multicenter cohort study.
Participants
Inclusion Criteria: Age ≥ 16 years with PTC >1 cm without preoperative evidence of lymph node disease (cN0).

Exclusion Criteria: Papillary microcarcinoma, subtotal or hemithyroidectomy as definitive procedure, preoperative evidence of nodal disease, lateral neck dissection performed at original surgery, distant metastatic disease.

Intervention: Thyroidectomy alone (group A) or CLND (group B). Of note, the study did not distinguish between ipsilateral and bilateral CLND; both were included in group B.

Sample Size: 606 patients from three centers in Australia, the United States, and England underwent surgery between 1995 and 2009, including 347 without CLND (group A) and 259 with CLND (group B).

Statistical Analysis: Fisher's exact test, Student's t-test, number needed to treat.

Results
Baseline Data: Group A was significantly older (mean age 48 vs. 44, p 0.002), and had significantly longer follow-up time (50 vs. 32 months, p <0.001). Group B had significantly higher rates of vascular invasion (50% vs. 36%, p 0.002). Tumor size was similar between the two groups.

Outcomes: Stimulated Tg values were lower in group B before initial radioiodine ablation (15.0 vs. 6.6 ng/mL; p 0.025). There was a trend toward a lower Tg at final follow-up in group B (1.9 vs. 7.2 ng/mL;

p 0.110). The rate of reoperation in the central compartment was lower in group B (1.5% vs. 6.1%; *p* 0.004). Though there was no difference in the incidence of permanent hypoparathyroidism or recurrent laryngeal nerve (RLN) palsy, group B had a significantly greater number of parathyroid autotransplantation (0.88 vs. 1.2; *p* 0.006) and temporary hypocalcemia (4.1% vs. 9.7%; *p* 0.026). Twenty CLND procedures were required to prevent one central compartment reoperation.

Discussion
Conclusion: The addition of routine CLND in cN0 papillary thyroid carcinoma is associated with lower postoperative Tg levels and reduces the need for reoperation in the central compartment.

Limitations: Retrospective study design with variable follow-up time, and lack of multivariate analysis. The data are from tertiary referral centers with high surgeon volume, which limits generalizability to lower-volume practices. The groups were not balanced for preoperative characteristics.

---

c. Central Compartment Neck Dissection for Locoregional Recurrence in PTC

A meta-analysis of the effect of prophylactic central compartment neck dissection on locoregional recurrence rates in patients with papillary thyroid cancer.

Wang TS, Cheung K, Farrokhyar F, Roman SA, Sosa JA

Ann Surg Oncol. 2013;20(11):3477–3483.

SYNOPSIS

Takeaway Point: This meta-analysis demonstrated a trend toward lower recurrence rates in patients with clinically node-negative PTC undergoing total thyroidectomy with prophylactic central node dissection (pCLND) compared to those undergoing total thyroidectomy alone.

Commentary: Most of the studies examining the effectiveness of prophylactic CLND are single-institution retrospective studies, and a prospective randomized trial is likely not feasible as it would require a prohibitively large sample size.[6] For these reasons, meta-analyses such as this study are important for evaluating optimal management algorithms for patients with DTC. The authors performed a meta-analysis of 11 studies involving more than 2300 patients to determine the impact of prophylactic CLND on recurrence rates after total thyroidectomy in the management of adult patients with PTC who are clinically node-negative. The authors showed a trend toward lower recurrence rate in patients undergoing prophylactic CLND for PTC compared to patients undergoing total thyroidectomy alone, although the difference did not reach statistical significance. The study is the first of its kind to exclude pediatric patients, those who underwent lobectomies, and those with microcarcinomas. However, it is limited by extent of follow-up data and exclusion of data regarding postoperative radioactive iodine administration. A subsequent consensus report by the European Society of Endocrine Surgeons[24] provides a critical appraisal of the studies and meta-analyses regarding prophylactic CLND to date and identifies a comprehensive list of bias sources. They conclude that prophylactic dissections should be risk-stratified and performed only by surgeons with the available expertise and experience.

ANALYSIS

Introduction: It is not known whether prophylactic central compartment lymph node dissection (pCLND) in conjunction with total thyroidectomy decreases rates of locoregional recurrence in patients with papillary thyroid cancer (PTC).

Objectives: To determine the effects of pCLND on locoregional recurrence rates in adult patients with PTC.

Methods
Trial Design: Meta-analysis of 11 studies.
Participants
Inclusion Criteria: Adults with PTC >1 cm who underwent total thyroidectomy with or without pCLND.

Exclusion Criteria: Age <18 years, no recurrence data, therapeutic lymph node dissection, microcarcinoma, review articles, letters to the editor, abstracts, or meeting proceedings.

Intervention: Included trials treated patients with clinically node-negative PTC with total thyroidectomy (TT) alone, or TT with pCLND.

Endpoints
Primary Endpoint: Locoregional recurrence.
Secondary Endpoints: Postoperative complications (calculated only for comparative studies).

Sample Size: 117 articles were initially reviewed; 58 were determined to be relevant and were reviewed in full text. Of these, 11 studies met the inclusion criteria for a pooled sample size of 2318 patients.

Statistical Analysis: Interclass correlation coefficient, fixed and random effects modeling, Cochran's Q-test, relative risk, and weighted pooled estimates of proportions.

Results

Baseline Data: Six included studies compared TT with TT/pCLND, and five were cohort studies of TT/pCLND. Assessment of study quality by two reviewers had an interrater reliability of 93.5%.

Outcomes: Pooled recurrence rates for all patients undergoing TT/pCLND was 4.7%, compared with 7.9% in the TT-alone group. The relative risk of recurrence for patients undergoing TT/pCLND was 0.59 (95% CI 0.33–1.07), favoring a lower recurrence rate in the TT/pCLND arm, but not reaching statistical significance. The number of patients who would need to be treated (NNT) in order to prevent a single recurrence is 31. The comparative studies were also analyzed for complication rates. The relative risk for permanent hypocalcemia after TT/pCLND was 1.82 (95% CI 0.51–6.5) and for permanent recurrent laryngeal nerve injury was 1.14 (95% CI 0.46–2.83).

Discussion

Conclusion: There was no difference in recurrence or long-term complication rates between patients undergoing TT or TT/pCLND. There was a trend toward lower recurrence rates in TT/pCLND patients, with a NNT of 31 patients.

Limitations: Limited and variable data on postoperative follow-up period, as well as variability in the designs and data collected in the studies included in the analysis. Single-institution cohort studies were included in the primary analysis.

---

d. Guidelines for the Management of Asymptomatic Primary Hyperparathyroidism

(1) Guidelines for the management of asymptomatic primary hyperparathyroidism: Summary statement from the Fourth International Workshop.

Bilezikian JP, Brandi ML, Eastell R, Silverberg SJ, Udelsman R, Marcocci C, Potts JT Jr.

J Clin Endocrinol Metab. 2014;99(10):3561–3569.

(2) The surgical management of asymptomatic primary hyperparathyroidism: Proceedings of the Fourth International Workshop.

Udelsman R, Åkerström G, Biagini C, Duh QY, Miccoli P, Niederle B, Tonelli F

J Clin Endocrinol Metab. 2014;99(10):3595–3606.

SYNOPSIS

Takeaway Point: Parathyroid surgery is safe and often curative for primary hyperparathyroidism when performed by an experienced surgeon. The revised guidelines for surgical management of asymptomatic primary hyperparathyroidism (PHPT) may lead to more patients undergoing parathyroid surgery.

Commentary: Surgery is the only potentially curative option for patients with primary hyperparathyroidism. All patients with symptomatic disease should be considered for surgery. However, patients more often present with asymptomatic disease. In light of evolving diagnostic and clinical information, criteria for the management of asymptomatic PHPT have been described and revised in several international workshops. Compared to previous guidelines, the 2014 version includes criteria based on radiographic evidence of PHPT (vertebral fractures and nephrocalcinosis/lithiasis). The 2014 guidelines also reintroduced elevated 24-hour urine calcium (>400 mg/day) as a criterion for surgical candidacy. Overall, the revised guidelines are expected to lead to an increase in parathyroid surgery. Whereas the revised guidelines reflect the evolving understanding of parathyroid disease, more studies are needed to further delineate biochemical thresholds and the role of genetic testing, as well as to determine the long-term effects of pharmacologic agents in managing PHPT.

ANALYSIS

Introduction: The surgical management of patients with asymptomatic primary hyperparathyroidism (PHPT) has undergone considerable advances in the past two decades. The last international workshop on this subject was in 2008, and since that time improved diagnostic modalities and intraoperative adjuncts have changed when and how to perform parathyroid surgery.

Methods

A group of international experts in asymptomatic PHPT participated in an open 3-day conference on September 19–21, 2013, in

Florence, Italy. A smaller subcommittee, the Expert Panel, then met in closed session to reach an evidence-based consensus on how to address the questions and data aired in the open forum.

Participants: Patients with primary hyperparathyroidism without symptoms or signs associated with excess parathyroid hormone (PTH) or hypercalcemia.

Results

1. All patients with PHPT who meet surgical criteria should be referred to an experienced endocrine surgeon. Surgical criteria include (a) symptomatic disease and (b) asymptomatic disease: age <50 years, serum calcium >1.0 mg/dL above normal limits, bone mass density by DXA with a T-score of <2.5, radiographic evidence of vertebral fracture, creatinine clearance <60 mL/min, radiographic evidence of nephrolithiasis or nephrocalcinosis, or 24-hour urine calcium >400 mg/day.

2. There are insufficient data at this time to recommend parathyroidectomy for the purpose of improving cardiovascular or neurocognitive endpoints.

3. The frequency of hereditary forms of PHPT may be underappreciated. Familial screening, when performed, should include testing for multiple endocrine neoplasia (MEN) types 1 and 2, familial hypocalciuric hypercalcemia (FHH), and the hyperparathyroidism–jaw tumor (HPT-JT) syndrome.

4. Imaging is not a diagnostic procedure; it is a localization procedure to help the surgeon optimize the operative plan. Cervical ultrasound, sestamibi scan, and four-dimensional (4D) CT scan are the most commonly employed modalities.

5. Operative approaches include traditional bilateral cervical exploration, minimally invasive parathyroidectomy, and endoscopic techniques. A focused approach requires the use of preoperative localization and intraoperative PTH assay. In experienced hands, both bilateral neck and focused approaches yield excellent cure rates with minimal complication rates.

6. Patients with familial hyperparathyroidism and those with sporadic or pharmacologically induced disease (lithium) who harbor multigland hyperplasia are suboptimal candidates for minimally invasive techniques and usually require bilateral exploration.

7. Asymptomatic patients who do not meet surgical criteria can be followed and managed medically. Follow-up entails yearly calcium and PTH levels and dual-energy x-ray absorptiometry

(DXA; also known as *bone densitometry*) scan every 1–2 years. The calcimimetic cinacalcet lowers serum calcium and is an approved drug for the medical management of PHPT. Bisphosphonate therapy may be used to improve bone mineral density.

Discussion

Conclusion: The revised 2014 guidelines expand the role of surgery in the management of asymptomatic PHPT, and provide more specific monitoring guidelines for patients who do not meet criteria for surgery.

Limitations: Lack of data from randomized controlled trials.

---

e. Limited versus Bilateral Exploration for Primary Hyperparathyroidism

Predicting the success of limited exploration for primary hyperparathyroidism using ultrasound, sestamibi, and intraoperative parathyroid hormone: Analysis of 1158 cases.

Siperstein A, Berber E, Barbosa GF, Tsinberg M, Greene AB, Mitchell J, Milas M

Ann Surg. 2008 Sep;248(3):420–428.

SYNOPSIS

Takeaway Point: Limited exploration (LE) for primary hyperparathyroidism (PHPT) with the use of localizing studies and intraoperative PTH (IOPTH) monitoring fails to identify additional parathyroid pathology in at least 16% of patients.

Commentary: The traditional surgical approach for primary hyperparathyroidism is a bilateral cervical exploration with excision of only the enlarged or abnormal-appearing glands. With the advent of the rapid intraoperative PTH assay (IOPTH) and utilization of preoperative localization studies in the 1990s, focused parathyroidectomy has become the favored approach for a suspected single adenoma.[25,26] Several large retrospective studies have demonstrated a cure rate equivalent to that of a four-gland exploration.[27,28] The potential benefits of focused parathyroidectomy include smaller incision, decreased extent of dissection, shorter operative time, lower incidence of postoperative hypocalcemia, decreased hospital stay, and reduced cost.[27] However, controversy still exists over which method is best; proponents of bilateral exploration claim that preoperative imaging studies and IOPTH can be misleading and that a focused approach will miss multigland disease in some patients and result in persistent or recurrent hyperparathyroidism.[29,30]

This is the largest study to date to evaluate the prevalence of additional parathyroid pathology in patients who are candidates for LE. The authors found that in patients with positive localizing studies [preoperative sestamibi and ultrasound] and IOPTH, LE fails to identify multiglandular disease in 16–22% of patients. The study therefore indicates a potential failure to detect abnormal glands in up to one in five patients in whom all currently available adjuncts to parathyroid surgery are used. This has implications for disease recurrence and persistence, and argues for routine bilateral exploration (BE) for primary hyperparathyroidism. The limitations of the study include its lack of long-term outcomes specifying recurrence rates, as well the fact that it is based on single-institution data, which limits generalizability.

ANALYSIS

Introduction: The introduction of adjunct studies has enabled a practice of limited neck exploration (LE) as an alternative to bilateral neck exploration (BE) in the surgical management of parathyroid disease.

Objectives: To evaluate the ability of sestamibi scintigraphy, neck ultrasound, and IOPTH to direct a LE that successfully eliminates all pathologic parathyroid tissue from the neck in cases of sporadic primary HPT.

Methods
Trial Design: Prospective cohort study.
Participants
Inclusion Criteria: Patients undergoing surgery for PHPT.

Exclusion Criteria: Previous neck surgery, familial or hereditary parathyroid disorders, secondary or tertiary hyperparathyroidism, lithium-induced hyperparathyroidism, parathyroid cancer, concomitant thyroid pathology requiring surgery, incomplete data.

Interventions: All patients underwent surgeon-performed ultrasound (US), sestamibi scan, single-photon emission computed tomography (SPECT)/CT of the neck and chest, and IOPTH. Intraoperatively, surgeons first performed either a focal (one-gland) or unilateral (two-gland) exploration based on preoperative imaging studies. If imaging studies were negative or discordant, patients had bilateral neck exploration at the outset. Regardless of

IOPTH, all patients had contralateral neck exploration. Abnormal glands were defined as grossly enlarged and hypercellular on pathology. Follow-up labs were drawn 2 weeks and 6 months after surgery.

Endpoints: Operative findings, gland histology, and follow-up serum calcium and PTH values as a marker of success of an operative approach. Failure of focused exploration was defined as additional pathology after the focal or unilateral exploration would have stopped (due to abnormal gland in the expected location with an appropriate IOPTH drop).

Sample Size: Between 1999 and 2007, 916 patients with first-time sporadic primary HPT and without concomitant thyroid pathology underwent bilateral neck exploration (BE) at one US center.

Statistical Analysis: χ^2 test, Student's *t*-test, and analysis of variance (ANOVA).

Results

Baseline Data: Mean follow-up was 28 ± 23 months. The population was 77% female; mean age was 59. At exploration, 68% had a single adenoma (SA), 16% had double adenomas, and 16% had hyperplasia.

Outcomes: For preoperative diagnosis of multiglandular disease (MGD), accuracy was 49% for sestamibi scan, 69% for US, and 62% when sestamibi and US were in concordance. In patients with negative sestamibi scans, SA was found in 50% and MGD in the remaining 50%. For patients with discordant preoperative studies, SA was present in 53%, and MGD in 47%. For preoperative diagnosis of SA, sestamibi scan was correct in 70% of cases, US in 75%, and concordance between the two in 77%. In patients with MGD, a subsequent gland identified was larger than the index gland in 23%. 98% of BE patients were cured of primary HPT. There was no relationship between success of focal exploration by sestamibi alone, US alone, both together, or preoperative level of serum calcium.

Discussion

Conclusion: Localizing studies and IOPTH fail to identify MGD in at least 16% of patients undergoing LE, and this has potential implications for future recurrence.

Limitations: The authors define an abnormal parathyroid gland by gland size and histopathology, which are not necessarily correlated with increased hormonal activity.

Nonrandomized single-institution data, lack of long-term outcomes.

---

f. Medical Guidelines for the Management of Adrenal Incidentalomas

The American Association of Clinical Endocrinologists and American Association of Endocrine Surgeons medical guidelines for management of adrenal incidentalomas.

Zeiger MA, Thompson GB, Duh QY, Hamrahian AH, Angelos P, Elaraj D, Fishman E, Kharlip J, American Association of Clinical Endocrinologists, American Association of Endocrine Surgeons

Endocr Pract. July–Aug. 2009;15(Suppl 1):1–20.

SYNOPSIS

Takeaway Point: Patients with adrenal incidentalomas (see definition in next paragraph) should undergo extensive multidisciplinary workup, and pheochromocytoma must be ruled out prior to any biopsy or resection. Adrenalectomy is indicated for lesions ≥4 cm; laparoscopic adrenalectomy is recommended for unilateral aldosteronoma, while open adrenalectomy is the approach of choice for suspected adrenocortical carcinoma.

Commentary: An adrenal *incidentaloma* is an adrenal mass 1 cm or more in diameter that is discovered serendipitously on radiology in the absence of symptoms or clinical findings suggestive of adrenal disease. The overall prevalence of adrenal adenomas based on autopsy studies is 6%, and prevalence increases with age. Prior to these 2009 recommendations, the only existing national practice guidelines for the management of adrenal incidentaloma was one developed by the National Institute of Health in 2002. The major difference is an updated recommendation for surgical resection of adrenal masses ≥4 cm (the threshold for resection according to the 2002 NIH guidelines was 6 cm).[31] As with the management of thyroid and parathyroid pathologies, the management of adrenal lesions is based largely on consensus guidelines due to the paucity of data from randomized controlled trials. As the majority of evidence is retrospective in nature, most of the recommendations articulated in the 2009 guidelines are graded as C or D. Best practice demands a multidisciplinary approach to management.

ANALYSIS

Introduction: In 2009, the American Association of Clinical Endocrinologists and American Association of Endocrine Surgeons convened a panel of experts to address the appropriate evaluation and treatment of adrenal incidentalomas. The Expert Panel conducted a literature review and set forth a total of 26 recommendations.

Methods

The panel recommendations were based on the available published data and formulated based on the American Association of Clinical Endocrinologists Protocol for Standardized Production of Clinical Practice Guidelines published in 2004.[32] Where data were lacking, the panel relied on their experience and judgment to provide recommendations.

Results

This document presents a detailed protocol regarding the workup and treatment of the adrenal incidentaloma, as well as separately addressing the possible etiologies (adrenocortical adenoma, pheochromocytoma, aldosteronoma, adrenocortical cancer) and management considerations for each entity.

The pertinent recommendations include the following:

1. **General**

   Patients with an adrenal incidentaloma should undergo evaluation clinically, biochemically, and radiographically for signs and symptoms of hypercortisolism, hyperaldosteronism, and the presence of a pheochromocytoma or a malignant tumor; those who do not fulfill criteria for surgical resection need radiographic evaluation at 3–6 months and then annually for 1–2 years (recommendations 1 and 2; grade C).

2. **Subclinical cushing syndrome**

   In patients with subclinical cortisol syndrome, surgical resection should be reserved for those with worsening hypertension, abnormal glucose tolerance, dyslipidemia, or osteoporosis (recommendation 6; grade D).

3. **Pheochromocytoma**

   Patients with suspected pheochromocytoma should undergo urine and/or plasma catecholamine measurement (recommendation 8; grade A); surgical resection should be performed for all pheochromocytomas, and an α-adrenergic blocking agent should be administered preoperatively. Long-term follow-up is necessary after resection as recurrence may occur (recommendations 10 and 11; grade C).

4. **Primary hyperaldosteronism**

   Adrenal venous sampling at an experienced center is recommended in most patients older than 40 years with a diagnosis of primary hyperaldosteronism; laparoscopic adrenalectomy is recommended for patients with unilateral disease (recommendations 15 and 16; grade C); those with bilateral idiopathic hyperaldosteronism and those not amenable to surgery should be treated with nonselective mineralocorticoid blockade (recommendation 17; grade A).

5. **Adrenal masses suspicious for malignancy**

   Any adrenal mass with concerning radiographic characteristics and lesions ≥4 cm should be resected, and the presence of a pheochromocytoma should be ruled out before attempted resection or biopsy of any adrenal mass (recommendations 18, 19, and 24; grade C).

6. **Adrenocortical carcinoma (ACC)**

   All patients with suspected ACC should have biochemical evaluation to identify potential hormone excess that may serve as a tumor marker and to determine need for preoperative steroid therapy (recommendation 20; grade D). Open adrenalectomy should be performed if ACC is suspected (recommendation 21; grade C).

7. **Metastatic adrenal lesions**

   Such should be suspected in patients with a history of cancer and an adrenal mass who do not fulfill criteria for an incidentaloma; adrenal metastasectomy is rarely indicated but may be considered in the case of an isolated adrenal metastatic lesion (recommendations 22 and 26; grade C).

Discussion

Conclusion: Patients with incidental adrenal lesions should undergo biochemical testing to rule out a functioning tumor. Hormonally active tumors and adrenal cortical cancer require surgical extirpation. Adrenalectomy should also be considered in nonfunctioning lesions >4 cm. Small incidentalomas can be monitored with interval biochemical and radiographic evaluation.

Limitations: Most of the studies informing the guidelines have weak evidence ratings, which are reflected in the recommendation grades (mostly C and D). In addition, the recommendations may reflect the bias of the experts on the task force.

g. Laparoscopic versus Open Adrenalectomy

Comparison of laparoscopic versus open adrenalectomy: Results from American College of Surgeons-National Surgery Quality Improvement Project.

Elfenbein DM, Scarborough JE, Speicher PJ, Scheri RP

J Surg Res. 2013;184(1):216–220.

SYNOPSIS

Takeaway Point: Laparoscopic adrenalectomy is associated with improved 30-day postoperative outcomes, including reduced length of stay, compared to open adrenalectomy.

Commentary: This retrospective study represents the largest comparison to date of laparoscopic versus open adrenalectomy for a variety of adrenal pathology. The authors demonstrated that patients undergoing open adrenalectomy have substantially higher rates of 30-day postoperative morbidity and an average length of stay that is 3 days longer than that of patients who undergo laparoscopic adrenalectomy. Although there was a trend toward lower mortality in patients who had a laparoscopic approach, there was no significant difference in 30-day mortality between the groups. Important limitations of the study include its retrospective nature, lack of detail regarding adrenal pathology including tumor size, information about conversion rates of laparoscopic to open approach, short-term follow-up, and a paucity of adrenal-specific complications such as adrenal insufficiency and tumor recurrence.

ANALYSIS

Introduction: Laparoscopic adrenalectomy was first described in 1992, and a large-scale analysis of laparoscopic versus open adrenalectomy in the Veterans Administration National Surgical Quality Improvement Program (VA NSQIP) database (2001–2004) demonstrated superior short-term outcomes with the laparoscopic approach. Despite this, the laparoscopic approach remains controversial, especially for malignant disease, where some studies have demonstrated worse oncologic outcomes.

Objectives:
To compare the 30-day outcomes after laparoscopic versus open adrenalectomy for malignant versus benign disease using the American College of Surgeons (ACS)-NSQIP database.

Methods

Trial Design: Retrospective database study.

Participants: All patients who underwent adrenalectomy for adrenal pathology captured in the ACS–NSQIP datasets.

Intervention: Adrenalectomy.

Endpoints

Primary Endpoint: 30-day mortality, overall complication rate, postoperative length of hospitalization.

Secondary Endpoints: 21 specific complications and overall morbidity, need for reoperation within 30 days.

Sample Size: 3100 patients from the 2005–2010 NSQIP database.

Statistical Analysis: χ^2 test, Wilcoxon rank sum test, multivariate regression.

Results

Baseline Data: 644 patients underwent open procedures, and 2456 underwent laparoscopic adrenalectomy. The open cohort was more likely to have nonindependent functional status (4.5% vs. 2%, p <0.01), disseminated disease (8.1% vs. 3.9%, p <0.01), and American Society of Anesthesiologists (ASA) classification ≥3 (68.9% vs. 60.6%, p <0.01). 37.6% of the open group had a malignant lesion versus 19.5% of the laparoscopic group (p <0.01).

Outcomes: Patients undergoing a laparoscopic procedure had significantly lower 30-day morbidity (6.4% vs. 18.8%, p <0.001) and shorter length of stay (2 vs. 5 days, p <0.001) than did patients undergoing an open procedure. Mortality was lower in the laparoscopic group, although this difference was not statistically significant (0.4% vs. 1.1%, p 0.18). Among patients with metastatic disease, 30-day morbidity was lower in the laparoscopic group (7.3% vs. 21.9%, p <0.001) but there was no significant difference in 30-day mortality (0.8% vs. 2.1%, p 0.31).

Discussion

Conclusion: The laparoscopic approach to adrenalectomy is associated with sizable reductions in postoperative morbidity and length of postoperative hospitalization. Short-term outcomes for patients with malignant disease are similar to those in the overall study population, although long-term data are needed to prove oncologic equivalency between the open and laparoscopic approach.

Limitations: Retrospective study, lack of detail regarding adrenal tumor, recurrence, and short-term follow-up. No long-term data are available to comment on oncologic outcomes.

REFERENCES

1. Halsted WS. The operative story of goiter. *Johns Hopkins Hosp Rev.* 1920;19:71–257.

2. Trohler U. Towards endocrinology: Theodor Kocher's 1883 account of the unexpected effects of total ablation of the thyroid. *J Roy Soc Med.* 2011;104(3):129–132.

3. Becker WF. Presidential address: Pioneers in thyroid surgery. *Ann Surg.* 1977;185(5):493–504.

4. Davies L, Welch HG. Current thyroid cancer trends in the United States. *JAMA Otolaryngol.* 2014;140(4):317–322.

5. Elaraj D, Sturgeon C. Operative treatment of primary hyperparathyroidism: Balancing cost-effectiveness with successful outcomes. *Surg Clin N Am.* 2014;94(3):607–623.

6. Carling T, Carty SE, Ciarleglio MM, et al. American Thyroid Association (ATA)–design and feasibility of a prospective randomized controlled trial of prophylactic central lymph node dissection for papillary thyroid carcinoma. *Thyroid.* 2011.

7. Field MJ, Lohr KN, Institute of Medicine (US). Committee to Advise the Public Health Service on Clinical Practice Guidelines, United States. Department of Health and Human Services. *Clinical Practice Guidelines: Directions for a New Program.* Washington, DC: National Academy Press; 1990.

8. Mechanick JI, Camacho PM, Cobin RH, et al. American Association of Clinical Endocrinologists Protocol for Standardized Production of Clinical Practice Guidelines–2010 update. *Endocrine Practice.* 2010;16(2):270–283.

9. Shekelle PG, Woolf SH, Eccles M, Grimshaw J. Clinical guidelines: Developing guidelines. *Br Med J.* 1999;318(7183):593–596.

10. Cooper DS, Doherty GM, Haugen BR, et al. Management guidelines for patients with thyroid nodules and differentiated thyroid cancer. *Thyroid.* 2006;16(2):109–142.

11. Lundgren CI, Hall P, Dickman PW, Zedenius J. Influence of surgical and postoperative treatment on survival in differentiated thyroid cancer. *Br J Surg.* 2007;94(5):571–577.

12. Podnos YD, Smith D, Wagman LD, Ellenhorn JD. The implication of lymph node metastasis on survival in patients with well-differentiated thyroid cancer. *Am Surgeon.* 2005;71(9):731–734.

13. Tisell LE, Nilsson B, Molne J, et al. Improved survival of patients with papillary thyroid cancer after surgical microdissection. *World J Surg.* 1996;20(7):854–859.

14. Scherl S, Mehra S, Clain J, et al. The effect of surgeon experience on the detection of metastatic lymph nodes in the central compartment and the pathologic features of clinically unapparent metastatic lymph nodes:

What are we missing when we don't perform a prophylactic dissection of central compartment lymph nodes in papillary thyroid cancer? *Thyroid.* 2014;24(8):1282–1288.

15. Kouvaraki MA, Shapiro SE, Fornage BD, et al. Role of preoperative ultrasonography in the surgical management of patients with thyroid cancer. *Surgery.* 2003;134(6):946–954; discussion 954–945.

16. Wang TS, Evans DB, Fareau GG, Carroll T, Yen TW. Effect of prophylactic central compartment neck dissection on serum thyroglobulin and recommendations for adjuvant radioactive iodine in patients with differentiated thyroid cancer. *Ann Surg–Oncol.* 2012;19(13):4217–4222.

17. Zetoune T, Keutgen X, Buitrago D, et al. Prophylactic central neck dissection and local recurrence in papillary thyroid cancer: A meta-analysis. *Ann Surg Oncol.* 2010;17(12):3287–3293.

18. So YK, Seo MY, Son YI. Prophylactic central lymph node dissection for clinically node-negative papillary thyroid microcarcinoma: Influence on serum thyroglobulin level, recurrence rate, and postoperative complications. *Surgery.* 2012;151(2):192–198.

19. Chisholm EJ, Kulinskaya E, Tolley NS. Systematic review and meta-analysis of the adverse effects of thyroidectomy combined with central neck dissection as compared with thyroidectomy alone. *Laryngoscope.* 2009;119(6):1135–1139.

20. Sosa JA, Bowman HM, Tielsch JM, Powe NR, Gordon TA, Udelsman R. The importance of surgeon experience for clinical and economic outcomes from thyroidectomy. *Ann Surg.* 1998;228(3):320–330.

21. Stavrakis AI, Ituarte PH, Ko CY, Yeh MW. Surgeon volume as a predictor of outcomes in inpatient and outpatient endocrine surgery. *Surgery.* 2007;142(6):887–899; discussion 887–899.

22. Goffredo P, Roman SA, Sosa JA. Have 2006 ATA practice guidelines affected the treatment of differentiated thyroid cancer in the United States? *Thyroid.* 2014;24(3):463–471.

23. Bilimoria KY, Bentrem DJ, Ko CY, et al. Extent of surgery affects survival for papillary thyroid cancer. *Ann Surg.* 2007;246(3):375–381; discussion 381–374.

24. Sancho JJ, Lennard Tw Fau-Paunovic I, Paunovic I Fau-Triponez F, Triponez F Fau-Sitges-Serra A, Sitges-Serra A. Prophylactic central neck disection in papillary thyroid cancer: A consensus report of the European Society of Endocrine Surgeons (ESES) (1435–2451; electronic).

25. Irvin GL 3rd, Dembrow VD, Prudhomme DL. Operative monitoring of parathyroid gland hyperfunction. *Am J Surg.* 1991;162(4):299–302.

26. Arici C, Cheah WK, Ituarte PH, et al. Can localization studies be used to direct focused parathyroid operations? *Surgery.* 2001;129(6):720–729.

27. Udelsman R, Lin Z, Donovan P. The superiority of minimally invasive parathyroidectomy based on 1650 consecutive patients with primary hyperparathyroidism. *Ann Surg.* 2011;253(3):585–591.

28. McGill J, Sturgeon C, Kaplan SP, Chiu B, Kaplan EL, Angelos P. How does the operative strategy for primary hyperparathyroidism impact the findings and cure rate? A comparison of 800 parathyroidectomies. *J Am Coll Surg.* 2008;207(2):246–249.

29. Norman J, Lopez J, Politz D. Abandoning unilateral parathyroidectomy: Why we reversed our position after 15,000 parathyroid operations. *J Am Coll Surg.* 2012;214(3):260–269.

30. Schneider DF, Mazeh H, Sippel RS, Chen H. Is minimally invasive parathyroidectomy associated with greater recurrence compared to bilateral exploration? Analysis of more than 1,000 cases. *Surgery.* 2012;152(6):1008–1015.

31. NIH State-of-the-Science Statement on management of the clinically inapparent adrenal mass ("incidentaloma"). *NIH Consens State Sci Statements.* 2002;19(2):1–23.

32. Mechanick JI, Bergman DA, Braithwaite SS, Palumbo PJ, American Association of Clinical Endocrinologists Ad Hoc Task Force for Standardized Production of Clinical Practice G. American Association of Clinical Endocrinologists protocol for standardized production of clinical practice guidelines. *Endocrine Practice.* 2004;10(4):353–361.

7

Hepatopancreaticobiliary Surgery

Rachel Beard • Tara Kent

INTRODUCTION

Surgical therapy for hepatopancreaticobiliary disease has a rich history with meteoric advances occurring over the last century. Perhaps surprisingly, it was not until 1848, and the description of pancreatic lipase by French physiologist Claude Bernard, that the exocrine function of the pancreas was recognized.[1] In 1899, William Stewart Halsted first successfully resected the head of the pancreas along with the duodenum for ampullary cancer. This evolved into the one-stage pancreaticoduodenectomy described by Allen Oldfather Whipple in 1940.[2] Puestow and Gillesby introduced the lateral pancreaticojejunostomy for the management of chronic pancreatitis in 1958, and Frey and Child introduced the 95% distal pancreatectomy in 1965. Carl Langenbuch performed the first successful cholecystectomy in 1882, and the first elective hepatic resection for tumor in 1888.[3] The modern era of hepatic resection was brought about in 1952 when Lortat-Jacob and Robert performed the first true anatomic liver resection with primary vascular control.[4]

Advances in technology over the next few decades were crucial in the evolution of hepatopancreaticobiliary surgery. The first laparoscopic cholecystectomy was performed by Mouret in 1987 and more widely described by Dubois in 1988.[5] Andrew Warshaw described the utility of laparoscopy in the diagnosis and staging of pancreatic cancer. The first endoscopic papillotomy for calculi removal was performed by Safrany in 1980, and this evolved into endoscopic retrograde cholangiopancreatography (ERCP), a crucial adjunct for management of biliary disease.[6] The development of new surgical instruments such as the harmonic scalpel and Liga-Sure vessel-sealing system made liver resections more expeditious and decreased transfusion requirements.

With improved surgical technique, the indications for pancreaticobiliary surgery have also expanded. Surgical resection of pancreatic cancer can now include portomesenteric venous resection if arterial inflow can be preserved.[7] Techniques for resection have also been refined and optimized. Pylorus-preserving pancreatoduodenectomy, for example, is equally effective from an oncologic perspective when compared to the standard Whipple procedure, with similar recovery and complication profiles.[8] The DISPACT trial examined stapled and hand-sewn closure for distal pancreatectomy and showed no difference in subsequent pancreatic fistula formation.[9] This chapter will also discuss nonoperative advancements in the field, including the utility of prophylactic octreotide to reduce pancreatic fistulas,[10,11] and new chemotherapeutic regimens for metastatic pancreatic cancer.[12] In addition to cancer, this chapter will also discuss the management of benign pancreatic disease, including pancreatic cysts[13] and severe pancreatitis.[14–16]

Despite advancements in management, pancreatic cancer remains a leading cause in cancer-related death, and pancreatic resection is still associated with significant complications.[1] The development of risk assessment tools and consensus statements has helped guide decision making and improve outcomes.[17] International study groups have also reached consensus on the definition of several of the more common postoperative complications. This consensus is essential for future research, as it enables accurate comparisons between trials. *Pancreatic fistula* is now defined as a drain output of any measurable volume of fluid over postoperative day 3, with amylase content greater than 3 times the serum amylase activity.[18] *Delayed gastric emptying* is defined as the inability to return to a standard diet by the end of the first postoperative week and includes prolonged nasogastric intubation.[19]

Advances continue in the realm of liver surgery as well. Hepatocellular carcinoma (HCC) is effectively treated with major hepatectomy.[20] For the treatment of centrally located tumors, postresection adjuvant radiation therapy is feasible and safe, but has no survival benefit versus surgery alone.[21] For patients with advanced HCC and no feasible surgical treatment option, sorafenib prolongs survival and time to progression.[22] We will also discuss the surgical management of colorectal cancer liver metastases, and the potential benefit of neoadjuvant chemotherapy.[23] Finally, we will review the new technique of associating liver partition and portal vein ligation for staged hepatectomy, which, although feasible in initial trials, still lacks outcome and safety data.[24]

The low number of randomized controlled trials limits further advancements in the treatment of hepatopancreatobiliary disease. Many prior efforts at trial development have been thwarted by poor accrual, due in part to the relative rarity of the diseases. Some progress has been made in this area with the more recent multi-institution and international collaborative efforts. In addition, the recent advent of the HPB-NSQIP and Pancreatectomy Project allows for more widespread and standardized data acquisition.[25]

Since its inception, hepatopancreaticobiliary surgery has become more widely practiced, although no less challenging. In 1978 Sir Andrew Watt Kay famously wrote "For me, the tiger country is removal of the pancreas. The anatomy is very complex and one encounters abnormalities."[26] Surgeons play a key role in the management of both benign and malignant hepatopancreaticobiliary diseases, and a thorough understanding of the anatomy, physiology, and ever-evolving treatment options is crucial.

---

a. Prophylactic Octreotide and Pancreatic Fistula after Whipple

Does prophylactic octreotide decrease the rate of pancreatic fistula and other complications after pancreaticoduodenectomy? Results of a prospective randomized placebo-controlled trial.

Yeo CJ, Cameron JL, Lillemoe KD, Sauter PK, Coleman J, Sohn TA, Campbell KA, Choti MA

Ann Surg. 2000;232(3):419–429.

SYNOPSIS

Takeaway Point: Prophylactic octreotide does not decrease rates of pancreatic fistula, postoperative complications, or mortality in patients undergoing pancreaticoduodenectomy (PD).

Commentary: This was a well-designed prospective, randomized, double-blinded trial that sought to clarify conflicting data from previous studies regarding the role of prophylactic octreotide therapy for preventing complications, specifically pancreatic fistula, in patients undergoing PD. Whereas other studies demonstrating a benefit to prophylactic octreotide included patients undergoing other types of pancreatic resection as well, this study solely included patients undergoing PD and clearly demonstrated that octreotide does not reduce overall complications, fistula formation, death, or hospital stay. Interestingly, those patients on octreotide therapy who did develop a fistula had longer hospital stays than those who developed a fistula with placebo therapy. The implication of this finding in a small patient group is not clear, and the trial was not powered for subgroup analyses. The study also specifically looked at patients considered at high risk of fistula formation secondary to a soft pancreas texture and did not show a benefit in those patients, either. The additional cost of octreotide in the prophylactic setting cannot be justified and should be eliminated from practice in patients undergoing PD. This study confirmed the findings of the study published 3 years earlier by Lowy et al, which also showed that routine use of perioperative octreotide in patients undergoing PD was not effective in decreasing the incidence of pancreatic fistula or any other complication.[11]

ANALYSIS

Introduction: Four previous randomized trials demonstrated the utility of prophylactic octreotide in reducing pancreatic fistula and overall complications rates in patients undergoing pancreatic resection. However, a fifth trial examining only patients undergoing PD showed no benefit.

Objectives: To evaluate the role of prophylactic octreotide in reducing pancreatic fistula, overall complications, and death in patients undergoing PD.

Methods
Trial Design: Double-blinded, randomized controlled trial.
Participants
Inclusion Criteria: All patients with anticipated elective PD.

Exclusion Criteria: After randomization patients who did not undergo PD or did not receive at least a 5-day course of the study drug were excluded from the outcome analysis.

Intervention: Patients received either 250 μg octreotide or saline placebo preoperatively and then every 8 hours after surgery for 7 days, for a total of 22 doses. Postoperative drains were left in place until at least postoperative day 4. Amylase levels were checked on days 3 and 7 and if no fistula was demonstrated, drains were removed.

Endpoints

Primary Endpoint: Pancreatic fistula, overall postoperative complications, and death.

Secondary Endpoint: Cost analysis.

Sample Size: 383 patients were enrolled between February 1998 and February 2000 at a single institution. 383 were randomized and 211 were analyzed for outcome analyses, with 107 in the control group and 104 in the octreotide group.

Statistical Analysis: Student t-test and χ^2 statistics for univariate comparisons, with multivariate stepwise regression of the variables found to be significant on univariate analysis. Sample size calculations predicted 129 patients per arm were needed to demonstrate 10% decrease in fistula rate.

Results

Baseline Data: There was no difference between the two groups in terms of gender, race, preoperative factors, intraoperative factors, or pathologic findings.

Outcomes: The most common complications in both groups were pancreatic fistula, wound infection, and early delayed gastric emptying. The complications rates were not significantly different between the two groups, nor were the lengths of hospital stay or mortality. Complications including fistula formation were stratified by surgeon-described pancreatic texture. Complications were more frequent with a soft texture, but octreotide had no effect on the rate in any group. The total cost of octreotide was $61 per dose and $1408 per patient for the course administered in this study.

Discussion

Conclusion: Prophylactic octreotide does not decrease the rate of postoperative pancreatic fistula, hospital length of stay, or death overall for all patients or for those considered high risk due to soft pancreatic texture. Eliminating the use of prophylactic octreotide would result in a cost savings of $1408 per patient.

Limitations: A higher dose of octreotide was used in this study (250 μg) than was reported in any of the previous studies (100 or 150 μg). Patients undergoing pancreatic resections other than PD were not examined in this study as they were in previous European trials. The trial was terminated early because of lack of demonstrated benefit, and was not powered for the subgroup analyses they report.

b. Pylorus-Preserving Pancreaticoduodenectomy

Pylorus preserving pancreaticoduodenectomy versus standard Whipple procedure: A prospective, randomized, multicenter analysis of 170 patients with pancreatic and periampullary tumors.

Tran KT, Smeenk HG, van Eijck CH, Kazemier G, Hop WC, Greve JW, Terpstra OT, Zijlstra JA, Klinkert P, Jeekel H

Ann Surg. 2004;240(5):738–745.

SYNOPSIS

Takeaway Point: The standard Whipple procedure (SW) and pylorus-preserving pancreaticoduodenectomy (PPPD) are equally effective for the treatment of pancreatic and periampullary carcinoma.

Commentary: This study compares PPPD with SW for clinical and oncologic outcomes. The authors hypothesized that PPPD would be associated with reduced operative times, lower blood loss, shorter hospital stays, and more physiologic food passage. On analysis, the two procedures were not statistically different by any measure, including perioperative data, postoperative complications, resection margins, or overall and disease-free survival. The trial demonstrated the acceptability of either approach for the treatment of periampullary and pancreatic cancer. It is worthwhile to note that the debate between PPPD or SW remains contentious, with different studies having conflicting results. Furthermore, many studies on this question use delayed gastric emptying as the primary outcome measure rather than estimated blood loss (EBL), operative time, and length of stay, perhaps explaining the conflicting conclusions. Additionally, adjuvant therapy protocols for pancreatic cancer in the Netherlands (where this trial was performed) typically consist of chemotherapy only, rather than the chemoradiation that would be used in the United States, and the patients in this trial received no adjuvant therapy. This may limit generalizability of the results. Finally, the average blood loss in this single-center trial was much greater than that observed in prior studies, raising the possibility that center-specific techniques might impact the primary outcomes of EBL and operative time. These and other limitations emphasize the still unsettled nature of the controversy regarding PPPD versus SW.

ANALYSIS

Introduction: The PPPD, a modification to the classic Whipple operation, was initially described in 1944 and reintroduced in the 1970s. Some potential benefits include improvement in postoperative gastrointestinal function, shorter operative times, and less intraoperative blood loss; however, some studies have also reported a higher incidence of complications and concern about resection margins.

Objectives: "To evaluate whether PPPD has an advantage over the standard Whipple (SW) procedure."

Methods
Trial Design: Prospective randomized controlled trial.
Participants

Inclusion Criteria: Suspected pancreatic or periampullary cancer determined to be resectable based on preoperative imaging (CT and/or MRI).

Exclusion Criteria: Previous gastric resection, distant metastasis, positive peripyloric lymph nodes, or local unresectability were excluded from the analysis for efficacy. Patients with lesions other than pancreatic or periampullary adenocarcinoma were excluded from the survival analysis.

Intervention: Patients were randomized to undergo either PPPD or SW. Follow-up evaluations were conducted every 3 months.

Endpoints

Primary Endpoints: Operative time, blood loss, duration of hospital stay.

Secondary Endpoints: Delayed gastric emptying, disease-free and overall survival rates.

Sample Size: 170 patients from seven Dutch hospitals enrolled between 1992 and 2000; 87 patients were randomized to PPPD and 83 to SW.

Statistical Analysis: Survival was calculated from the date of surgery using the Kaplan–Meier method and compared with the log-rank test. Percentages were compared between groups using the Fisher exact test or the χ^2 test, and other data were compared using the Mann–Whitney U-test. Sample size calculations estimated 65 patients per arm to demonstrate a 30% reduction in blood loss and 20% reduction in operative time.

Results

Baseline Data: Treatment groups were similar in terms of patient characteristics and pathologic diagnoses.

Outcomes: Follow-up was up to 115 months, median 18.5 months, range 1–115 months. There was no statistically significant difference in procedure-related outcomes or postoperative complications including blood loss, hospital stay, incidence of delayed gastric emptying (DGE), margin positivity, or mortality. Differences in the median disease-free survival (49 months in SW group and 23 months in PPPD group, p 0.60) and overall survival rates (17 months in SW group and 29 months in PPPD group, p 0.50) were not statistically significant.

Discussion

Conclusion: The two operations are comparable with respect to short-term recovery and complications, as well as long-term and disease-free survival.

Limitations: Both small- and large-volume centers were included. No adjuvant chemotherapy or radiotherapy was provided to the patients.

---

c. Sorafenib in Advanced Hepatocellular Carcinoma
Sorafenib in advanced hepatocellular carcinoma.

Llovet JM, Ricci S, Mazzaferro V, Hilgard P, Gane E, Blanc J-F, de Oliveira AC, Santoro A, Raoul J-L, Forner A, Schwartz M, Porta C, Zeuzem S, Bolondi L, Greten TF, Galle PR, Seitz J-F, Borbath I, Häussinger D, Giannaris T, Shan M, Moscovici M, Voliotis D, Bruix J, for the SHARP Investigators Study Group

NEJM. 2008;359(4):378–390.

SYNOPSIS

Takeaway Point: Sorefenib prolongs survival and time to progression by nearly 3 months in patients with advanced HCC.

Commentary: This important study was the first to demonstrate a survival benefit from treatment with a systemic therapy for locally advanced HCC. Sorafenib was well tolerated and improved survival and time to progression by nearly 3 months, and is now considered first line treatment in patients with HCC who are not candidates for surgical resection. This is a promising treatment, and its utility in the adjuvant setting should be explored as well.

ANALYSIS

Introduction: HCC remains a major world health problem, and when surgical resection is not an option, prognosis is dismal. No systemic therapy to date has demonstrated improved survival in patients with advanced HCC. An uncontrolled phase 2 study of sorafenib, a small-molecule inhibitor that inhibits tumor cell proliferation, showed a beneficial effect in extending survival and time to progression.

Objectives: To assess the efficacy and safety of sorafenib in patients with advanced HCC.

Methods

Trial Design: A multicenter, phase 3, double-blind, placebo-controlled trial.

Participants

Inclusion Criteria: Patients with pathology-proven advanced-stage HCC who had not received previous systemic therapy; Eastern Cooperative Oncology Group (ECOG) score of ≤2; Child–Pugh class A; life expectancy of ≥12 weeks; adequate hematologic, renal, and liver function; and at least one untreated target lesion.

Exclusion Criteria: Patients who had previously received molecular target therapies or other systemic treatment.

Intervention: Randomization to either sorafenib (400 mg twice daily) or placebo. Randomization was stratified by region, ECOG status, and presence of macrovascular invasion. Treatment was continued until radiologic progression, unacceptable adverse events, or death.

Endpoints

Primary Endpoint: Overall survival and time to symptomatic progression.

Secondary Endpoints: Time to radiologic progression, disease control rate, and safety.

Sample Size: 121 centers in 21 countries; 602 patients randomized from March 2005 to April 2006, with 299 to sorafenib and 303 to placebo.

Statistical Analysis: A Cox proportional-hazards model for overall survival. A stratified log-rank test was used for analysis of radiologic progression, disease control rates using the Cochran–Mantel–Haenszel test. Adverse events were compared with Fisher's exact test.

Results

Baseline Data: There were no relevant differences between the two groups in terms of demographics, cause of liver disease, previous therapy, prognostic indicators, or tumor stage.

Outcomes: Overall median survival was significantly longer in the sorafenib group (10.7 vs. 7.9 months, hazard ratio 0.69, 95% CI 0.55–0.87, p <0.001), and at one year there was a 31% relative reduction in the risk of death. After adjustment for other prognostic indicators, the effect of sorafenib on overall survival remained significant (hazard ratio 0.73, 95% CI, 0.58–0.92, p 0.004). The median time to progression was significantly longer in the sorafenib group than in the placebo group (5.5 vs. 2.8 months, hazard ratio 0.58, 95% CI, 0.45–0.74, p <0.001). The overall incidence of treatment-related adverse events was 80% and in the sorafenib group consisted mainly of grade 1 or 2 gastrointestinal, constitutional, and dermatologic side effects. The study was stopped at the second planned interim analysis because of the significant reduction in risk of death in the sorafenib group.

Discussion

Conclusion: In patients with advanced HCC, median survival and the time to radiologic progression were nearly 3 months longer for patients treated with sorafenib than for those given placebo.

Limitations: Quality of life was not well assessed. Symptomatic progression was evaluated using a self-reported functional health status questionnaire, which may have been influenced by the adverse effects of the drug, tumor-related symptoms, and symptoms attributable to liver failure, which persisted regardless of whether the tumor responded to therapy.

---

d. ERCP versus Conservative Management in Pancreatitis

Early endoscopic retrograde cholangiopancreatography in predicted severe acute biliary pancreatitis: A prospective multicenter study.

van Santvoort HC, Besselink MG, de Vries AC, Boermeester MA, Fischer K, Bollen TL, Cirkel GA, Schaapherder AF, Nieuwenhuijs VB, van Goor H, Dejong CH, van Eijck CH, Witteman BJ, Weusten BL, van Laarhoven CJ, Wahab PJ, Tan AC, Schwartz MP, van der Harst E, Cuesta MA, Siersema PD, Gooszen HG, van Erpecum KJ, Dutch Acute Pancreatitis Study Group

Ann Surg. 2009;250(1):68–75.

SYNOPSIS

Takeaway Point: Early endoscopic retrograde cholangiopancreatography (ERCP) reduces complications in patients with acute biliary pancreatitis (ABP) and concurrent cholestasis [defined as total bilirubin > 2.3 and/or dilated common bile duct (CBD), without fever].

Commentary: This study examined a subset of patients that were enrolled in the Probiotics in Pancreatitis Trial (PROPATRIA) from the Dutch Acute Pancreatitis Study Group. That trial enrolled adult patients presenting with their first episode of predicted severe acute pancreatitis of all causes. This study looked specifically at patients with ABP, excluding those with concurrent cholangitis, to determine whether early ERCP is also beneficial for patients without cholangitis. When compared to conservative management, early ERCP in patients with ABP with cholestasis reduces complications overall and reduces serious complications such as substantial pancreatic necrosis, and should be recommended in this subset. The same benefit was not seen in patients with ABP in the absence of cholestasis, for whom conservative management and early ERCP yielded similar clinical outcomes.

ANALYSIS

Introduction: Gallstones are the most common etiology of acute pancreatitis in the western world. Severe complications occur in 20% of patients with ABP, with a subsequent 30% mortality. Previous studies have concluded that early ERCP is indicated for patients with ABP and cholangitis; however, the role of early ERCP for patients with predicted severe ABP without cholangitis remains unclear.

Objectives: To determine whether early ERCP, as compared to conservative treatment, reduces the risk of complications and mortality for patients with predicted severe ABP without cholangitis.

Methods
Trial Design: A prospective, observational, multicenter study of a subset of patients from a larger cohort enrolled in the Probiotics in Pancreatitis Trial (PROPATRIA).
Participants
Inclusion Criteria: Adult patients with primary episode of severe acute pancreatitis who developed ABP [defined as gallstones and/or sludge, or dilated CBD, or two of the following

laboratory abnormalities: serum bilirubin >1.3 mg/dL; alanine transaminase (ALT) >100 U/L and greater than aspartate aminotransferase (AST); or alkaline phosphatase >195 U/L with γ-glutamyltransferase (GGT) >45 U/L].

Exclusion Criteria: Chronic pancreatitis and potential cholangitis.

Intervention: Patients were stratified as having potential cholangitis (bilirubin >1.2 mg/dL and/or dilated CBD and fever), cholestasis (bilirubin >2.3 mg/dL and/or dilated CBD and afebrile), or neither cholestasis nor potential cholangitis. The decision to perform ERCP was left to the treating physician. Patients who underwent ERCP within 72 hours were considered in the early ERCP group and those that did not constituted the conservative treatment group. Patients with potential cholangitis were excluded from the analysis.

Endpoints

Primary Endpoint: Mortality and overall complications during admission and during 90-day follow-up.

Secondary Endpoints: CT severity index, the need for percutaneous drainage or operative intervention for infected necrosis, hospital stay, and ICU stay.

Sample Size: Of the 296 patients from 15 Dutch hospitals enrolled on the PROPATRIA trial between March 2004 and March 2007, this trial included 153 patients, 81 who underwent early ERCP and 72 who were treated conservatively.

Statistical Analysis: Continuous data by Student's t-test or Mann–Whitney U-test. Proportions were compared by the Fisher exact test. Multivariate logistic regression to adjust for cofounders.

Results

Baseline Data: For patients with cholestasis, the APACHE II score on admission was slightly higher in the conservative treatment group (p 0.064). For patients without cholestasis, the ASA class was significantly higher in the conservative treatment group (p 0.016).

Outcomes: For patients with cholestasis, 67% underwent early ERCP and had significantly fewer overall complications (25% vs. 54%, p 0.02) and fewer substantial complications, including >30% pancreatic necrosis (8% vs. 31%, p 0.01). On multivariate analysis early ERCP remained associated with a lower risk of overall complications (OR 0.35; 95% CI; 0.13–0.99, p 0.049). Mortality was not significantly different. For patients without cholestasis, 39% underwent early ERCP and no benefit was demonstrated when compared to conservative treatment. Differences in secondary endpoints were not demonstrated in either group.

Discussion

Conclusion: Early ERCP is associated with fewer complications in predicted severe ABP if cholestasis is present.

Limitations: This study was not randomized, and there was variation in indication for ERCP amongst the different centers.

---

e. PANTER Trial

A step-up approach or open necrosectomy for necrotizing pancreatitis.

van Santvoort HC, Besselink MG, Bakker OJ, Hofker HS, Boermeester MA, Dejong CH, van Goor H, Schaapherder AF, van Eijck CH, Bollen TL, van Ramshorst B, Nieuwenhuijs VB, Timmer R, Laméris JS, Kruyt PM, Manusama ER, van der Harst E, van der Schelling GP, Karsten T, Hesselink EJ, van Laarhoven CJ, Rosman C, Bosscha K, de Wit RJ, Houdijk AP, van Leeuwen MS, Buskens E, Gooszen HG, Dutch Pancreatitis Study Group

NEJM. 2010;362(16):1491–1502.

SYNOPSIS

Takeaway Point: For patients with necrotizing pancreatitis and secondary infection, a step-up approach reduces both short- and long-term complications as well as overall healthcare costs when compared to upfront open necrosectomy.

Commentary: The trial compared two treatment approaches for necrotizing pancreatitis: primary open necrosectomy, and a step-up approach of initial percutaneous or endoscopic drainage with subsequent additional drainage or necrosectomy if needed. The aims of these approaches differed; the goal of open necrosectomy is complete debridement of necrotic tissue, whereas the step-up approach aims to control the source of infection. Although some patients in the step-up approach ultimately required necrosectomy, 40% avoided an open operation and were sufficiently treated with less invasive procedures. Major short- and long-term complications and healthcare costs were reduced in the step-up approach group. This trial supports the step-up approach as the standard of care for necrotizing pancreatitis; however, several subsequent letters to the editor and an editorial by Dr. Andrew Warshaw expressed concern over the high mortality rates that did not differ between groups, as well as the limited applicability of the step-up approach as it mandates a retroperitoneal access route, and cautioned against using this approach as a default therapy for all necrotizing pancreatitis patients.[27-29]

ANALYSIS

Introduction: Necrotizing pancreatitis has traditionally been treated with open necrosectomy to remove infected necrotic tissue, an operation with high morbidity and mortality. Less invasive approaches, including percutaneous and endoscopic drainage and minimally invasive necrosectomy, have been explored, and can be performed in a so-called step-up approach with subsequent open necrosectomy if needed.

Objectives: To compare open necrosectomy to a minimally invasive step-up approach for the treatment of necrotizing pancreatitis.

Methods
Trial Design: A multicenter, randomized controlled trial.
Participants
Inclusion Criteria: Adults with acute pancreatitis and signs of pancreatic or peripancreatic necrosis.

Exclusion Criteria: Patients with chronic pancreatitis, previous exploratory laparotomy during the current episode of pancreatitis, previous surgery for pancreatic necrosis, or pancreatitis secondary to abdominal surgery or an acute intraabdominal event.

Intervention: Patients were randomly assigned to either primary open necrosectomy or the minimally invasive step-up approach. Randomization occurred once a decision to perform a surgical intervention had been made, and if percutaneous or endoscopic drainage of the fluid collection was deemed possible.

Endpoints
Primary Endpoint: Composite of major complication or death during admission or within 3 months of discharge.

Secondary Endpoints: Individual components of the primary endpoint, other complications, healthcare resource utilization, and total medical costs.

Sample Size: 88 patients were randomized from 19 Dutch hospitals between November 2005 and October 2008; 45 to open necrosectomy and 43 to step-up approach.

Statistical Analysis: Occurrences of endpoints were compared between treatment groups, and results are presented as risk ratios with 95% confidence intervals. Differences in other outcomes were assessed with the use of the Mann–Whitney U-test. Power analysis estimated 88 patients needed to detect a 64% relative reduction in the composite primary endpoint. Intention-to-treat analysis.

Results

Baseline Data: Baseline characteristics of the treatment groups were similar.

Outcomes: In the primary necrosectomy group, patients underwent a median of one necrosectomy with 42% requiring at least one additional operation and 33% requiring additional percutaneous drainage after laparotomy. In the step-up group, 44% of patients required a second drainage procedure and 60% ultimately underwent necrosectomy, with 33% requiring one or more additional operations and 27% undergoing subsequent percutaneous drainage after laparotomy. The composite primary endpoint of major complications or death occurred in 69% of the necrosectomy group and 40% of the step-up approach group (RR 0.57, 95% CI 0.38–0.87, p 0.006). Mortality was not significantly different between the two groups. After 6 months, patients in the necrosectomy group had significantly more incisional hernias (7% vs. 24%, p 0.03), new-onset diabetes (16% vs. 38%, p 0.02), and pancreatic enzyme requirement (16% vs. 38%, p 0.02). Utilization of healthcare resources was lower for the step-up group (p 0.004) and at 6-month follow-up the step-up approach had reduced costs by 12%.

Discussion

Conclusion: A minimally invasive step-up approach, as compared with open necrosectomy, reduced the rate of the composite end points of major complications or death among patients with necrotizing pancreatitis and infected necrotic tissue.

Limitations: The study was not designed or powered to demonstrate a difference in death rate alone. Initial power analysis assumed a very large relative reduction in primary endpoint.

---

f. Consensus Guidelines for Management of Pancreatic Cysts

International consensus guidelines 2012 for the management of IPMN and MCN of the pancreas.

Tanaka M, Fernández-del Castillo C, Adsay V, Chari S, Falconi M, Jang JY, Kimura W, Levy P, Pitman MB, Schmidt CM, Shimizu M, Wolfgang CL, Yamaguchi K, Yamao K, International Association of Pancreatology

Pancreatology. 2012;12(3):183–197.

SYNOPSIS

Takeaway Point: In the absence of randomized controlled trials and high-grade evidence, these consensus guidelines offer the best recommendations for the management of intraductal papillary mucinous neoplasm (IPMN) and mucinous cystic neoplasm (MCN) of the pancreas.

Commentary: These guidelines summarize the first updated recommendations since the initial publication 6 years prior. As resection remains the recommendation of main duct (MD)-IPMN and MCN, the natural history of these lesions is still largely unknown and there is a great need for more prospective studies with long-term follow-up. The known malignant potential of these lesions, however, makes constructing a randomized trial comparing resection to observation ethically questionable.

ANALYSIS

Introduction: Since the initial publication of international consensus guidelines for management of IPMN and MCN of the pancreas in 2006, a considerable amount of new data has been generated regarding preoperative diagnosis and management. In particular, the role of endoscopic ultrasonography-guided fine-needle aspiration (EUS-FNA) and indications for resection of side-branch IPMN have evolved. A symposium was held at the 14th meeting of the International Association of Pancreatology (IAP), where these new data were presented and new guidelines were generated.

Objectives: To summarize new international consensus guidelines for management of IPMN and MCN of the pancreas as agreed upon during the 14th meeting of the IAP in 2010.

Recommendations

Classification: The threshold of main pancreatic duct (MPD) dilation for characterization of main duct IPMN (MD-IPMN) has been lowered to >5 mm without other cause of obstruction. Ductal dilation of 5–9 mm is considered a worrisome feature, and ductal dilation of ≥10 mm is considered a high-risk feature.

Investigation: For cysts ≥1 cm, CT or MRI with magnetic resonance cholangiopancreatography (MRCP) is recommended to check for worrisome features. EUS is recommended for those with worrisome features or size >3 cm, and those with high-risk stigmata should undergo resection.

Indications for Resection: Resection is recommended for MD-IPMN, and if high-grade dysplasia is present at margins then resection should be extended to at least moderate-grade dysplasia. For branch duct IPMN (BD-IPMN), patients can be observed for lesions >3 cm but without high-risk stigmata. Resection is recommended for all patients with MCN, and laparoscopic and limited resections can be done if MCN is <4 cm.

Methods of Resection: Pancreatectomy with lymph node dissection remains the standard for invasive and noninvasive MCNs and IPMNs. If there is no suspicion for malignancy, then more limited resection can be considered. Multifocal BD-IPMN carry a similar risk of malignancy as unifocal BD-IPMN, but the threshold for total pancreatectomy be lower in patients with a strong family history.

Histology: IPMNs should be reported as colloid versus tubular invasive carcinoma, as colloid carcinomas carry a better prognosis than tubular. Minimally invasive carcinomas should be further staged as T1 category per the conventional staging protocols and subdivided into T1a ($\leq$0.5 cm), T1b (>0.5 cm and $\leq$1 cm), and T1c (1–2 cm). For IPMN: the gastric subtype is usually low-grade, although if carcinoma does develop it is usually tubular and aggressive. Large intestinal-type IPMNs may develop invasive colloid carcinoma with indolent behaviors. If high-grade dysplasia is present on frozen section at resection, further resection is warranted, including total pancreatectomy if needed.

Follow-up: The decision can be made to observe a BD-IPMN if no high-risk stigmata are present. MR/MRCP (or CT) should be performed at short intervals (3–6 months) to establish stability if no prior imaging is available. Frequency of imaging is then dependent on cyst size. If <1 cm, then CT/MRI can be repeated in 2–3 years. If 1–2 cm, then imaging should be performed annually for 2 years and then at a lengthened interval if stable. If 2–3 cm, then a repeat EUS should be performed in 3–6 months followed by alternating MRI and EUS at lengthened intervals. If >3 cm, surgery should be strongly considered. Following resection, noninvasive MCNs require no surveillance after resection as they are almost always solitary. IPMNs need surveillance based on margin status.

Discussion
Conclusion: Resection is still recommended for MD-IPMN or MCN; the indications for resection for BD-IPMN are more conservative, and those >3 cm without high-risk stigmata can be

observed. The criteria for characterization of MD-IPMN has been lowered to MPD dilation of >5 mm. Pancreatectomy with lymph node dissection remains the standard for invasive and noninvasive MCNs and IPMNs; limited resections are reserved for those without suspicion of malignancy. Frozen section analysis of margin should be done to ensure that there is no high-grade dysplasia or invasive cancer. Recommendations for postoperative surveillance are dependent on resection margin status.

Limitations: The majority of publications are still retrospective or uncontrolled trials with limited long-term follow-up. The levels of evidence and the grade of recommendations are overall low (4 or 5, and grade C).

g. DISPACT Trial

Efficacy of stapler versus hand-sewn closure after distal pancreatectomy (DISPACT): A randomised, controlled multicentre trial.

Diener MK, Seiler CM, Rossion I, Kleeff J, Glanemann M, Butturini G, Tomazic A, Bruns CJ, Busch OR, Farkas S, Belyaev O, Neoptolemos JP, Halloran C, Keck T, Niedergethmann M, Gellert K, Witzigmann H, Kollmar O, Langer P, Steger U, Neudecker J, Berrevoet F, Ganzera S, Heiss MM, Luntz SP, Bruckner T, Kieser M, Büchler MW

Lancet. 2011;377(9776):1514–1522.

SYNOPSIS

Takeaway Point: Stapled and hand-sewn closure of the pancreatic remnant result in equivalent clinical outcomes, including rates of pancreatic leak and mortality.

Commentary: This prospective, randomized, multicenter trial compared stapled to hand-sewn techniques for closure of the pancreatic remnant after distal pancreatectomy. The study demonstrated no difference in any clinical outcome, including pancreatic leak, short- or long-term mortality, hospital stay, or any other postoperative complication. Both stapled and hand-sewn closure were found to be equally safe. This trial supports surgeons using stapled or hand-sewn approaches according to their preference, taking into account characteristics of the patient, the pancreas, and their own comfort with the two approaches. As minimally invasive approaches to distal pancreatectomy have become more standard, stapled division of the pancreas may grow in popularity, but hand-sewn division and closure of the pancreatic remnant remain appropriate options, particularly when the pancreas is too bulky to accommodate the stapler.

ANALYSIS

Introduction: The rate of pancreatic fistula formation following distal pancreatectomy is 13–64%, and is a major source of morbidity. Multiple techniques to prevent this complication have been proposed, including hand-sewn and stapled closure, the use of mesh, sealing with fibrin glue, and patching with seromusculature or serosa.

Objectives: To assess the effect of stapled versus hand-sewn closure on formation of postoperative pancreatic fistula after distal pancreatectomy.

Methods

Trial Design: A randomized controlled trial with a two-group parallel group-sequential superiority design.

Participants

Inclusion Criteria: Patients with diseases of the pancreatic body and tail undergoing elective open distal pancreatectomy for malignant, benign, or neuroendocrine tumors (classified as high risk for pancreatic fistula formation), or undergoing resection for chronic pancreatitis or pseudocyst (classified as low risk).

Exclusion Criteria: Of 450 patients randomized, 98 were excluded because no left resection was done or informed consent was withdrawn, and another 56 were excluded from the intention-to-treat population because they were not treated according to protocol, resulting in 296 patients in the per protocol population.

Intervention: Patients were randomly assigned to stapled or hand-sewn closure of the pancreatic remnant. Randomization was stratified by participating centers and risk level (low or high).

Endpoints

Primary Endpoint: Combination outcome of pancreatic fistula or death until postoperative day 7.

Secondary Endpoints: Mortality by postoperative day 30 and within 12 months, persistent pancreatic fistula, wound dehiscence, wound infection, intraabdominal fluid collection (sterile) or abscess (infected), total operating time, time for distal pancreatectomy, length of hospital stay, new-onset diabetes mellitus.

Sample Size: 450 patients were enrolled from 21 European centers (participating centers had to perform at least 10 pancreatic resections per year) between November 2006 and July 2009, 221 randomized to stapler and 229 to hand-sewn. Of these, 352 patients were analyzed (177 stapler, 175 hand-sewn).

Statistical Analysis: Cochran–Mantel–Haenszel test to null hypothesis of equal fistula rates for two techniques, binary logistic regression model with primary endpoint as a dependent variable.

Results

Baseline Data: The study groups were similar in terms of all patient and procedure characteristics. Most cases (71.3%) were done by highly experienced surgeons, and most included splenectomy (83%) and lymph node dissection (63%).

Outcomes: The rate of pancreatic fistulas (32% in stapler and 28% in hand-sewn, p 0.56) and mortality at postoperative day 7 (0 in stapler group vs. 1 in hand-sewn, p 0.31) did not differ between the two groups. None of the primary or secondary endpoints, including overall operative time, differed to a statistically significant degree.

Discussion

Conclusion: Stapled and hand-sewn closure are equally safe after distal pancreatectomy.

Limitations: Randomization was done preoperatively rather than intraoperatively to avoid delays; however, this practice led to the loss of some patients because disease was unresectable by distal pancreatectomy. Significant number of patients eliminated because of failure of protocol or failure of consent.

---

h. Adjuvant Radiotherapy for Central Liver Hepatoma

Adjuvant radiotherapy in centrally located hepatocellular carcinomas after hepatectomy with narrow margin (<1 cm): A prospective randomized study.

Yu W, Wang W, Rong W, Wang L, Xu Q, Wu F, Liu L, Wu J

J Am Coll Surg. 2014;218(3):381–392.

SYNOPSIS

Takeaway Point: For patients with centrally located HCC, there is no evidence to suggest that postresection adjuvant radiation therapy (XRT) improves local control, reduces recurrence, or confers a survival benefit.

Commentary: XRT has demonstrated a clear benefit in other malignancies such as rectal cancer in improving local control and extending survival. Centrally located HCC is difficult to resect with clear margins because of the proximity of major vascular structures, and an adjuvant therapy such as XRT to improve local control would be ideal. This study, however, did not demonstrate a benefit in either improved recurrence-free or overall survival for patients treated postoperatively after resection. A post hoc nonrandomized subgroup comparison of patients with small HCC tumors (≤ 5 cm) demonstrated a statistically significant improvement in recurrence free survival for patients who received adjuvant XRT compared to those who did not; however, this finding should be interpreted with caution, as there was no significant different in overall survival. Moreover, this study was not adequately powered to demonstrate a difference in this subgroup analysis.

ANALYSIS

Introduction: Surgical resection offers the best chance of cure for HCC, but recurrence rates remain high. Adjuvant XRT for HCC has not been well studied. Centrally located HCC, in Couinaud segments IV, V, or VIII, presents a challenge for resection with a high frequency of narrow (<1 cm) margins given the proximity of major vasculature.

Objectives: To evaluate the safety and efficacy of adjuvant RT for centrally located HCC after narrow-margin (<1-cm) hepatectomy.

Methods
Trial Design: A randomized, open-label, single-center trial.
Participants
Inclusion Criteria: Patients with centrally located HCC with no preoperative XRT, resectable lesion, compensated or no cirrhosis, Child–Pugh class A, ECOG status 0 or 1, no prior transcatheter arterial chemoembolization (TACE) therapy within 4 weeks of study entry.

Exclusion Criteria: Patients with presence of distant metastases, resection margin ≥ 1 cm, palliative resection with residual tumor, and non-HCC on surgical pathology.

Intervention: Following resection, patients were randomized to receive adjuvant XRT or assigned to a control group. XRT consisted of a target total dose of 60 Gy delivered using 2 Gy/fraction, 5 days per week.

Endpoints

Primary Endpoint: Recurrence-free survival.

Secondary Endpoint: Overall survival.

Sample Size: 119 patients at a single center in China from July 2007 to March 2012, with 58 randomized to adjuvant RT and 61 to control group.

Statistical Analysis: χ^2 test, Fisher's exact test, and Student's t-test. Survival rates were evaluated by the Kaplan–Meier method, and compared using the stratified log-rank test. Sample size calculations estimated that 199 patients would demonstrate a 30% improvement in recurrence-free survival with 90% power.

Results

Baseline Data: Patients in the adjuvant XRT group had increased alcohol intake (p 0.03) and higher mean serum albumin (p 0.02). Baseline characteristics, including operative variables, were otherwise not significantly different.

Outcomes: 51 of the 58 patients allocated to adjuvant XRT completed their treatment. Fatigue, nausea, and myeloid suppression were the most common toxicities, but overall these were not severe. Recurrence occurred in 41.3% (24) of patients in the adjuvant RT group and in 50.8% (31) of patients in the control group (p 0.30). Recurrence-free and overall survival rates through 5 years' follow-up were not significantly different between the two groups (p 0.06 and p 0.48, respectively). In a subset of patients with small HCC tumors (≤ 5 cm), recurrence-free survival was significantly better after adjuvant XRT (p 0.03), although overall survival was still not significantly different (p 0.92).

Discussion

Conclusion: Adjuvant XRT for centrally located HCC after narrow-margin hepatectomy is technically feasible and relatively safe but does not improve recurrence-free or overall survival. A post hoc subgroup comparison showed that adjuvant XRT improved recurrence-free survival but not overall survival for patients with small HCCs (≤ 5 cm).

Limitations: Patients who had undergone other adjuvant therapies including TACE or systemic therapies were not excluded. The study lacked a standardized approach to guide the management of patients with recurrence. No blinding for evaluation of outcomes. The study was not powered for subgroup analyses.

i. Consensus Statement on Colorectal Cancer Liver Metastases

Locoregional surgical and interventional therapies for advanced colorectal cancer liver metastases: Expert consensus statements.

Abdalla EK, Bauer TW, Chun YS, D'Angelica M, Kooby DA, Jarnagin WR

HPB. 2013;15(2):119–130.

SYNOPSIS

Takeaway Point: Resection strategies can be employed for multiple different disease scenarios, including bilateral liver metastases and synchronous presentation of primary and metastatic disease. Hepatic arterial infusion of chemotherapy is a valid option for liver-only disease, and ablation strategies continue to be studied but should not be employed as first-line therapy.

Commentary: Liver resection for hepatic colorectal metastases is now well established and supported by strong evidence. It has improved patient survival and should continue to be employed for lesions that are clearly resectable at presentation. The remaining open questions now focus on lesions that are deemed either borderline resectable or unresectable at presentation. The employment of novel and aggressive therapies to downsize these, including transarterial and chemoembolization and radiation therapies, show promise, but more in-depth trials are needed to establish their safety and efficacy.

ANALYSIS

Introduction: Multiple treatment strategies are available for the treatment of colorectal liver metastases (CRLM). Treatment strategies should be determined by a multidisciplinary approach and individualized for each patient. Options include resection, in either one or multiple stages and with or without portal vein embolization, downstaging preoperatively with systemic or regional therapies, simultaneous resection of the primary and metastatic disease, staged resections, chemotherapy by hepatic arterial infusion, and ablation.

Objectives: This article reports an expert consensus on locoregional and interventional therapies for the treatment of CRLM and synchronous presentation of primary and metastatic cancer.

Recommendations

Approaches to Bilateral Colorectal Cancer Liver Metastases:
Resection is the reference standard treatment for bilateral CRLM.
One-stage surgery with multiple resections is effective. Two-stage
hepatectomy with perioperative chemotherapy with or without
portal vein ligation may allow for complete resection in patients
who would otherwise be considered unresectable.

**Approaches to the Synchronous Presentation of Colorectal
Cancer and CRLM:** For such patients, pretreatment evaluation
should be multidisciplinary by colorectal and hepatic surgeons
and medical oncologists. In many patients simultaneous resection
of the primary colorectal cancer and liver metastases is feasible,
safe, and effective, providing patients adequate functional liver
reserve (FLR). If not, or if they would be higher risk secondary
to morbidities or to the extent or surgery required at both sites,
a staged resection should be considered. In staged resections, the
risk of complications from the primary tumor and the risk of progression of marginally resectable CRLM during treatment should
be considered when prioritizing one site or the other. If disease is
synchronous and the primary tumor is relatively asymptomatic,
preoperative chemotherapy of 2–3 months' duration is relatively
safe and should be considered for those at high risk of recurrent
disease base on clinical risk score.

Intraarterial Therapies: Hepatic arterial infusion (HAI) therapy
is a promising option for the provision of palliative or adjuvant
therapy in patients with CRLM, but is best administered in experienced centers. In patients with unresectable CRLM, floxuridine-
based HAI improves tumor response and hepatic progression-free
survival, but does not demonstrate a clear survival advantage compared to systemic chemotherapy. Randomized controlled trials are
warranted to clarify advantages and indications for HAI.

Radioembolization: Yttrium-90 transarterial radioembolization
is effective and has shown promising early results in the palliative management of unresectable CRLM. It can be considered for
patients with liver-only disease after failure of systemic chemotherapy. It should not be considered as first-line therapy except in
clinical trials.

Chemoembolization: Traditional transcatheter arterial chemoembolization (TACE) lacks data for CRLM. Drug-eluting beads
delivering irinotecan is a new therapy that is being explored and
shows promising early results.

Ablation Strategies (Radiofrequency, Microwave, and External Beam): Ablation strategies are inadequately studied and have high local failure rates. These modalities tend to be limited by tumor size, multiplicity, and location. They are not recommended as first-line treatments for resectable disease, but play a second-line role in highly select patients.

Discussion

Conclusion: Resection remains the reference treatment for bilateral CRLM and synchronous primary cancer and liver metastases. For bilateral disease, one-stage resections are acceptable, although two-stage procedures with portal vein ligation may allow for resection of more advanced disease. Simultaneous resection is possible for synchronous disease, although staged resections are recommended if the FLR is marginal. If staged resection is done, the order is dependent on the degree of symptoms of the primary tumor and the concern for progression of marginally resectable liver metastases. TACE is a valid option for liver-only disease, while ablation strategies are still being studied.

---

j. Improved Survival after Liver Resection for Hepatocellular Carcinoma

Improved long-term survival after major resection for hepatocellular carcinoma: A multicenter analysis based on a new definition of major hepatectomy.

Andreou A, Vauthey JN, Cherqui D, Zimmitti G, Ribero D, Truty MJ, Wei SH, Curley SA, Laurent A, Poon RT, Belghiti J, Nagorney DM, Aloia TA, International Cooperative Study Group on Hepatocellular Carcinoma

J Gastrointest Surg. 2013;17(1):66–77.

SYNOPSIS

Takeaway Point: Major hepatectomy of four or more segments is an accepted treatment for locally advanced hepatocellular carcinoma (HCC) and can offer long-term survival.

Commentary: This large multicenter study included patients with HCC from three countries undergoing a major hepatic resection, defined as resection of four or more contiguous segments. It compared outcomes among different countries and also looked at how outcomes have changed over a three-decade period. Patients undergoing extended hepatectomy had comparable

90-day and long-term survival when compared to patients undergoing less extensive resections. The exception was patients with underlying fibrosis or cirrhosis, who fared worse after undergoing extended hepatectomy than after undergoing right hepatectomy. If appropriate, such patients should be referred for transplantation instead of extensive resection. Outcomes have improved over time as preoperative imaging, patient selection, and surgical techniques have all become increasingly sophisticated. Although this is a retrospective database study, it provides compelling evidence that major hepatectomy is a valid treatment for HCC in appropriately selected patients. It is important to note that many studies have shown that liver transplantation offers the best long-term outcomes for HCC in terms of lower recurrence rates and improved survival, therefore hepatic resections cannot be considered optimal care.[30,31]

ANALYSIS

Introduction: HCC remains one of the most common malignancies worldwide, and surgery offers the only chance for cure. Hepatic resection is the preferred treatment for patients with preserved liver function and the only option for patients with large or multifocal tumors who are not candidates for transplantation. Major hepatectomy, defined as four or more liver segments according to Couinaud's classification, is often required, but the outcomes of such a large resection are not well studied.

Objectives: To examine long-term survival trends for patients treated with major hepatectomy for HCC.

Methods
Trial Design: Multicenter retrospective database study.
Participants
Inclusion Criteria: Patients with HCC who underwent major hepatectomy.

Exclusion Criteria: None.

Intervention: None; retrospective database analysis.

Endpoints

Primary Endpoint: Overall survival and postoperative mortality rates (within 90 days) after hepatic resection.

Secondary Endpoint: Identification of clinical factors associated with survival.

Sample Size: 539 patients between April 1981 and January 2008 at five major hepatobiliary centers in three countries (USA, China, France). 332 underwent right hepatectomy and 207 underwent extended hepatectomy.

Statistical Analysis: Patients were stratified according to extent of hepatectomy (right vs. extended), country of origin, and time period in which procedure was performed (1981–1989, 1990–1999, 2000–2008). χ^2 or Fisher's exact test for categorical variables and the Mann–Whitney U- or Kruskal–Wallis H-test for continuous variables. Survival was calculated using the Kaplan–Meier method. Log-rank tests were used to assess significance for univariate analyses.

Results

Baseline Data: Patients who underwent extended hepatectomy had larger median tumor size (12 vs. 8 cm, $p < 0.0001$), higher incidence of bilateral HCC ($p < 0.001$), more frequent positive surgical margins (16% vs. 10%, p 0.042), and were less frequently cirrhotic (28% vs. 40%, p 0.005) than patients who underwent right hepatectomy.

Outcomes: The 90-day postoperative mortality for all patients who underwent major hepatectomy was 4% and did not differ according to the extent of resection (p 0.976). Patients with fibrosis or cirrhosis had a worse 90-day mortality when undergoing extended hepatectomy (p 0.002) and worse overall survival (p 0.006). Median long-term follow-up was 63 months, and 5-year survival was 40%. Overall survival did not significantly differ by the extent of resection when comparing right versus extended hepatectomy (p 0.523). After multivariate analysis, predictors of diminished overall survival included α-fetoprotein (AFP) >1000 ng/mL, tumor size >5 cm, major vascular invasion, extrahepatic metastases, positive surgical margins and earlier time period, while predictors of 90-day mortality included major vascular invasion and earlier time period.

Discussion

Conclusion: This multinational, long-term HCC survival analysis indicates that expansion of surgical indications to include resection of four or more liver segments is justified by the significant improvement in outcomes over the past three decades.

Limitations: Variation in selection of surgical candidates amongst the different centers, morbidity not analyzed because of variability of reporting postoperative complications. Retrospective, observational study.

k. EORTC 40983: Colorectal Liver Metastases

Perioperative FOLFOX4 chemotherapy and surgery versus surgery alone for resectable liver metastases from colorectal cancer (EORTC 40983): Long-term results of a randomised, controlled, phase 3 trial.

Nordlinger B, Sorbye H, Glimelius B, Poston GJ, Schlag PM, Rougier P, Bechstein WO, Primrose JO, Walpole ET, Finch-Jones M, Jaeck D, Mirza D, Parks RW, Mauer M, Tanis E, Van Cutsem E, Scheithauer W, Gruenberger T, EORTC Gastro-Intestinal Tract Cancer Group, Cancer Research UK, Arbeitsgruppe Lebermetastasen und–tumoren in der Chirurgischen Arbeitsgemeinschaft Onkologie (ALM-CAO), Australasian Gastro-Intestinal Trials Group (AGITG), Fédération Francophone de Cancérologie Digestive (FFCD)

Lancet Oncol. 2013;14(12):1208–1215.

SYNOPSIS

Takeaway Point: Preoperative chemotherapy with FOLFOX4 for the treatment of resectable colorectal cancer liver metastases improves progression-free survival (PFS); however, an overall survival benefit was not seen.

Commentary: This trial presents the long-term follow-up of the EORTC 40983 trial, comparing surgery alone to perioperative chemotherapy plus surgery for patients with colorectal cancer liver metastases. The prior analysis had shown a progression-free survival benefit to perioperative chemotherapy. In this long-term analysis, no overall survival benefit was demonstrated. It is important to note that this trial was not powered to detect a survival difference among groups that were either treated preoperatively with FOLFOX4 or went straight to surgery. Because of long survival times in both groups, such a study would require extremely long follow-up and large numbers. This surgery demonstrated that preoperative FOLFOX4 therapy was well tolerated overall and is compatible with major liver surgery, and given the improvement in progression-free survival, it should be considered for this patient population.

ANALYSIS

Introduction: Surgical resection is curative for colorectal liver metastases; however, following resection, a significant number of patients suffer recurrence of disease in the remnant liver. There has been suggestion in some studies that chemotherapy may improve prognosis in such patients by treating micrometastatic disease. The EORTC 40983 study previously published data showing increased PFS for perioperative chemotherapy with surgery in comparison to surgery alone, but those data were published while overall long-term survival was still being monitored.

Objectives: To compare overall survival data after long-term follow-up in patients with resectable liver metastases from colorectal cancer treated with FOLFOX4 chemotherapy plus surgery versus surgery alone.

Methods
Trial Design: A randomized, controlled, parallel-group phase 3 trial.

Participants

Inclusion Criteria: Age 18–80 with histologically proven colorectal cancer, one to four resectable liver metastases, no detectable extrahepatic tumors, primary tumor previously resected or deemed to be resectable.

Exclusion Criteria: Previous oxaliplatin, other cancer in past 10 years, hepatic insufficiency, absolute neutrophil count (ANC) <1.5, serum creatinine greater than twice upper limit of normal, grade of common toxicity criteria more than 1 for peripheral neuropathy, congestive heart failure (CHF), angina, arrhythmia, hypertension, neurological or psychiatric disorders, active infection, pregnant or breastfeeding women.

Intervention: Randomization to surgery alone, or perioperative FOLFOX4, dosed at six 14-day cycles of oxaliplatin, folinic acid, and fluorouracil, before and after surgery.

Endpoints

Primary Endpoint: Progression-free survival.

Secondary Endpoints: Tumor resectability and tumor response.

Sample Size: 364 patients from 78 hospitals in Europe, Australia, and Hong Kong between October 2000 and July 2004, with 182 randomized to each group, 171 per group were eligible and 152 per group underwent resection.

Statistical Analysis: Survival was compared with a two-sided nonstratified log-rank test and the Kaplan–Meier method. A competing risk analysis to investigate the effects of deaths from other causes was done using a Gray test. Trial was powered to detect a 40% increase in median PFS, requiring 278 deaths; an a posteriori calculation estimated that 194 deaths would reach 80% power to detect an increase in 10% of proportion of patients alive at 3 years.

Results

Baseline Data: Baseline tumor and patient characteristics were similar between the two groups.

Outcomes: Median follow-up was 8.5 years, and at that time 59% of patients in the preoperative chemotherapy group and 63% in the surgery-only group had died (hazard ratio 0.88, 95% CI 0.68–1.14, p 0.34). Median overall survival was 61.3 (51.0–83.4) months in the perioperative chemotherapy group and 54.3 (41.9–79.4) months in the surgery-only group. Six patients per group were determined to have died from toxicity of protocol treatment, complications of protocol surgery, or toxicity of further cancer treatments.

Discussion

Conclusion: No difference was found in overall survival with the addition of perioperative chemotherapy with FOLFOX4 compared with surgery alone for patients with resectable liver metastases from colorectal cancer. However, the previously observed benefit in PFS means that perioperative chemotherapy with FOLFOX4 should remain the reference treatment for this population of patients.

Limitations: The trial was not powered to detect an increase in overall survival. Treatments for recurrences were not systemic and differed between groups (ie, chemotherapy was administered more frequently at first progression to patients in the surgery-only group), and this may have affected survival results.

I. Paclitaxel plus Gemcitabine for Metastatic Pancreatic Cancer

Increased survival in pancreatic cancer with nab-paclitaxel plus gemcitabine.

Von Hoff DD, Ervin T, Arena FP, Chiorean EG, Infante J, Moore M, Seay T, Tjulandin SA, Ma WW, Saleh MN, Harris M, Reni M, Dowden S, Laheru D, Bahary N, Ramanathan RK, Tabernero J, Hidalgo M, Goldstein D, Van Cutsem E, Wei X, Iglesias J, Renschler MF

NEJM. 2013;369(18):1691–1703.

SYNOPSIS

Takeaway Point: For patients with metastatic pancreatic cancer, nab-paclitaxel combined with gemcitabine improves overall and progression-free survival compared to gemcitabine alone.

Commentary:

This large, multicenter, randomized phase 3 trial showed that nab-paclitaxel plus gemcitabine improved overall survival in patients with metastatic pancreatic cancer as compared to gemcitabine alone. Progression-free survival and response rate were also improved. The proportion of patients with serious adverse events was similar in the two treatment groups, and the rate of seriously life-threatening adverse events was not increased. Notably, some adverse events-peripheral neuropathy and myelosuppression were increased with combination therapy, but these seemed to be reversible. Overall, this important study points toward a potentially beneficial therapy for metastatic pancreatic cancer patients. It is important to note that the experimental regimen of nab-paclitaxel plus gemcitabine was compared to gemcitabine monotherapy rather than the gemcitabine plus erlotinib combination or FOLFIRINOX, both of which have demonstrated previous benefit.

ANALYSIS

Introduction: The prognosis for metastatic pancreatic cancer remains dismal, and although several phase 2 chemotherapy studies have shown promise, only two (gemcitabine plus erlotinib and FOLFIRINOX) have shown improved survival in phase 3 studies. In preclinical studies, nab-paclitaxel acted synergistically with gemcitabine and demonstrated promising efficacy with manageable side effects.

Objectives: This is a phase 3 study of the efficacy and safety of the combination of albumin-bound paclitaxel (nab-paclitaxel) plus gemcitabine versus gemcitabine monotherapy in patients with metastatic pancreatic cancer.

Methods

Trial Design: Phase 3 randomized controlled trial.

Participants

Inclusion Criteria: Age ≥18 years with metastatic pancreatic adenocarcinoma and Karnofsky performance status score of ≥70, no prior chemotherapy. Metastatic disease diagnosed within 6 weeks of randomization.

Exclusion Criteria: Patients could have received flurouracil or gemcitabine as radiation sensitizer, but those who had received cytotoxic doses of any chemotherapy were excluded. Also excluded were patients with islet cell neoplasm; locally advanced disease; and those without adequate hematologic, hepatic, and renal function to tolerate chemotherapy.

Intervention: Patients were treated with nab-paclitaxel (125 mg/m^2) followed by gemcitabine (1000 mg per square meter) on days 1, 8, and 15 every 4 weeks, or gemcitabine monotherapy at the same dose weekly for 7 or 8 weeks (cycle 1) and then on days 1, 8, and 15 every 4 weeks. Treatment was continued until disease progression or unacceptable adverse events. Crossover was not allowed. Tumor response was evaluated by cross-sectional imaging every 8 weeks by response evaluation criteria in solid tumors (RECIST) criteria, and safety was monitored. Patients were stratified by performance status, presence of liver metastases, and geographic region.

Endpoints

Primary Endpoint: Overall survival.

Secondary Endpoints: Progression-free survival and overall response rate.

Sample Size: Multicenter trial between May 2009 and April 2012, including 151 community and academic centers in 11 countries throughout North America (63%), eastern Europe (15%), Australia (14%), and western Europe (9%); 861 patients were randomized (431 in nab-paclitaxel plus gemcitabine arm and 430 in gemcitabine monotherapy arm), and 823 were treated (421 in nab-paclitaxel plus gemcitabine arm and 402 in gemcitabine monotherapy arm).

Statistical Analysis: Kaplan–Meier and stratified log-rank test, multivariate analysis with Cox proportional-hazards model. Comparison of response rates was performed with χ^2 test. Correlation between changes in CA19-9 levels and survival was evaluated with Cox regression model. Sample size calculation demonstrated 842 patients with 608 deaths needed to detect a hazard ration of 0.769 with combination therapy.

Results

Baseline Data: All demographic and clinical characteristics were balanced between the two groups.

Outcomes: Median survival was 8.5 months with combination therapy compared to 6.7 months with gemcitabine monotherapy ($p < 0.001$). Both 1- and 2-year survival rates were significantly higher with combination therapy compared to monotherapy, and progression-free survival was also longer (5.5 vs. 3.7 months, $p < 0.001$). Performance score and the absence of liver metastases were independent predictors of survival. The most common adverse events with grade ≥ 3 were neutropenia, fatigue, and neuropathy, and these were increased in the nab-paclitaxel group.

Discussion

Conclusion: Nab-paclitaxel plus gemcitabine significantly improved overall survival, progression-free survival, and response rate compared with gemcitabine alone, but rates of peripheral neuropathy and myelosuppression were increased.

Limitations: Quality of life was not measured.

---

m. Borderline Resectable Pancreatic Cancer

Borderline resectable pancreatic cancer: A consensus statement by the International Study Group of Pancreatic Surgery (ISGPS).

Bockhorn M, Uzunoglu FG, Adham M, Imrie C, Milicevic M, Sandberg AA, Asbun HJ, Bassi C, Büchler M, Charnley RM, Conlon K, Cruz LF, Dervenis C, Fingerhutt A, Friess H, Gouma DJ, Hartwig W, Lillemoe KD, Montorsi M, Neoptolemos JP, Shrikhande SV, Takaori K, Traverso W, Vashist YK, Vollmer C, Yeo CJ, Izbicki JR, International Study Group of Pancreatic Surgery

Surgery. 2014;155(6):977–988.

SYNOPSIS

Takeaway Point: In patients with borderline resectable pancreatic cancer (BRPC), portomesenteric venous resection is justified from an oncologic perspective, whereas arterial resection is not.

Commentary: This article describes an expert consensus statement that was issued by the ISGPS after an extensive literature review, which provided a much-needed definition of and treatment guidelines for BRPC. The authors validated previously described criteria for borderline resectability as established by the National Comprehensive Cancer Network (NCCN) guidelines issued in 2013. Borderline resectable pancreatic ductal adenocarcinoma is defined as: venous involvement of the superior mesenteric vein (SMV) or portal vein (PV) with suitable proximal and distal margins, allowing for resection and replacement; involvement of the gastroduodenal artery (GDA) up to the hepatic artery with short segment encasement or direct abutment of the hepatic artery with extension into the celiac axis; or tumor abutment of the superior mesenteric artery (SMA) of <180°. The authors conclude that patients with BRPC with limited venous involvement of the SMV or PV will benefit from more extensive resection, while those with arterial involvement will not. They further emphasize the importance of treating such patients at high-volume centers with a multidisciplinary approach. Although these data are based on expert consensus rather than prospective randomized data, this article incorporated both an exhaustive literature review and a large group of experts who practice in varied settings across multiple continents. Data were reviewed individually, and via an in-person meeting. This current effort reflects a well-rounded, serious review of available data by worldwide experts in the field. Randomized studies are needed; however, given the limited available population and difficulty obtaining good prospective data, this article provides a strong summary of the best available evidence at the time.

ANALYSIS

Introduction: Pancreatic cancer is a leading cause of cancer-related death and is one of few cancers with an increasing mortality. Up to 25% of patients are considered potentially inoperable at diagnosis because of involvement of surrounding vessels. With the improvement in operative techniques and perioperative care over the past several decades, the criteria for resectability have expanded and the term *borderline resectable pancreatic cancer* (BRPC) has become increasingly used.

Objectives: To expedite an internationally agreed-on definition and treatment consensus for patients with BRPC.

Methods

Trial Design: A computerized search of PubMed and Embase databases was carried out in February 2013 using the following key terms: pancreatic cancer, borderline resectable, extended resection, superior mesenteric vein, portal vein, celiac axis, superior mesenteric artery, common hepatic artery, irresectability, morbidity, mortality, and survival.

Participants

Inclusion Criteria: All levels of evidence were included and rated. Only studies published in English were included.

Exclusion Criteria: Case studies were excluded.

Intervention: All relevant literature was reviewed by the ISGPS study subgroup, who created a first draft of the consensus definitions and statement. This was reviewed by members of the ISGPS at a consensus meeting in April 2013, and a final consensus was formulated.

Results

Outcomes: The essential conclusions of the consensus statement are summarized below:

1. The ISGPS supports the imaging-based NCCN criteria for borderline resectability; CT findings of distortion of the SMV/ portal venous axis including short segment occlusion allowing reconstruction; encasement of the GDA to the hepatic artery with either short segment encasement or abutment without extension into the celiac axis; and tumor abutment of the SMA with ≤180° of vessel wall circumference.

2. There is clear evidence supporting operative exploration and resection in the presence of reconstructable mesentericoportal axis involvement if complete tumor excision (R0) is possible.

3. There is *no* good evidence that arterial resections during right-sided pancreatic resections are of benefit. In case of verification of arterial involvement, palliative treatment is the standard of care.

4. Patients with BRPC with suspected but not proven distant metastases and patients ineligible for surgery because of comorbidity should be reevaluated for operative intervention after neoadjuvant treatment; these patients should be offered exploration for potential resection only in the absence of disease progression.

Discussion

Conclusion: Current evidence supports portomesenteric resection in patients with BRPC, but there is no good evidence that arterial resections during right-sided, proximal pancreatic resections are of benefit; therefore, arterial resection should not be recommended in most cases. Multimodal therapy comprising neoadjuvant chemotherapy, radiation, and surgery may in the future provide the most favorable outcome in patients with BRPC.

Limitations: There is a paucity of multi-institutional and multinational studies on the topic, and further prospective studies are mandatory.

n. Pancreaticoduodenectomy with and without Intraperitoneal Drainage

A randomized prospective multicenter trial of pancreaticoduodenectomy with and without routine intraperitoneal drainage.

Van Buren II G, Bloomston M, Hughes SJ, Winter J, Behrman SW, Zyromski NJ, Vollmer C, Velanovich V, Riall T, Muscarella P, Trevino J, Nakeeb A, Schmidt CM, Behrns K, Ellison EC, Barakat O, Perry KA, Drebin J, House M, Abdel-Misih S, Silberfein EJ, Goldin S, Brown K, Mohammed S, Hodges SE, McElhany A, Issazadeh M, Jo E, Mo Q, Fisher WE

Ann Surg. 2014;259(4):605–612.

SYNOPSIS

Takeaway Point: Eliminating routine intraperitoneal drain placement for patients undergoing pancreaticoduodenectomy (PD) is associated with increased postoperative morbidity and mortality.

Commentary: This is the first prospective, randomized trial to address the question of whether routine peritoneal drainage following PD can be safely eliminated. The answer was a resounding no, with patients undergoing PD without drainage demonstrating an increased rate of complications, increased severity of complications, a trend toward increased mortality and ultimately the early closing of the trial prior to reaching goal accrual. These findings were largely attributable to sepsis, multiorgan system failure, and hemorrhage secondary to undiagnosed pancreatic fistulae. The elimination of routine intraperitoneal drainage in all comers is not safe and cannot be advocated. By employing more sophisticated and validated methods of predicting the likelihood of pancreatic leak, it may soon be possible to select a lower-risk group of patients who can forego intraperitoneal drainage, and the authors are currently retrospectively analyzing their data using a fistula risk score to explore this issue.[32] The issue of whether it was even ethical to randomize all patients undergoing PD, including those with well-established risk factors for developing a pancreatic leak including a soft pancreas and small duct, was raised in letters to the editor after the trial was published.[33]

ANALYSIS

Introduction: Routine placement of intraperitoneal drains following pancreaticoduodenectomy (PD) has traditionally been considered mandatory, most importantly to prevent the morbidity from an unrecognized pancreatic leak. This has been called into question, however, because the majority of patients do not develop a pancreatic leak and because drains have been shown to be unnecessary or harmful in other operations, including splenectomy and gastrectomy.

Objectives: To test the hypothesis that PD without the use of routine intraperitoneal drainage does not increase the frequency or severity of complications.

Methods

Trial Design: Prospective randomized controlled trial.

Participants

Inclusion Criteria: All patients undergoing PD.

Exclusion Criteria: Patient refusal.

Intervention: Intraperitoneal drain or no drain. Randomization was substratified for anticipated diagnosis to account for a soft or hard pancreas. If drains were used, a drain amylase was sent on postoperative day 3 and on other days if desired by the surgeon. Drains were left in place until either (1) the amylase value was <3 times the upper limit of normal serum amylase and/or (2) the output was ≤20 cm^3/day for 2 consecutive days.

Endpoints

Primary Endpoint: Difference in grade II or greater complication rate at 60 days.

Secondary Endpoints: Included overall complication rates, occurrence of specific complications, and mortality.

Sample Size: 137 patients from nine high-volume academic centers in the United States between September 2011 and December 2012, with 68 randomized to the drainage group and 69 in the no-drainage group.

Statistical Analysis: Primary endpoint was compared using the χ^2 test, and secondary endpoints were compared using the Fisher exact test, χ^2 test, or the *t*-test or Wilcoxon rank sum test. Sample size estimates required 376 patients per group to detect a 10% change in complication rate.

Results

Baseline Data: There were no significant differences between the two cohorts in demographics, comorbidities, indications for surgery, pancreas texture or duct size, and operative technique.

Outcomes: PD without drainage was associated with a higher morbidity, including a significantly increased rate of at least grade 2 complications at 30 days (64% vs. 47%, *p* 0.049) and 60 days (68% vs. 52%, *p* 0.047). Complications that were significantly different included gastroparesis, intraabdominal abscess, diarrhea, and abdominal fluid collection. The study was stopped early because of excess rates of mortality in the patients undergoing PD without routine intraperitoneal drainage (12% vs. 3%, p 0.097) at 90 days.

Discussion

Conclusion: Elimination of intraperitoneal drainage for PD increases the severity and frequency of complications and contributed to a fourfold increase in mortality in the group that was not drained.

Limitations: The trial was stopped early owing to the statistically significant increased morbidity demonstrated at 30 and 60 days and the trend toward increased mortality in the no-drainage group at 90 days.

---

o. PYTHON Trial

Early versus on-demand nasoenteric tube feeding in acute pancreatitis.

Bakker OJ, van Brunschot S, van Santvoort HC, Besselink MG, Bollen TL, Boermeester MA, Dejong CH, van Goor H, Bosscha K, Ahmed Ali U, Bouwense S, van Grevenstein WM, Heisterkamp J, Houdijk AP, Jansen JM, Karsten TM, Manusama ER, Nieuwenhuijs VB, Schaapherder AF, van der Schelling GP, Schwartz MP, Spanier BW, Tan A, Vecht J, Weusten BL, Witteman BJ, Akkermans LM, Bruno MJ, Dijkgraaf MG, van Ramshorst B, Gooszen HG, Dutch Pancreatitis Study Group

NEJM. 2014;371(21):1983–1993.

SYNOPSIS

Takeaway Point: For patients with high-risk acute pancreatitis, early nasoenteric feeding demonstrated no clinical benefit when compared with 72 hours of NPO (nil per os) followed by oral diet as tolerated.

Commentary: This study failed to demonstrate the benefits that previous trials and observational studies have associated with early enteric feeding for patients with high-risk acute pancreatitis.[34–36] The trophic effect of early feeding is thought to stabilize the gut mucosa and prevent bacterial overgrowth, thereby reducing inflammation and infectious complications; however, this outcome was not observed in the current trial. Similar outcomes were observed between early enteric feeding and NPO status for at least 72 hours with subsequent oral diet (the on-demand group). Moreover, only a third of patients in the on-demand group ultimately required tube feeding, leading the authors to conclude that nasoenteric feeds, and the associated discomfort, expense, and complications, could be avoided in the majority of patients in this population. This trial remains controversial and difficult to interpret, given that most patients with "high-risk pancreatitis" are unable to tolerate oral intake after 72 hours. In fact, the median days to toleration of a full oral diet was 9 in the early tube feeding group and 6 in the on-demand group. Certain patients, such as those requiring intubation, are not eligible for an early oral diet and would still require early enteral nutrition within 24–48 hours. Additionally, standard guidelines [Italian Association for Study of the Pancreas (AISP) and American Society for Parenteral and Enteral Nutrition (ASPEN)] continue to recommend enteral feeding within 24–48 hours for all patients, emphasizing the controversial nature of the topic.[37,38]

ANALYSIS

Introduction: In the treatment of acute pancreatitis, meta-analyses have demonstrated that early nasoenteric tube feeding compared to total parenteral nutrition results in reduced infection rates. Tube feeding is recommended when patients will be unable to tolerate an oral diet for 7 days, but it takes 3–4 days to make this assessment, by which time the patient is outside of the window for early enteric feeding and the benefits it confers.

Objectives: To compare the effects of early nasojejunal tube feeding with those of an oral diet started at 72 hours in patients with acute pancreatitis.

Methods

Trial Design: A multicenter, randomized controlled superiority trial.

Participants

Inclusion Criteria: Adults with their first episode of acute pancreatitis who were considered at high risk for complications [defined by an elevated APACHE II score, a high modified Glasgow score, or elevated C-reactive protein (CRP)]. Pancreatitis was diagnosed if at least two of the following conditions were present: typical abdominal pain, serum amylase or lipase >3 times normal, or characteristic findings on cross-sectional imaging.

Exclusion Criteria: Recurrent or chronic pancreatitis, or secondary to ERCP or malignancy. Pregnancy, preexisting enteral or parenteral nutrition, >24 hours since presentation, or >96 hours since symptom onset.

Intervention: Randomization to nasojejunal tube feeding initiated within 24 hours (the early group) or to an oral diet starting at 72 hours (the on-demand group). If oral diet was not tolerated by 96 hours, then nasojejunal feeding was started.

Endpoints

Primary Endpoint: Composite endpoint of major infection (infected pancreatic necrosis, bacteremia, or pneumonia) or death within 6 months after randomization.

Secondary Endpoints: Development of necrotizing pancreatitis as diagnosed on CT scan performed 5–7 days after admission, organ failure.

Sample Size: Patients enrolled from August 2008 to June 2012 from 19 Dutch hospitals; 208 patients were randomized, with 102 patients to early group and 106 patients to on-demand group; 3 patients were excluded from the analysis for incorrect diagnosis (1 in early group, 2 in on-demand group).

Statistical Analysis: Fischer's exact test for dichotomous data, Mann–Whitney U-test for continuous data, linear-by-linear association test with categorical data. Sample size calculation based on expected reduction in the composite endpoint from 40% to 22% estimated a necessary sample size of 208 patients.

Results

Baseline Data: The only baseline characteristic that differed between the two groups was mean body mass index (BMI) (29 in early group vs. 27 in on-demand group, p 0.01).

Outcomes: Major infection or death occurred in 30% of the early group and 27% of the on-demand group (p 0.76). Necrotizing pancreatitis developed in 63% of the early group and in 62% of the on-demand group. 18% of patients in the early group required ICU admission, compared to 19% of patients in the on-demand group. 31% of patients in the on-demand group required nasoenteric feeding.

Discussion

Conclusion: This trial did not show superiority of early nasoenteric tube feeding, as compared with an oral diet or on-demand tube feeding after 72 hours, in reducing the rate of infection or death in patients with acute pancreatitis at high risk for complications.

Limitations: The confidence interval of the primary endpoint was wide, indicating that the trial may have been too small to detect a difference between two groups. Tube feeding perhaps should have been started earlier or at a higher rate as with other trials in which a benefit of early tube feeding was demonstrated. The study also reported 44% and 38% dislodgement rates and 11% and 12% obstruction rates of the feeding tubes in the early tube feeding and on-demand tube feeding groups, respectively, making it unclear how adherent the groups actually were to their feeding plans.

p. Liver Partition and Portal Vein Ligation for Staged Hepatectomy

Systematic review and meta-analysis of feasibility, safety, and efficacy or a novel procedure: Associating liver partition and portal vein ligation for staged hepatectomy.

Schadde E, Schnitzbauer AA, Tschuor C, Raptis DA, Bechstein WO, Clavien PA

Ann Surg Oncol. 2015;22(9):3109–3120.

SYNOPSIS

Takeaway Point: Associating liver partition and portal vein ligation for staged hepatectomy (ALPPS) is technically feasible with successful increase in liver volume, but mortality and morbidity are significant, and evidence supporting use remains low.

Commentary: This systematic review attempted to answer questions regarding the safety, efficacy, and feasibility of ALPPS; however, few studies are available, and the overall level of evidence is low. The technique is promising owing to its clear technical feasibility and the variety of pathologies for which it can be employed. Mortality is significant but appears to be comparable to conventional two-stage hepatectomy. Currently, this technique remains somewhat controversial, given its high resource use and need for two operations. Although anecdotally it seems that the number of surgeons performing ALPPS is growing, many surgeons do not perform this operation at all, choosing to employ alternate means of achieving portal vein ligation such as portal vein embolization. In this setting, it would be difficult to accrue patients to a randomized trial. ALPPS surgeons are actively working to improve the level of evidence by tracking patients in an international registry.

ANALYSIS

Introduction: ALPPS is a new technique that allows for completion of a trisectionectomy when the liver remnant is marginal through a two-stage approach. Initially, portal vein ligation (PVL)

and parenchymal transection are performed, resulting in hypertrophy of the remnant liver, so that resection of the diseased liver can safely follow in a delayed fashion. Liver growth was observed at the rate of a 10-fold increase in only a few weeks, but concerns have been raised about morbidity and mortality.

Objectives: This systematic review was performed to assess the published evidence for feasibility, safety and oncological efficacy of ALPPS.

Methods
Trial Design: PubMed, the Cochrane Database, Embase, and SCOPUS were all searched for articles relevant to ALPPS. Manuscripts were tabulated in a qualitative synthesis and categorized into levels of evidence in accordance with the definition of the Centre of Evidence in Medicine in Oxford. A quantitative synthesis/meta-analysis was performed.

Participants
Inclusion Criteria: Full-text articles in all languages were screened for eligibility. Patients who were reported twice were excluded.

Exclusion Criteria: Studies unrelated to ALPPS, abstracts, letters, editorials, and opinion articles were excluded. Studies of up to three patients were considered case reports and excluded.

Intervention: Information on baseline descriptors of the patient population undergoing ALPPS was extracted from the studies. Indication to perform ALPPS was evaluated.

Endpoints: Data collection focused on three questions:

1. How feasible is ALPPS?
2. How safe is ALPPS?
3. How effective is ALPPS?

Sample Size: In total, 13 studies were included, 10 were case series (evidence level 4), two were comparative studies with a total of 55 patients [one comparing 7 patients undergoing ALPPS to 15 patients with portal vein embolization (PVE) and considered evidence level 4], and one with 48 ALPPS patients and 86 PVE or PVL patients considered evidence level 3b. The final study was an analysis of the 202 patients in the ALPPS registry and is considered level 2c evidence.

Statistical Analysis: Comprehensive meta-analysis software was used to generate meta-analysis and forest plots using the random effects model.

Results

Baseline Data: The indications for ALPPS were CRLM (199 patients), HCC (22 patients), perihilar cholangiocarcinoma (21 patients), intrahepatic cholangiocarcinoma (14 patients), gallbladder cancer (7 patients), non-CRLM (25 patients), and not reported in 7 patients.

Outcomes: The feasibility for completion of both stages of resection was 97%. The increase in liver volume was reported in two studies at 84% (CI 78–91%). The majority of studies reported a waiting interval of one week between the two stages. The meta-analysis shows an 11% (CI 8–16%) 90-day or in-hospital mortality. 44% (CI 38–50%) of patients experienced a complication of grade IIIa or higher. Complete oncologic resection was achieved in 91% (CI 87–94%) of patients. Overall survival and disease-free survival were rarely reported adequately. The most common study biases found were related to single-center case series and retrospective analyses, followed by the reporting bias of a voluntary registry and lack of a control group.

Discussion

Conclusion: ALPPS appears to offer a high feasibility of resecting primarily unresectable liver tumors, and a mortality comparable to conventional two-stage hepatectomies; however, data on oncologic outcomes are lacking.

Limitations: The systematic review was limited because of the small numbers of original publications, with those included offering low levels of evidence.

REFERENCES

1. de Romo AC. Tallow and the time capsule: Claude Bernard's discovery of the pancreatic digestion of fat. *Hist Philos Life Sci.* 1989;11(2):253–274.

2. Are C, Dhir M, Ravipati L. History of pancreaticoduodenectomy: Early misconceptions, initial milestones and the pioneers. *HPB.* 2011;13(6):377–384.

3. Morgenstern L. Carl Langenbuch and the first cholecystectomy. *Surg Endosc.* 1992;6(3):113–114.

4. Lortat-Jacob JL, Robert HA, Henry C. Excision of the right lobe of the liver for a malignant secondary tumor. *Arch Maladies l'Appareil Digestif Maladies Nutrition.* 1952;41(6):662–667.

5. Litynski GS. Profiles in laparoscopy: Mouret, Dubois, and Perissat: the laparoscopic breakthrough in Europe (1987-1988). *J Soc Laparoendosc Surgeons.* 1999;3(2):163–167.

6. Safrany L, Cotton PB. Endoscopic management of choledocholithiasis. *Surg Clin N Am.* 1982;62(5):825–826.

7. Bockhorn M, Uzunoglu FG, Adham M, Imrie C, Milicevic M, Sandberg AA, et al. Borderline resectable pancreatic cancer: A consensus statement by the International Study Group of Pancreatic Surgery (ISGPS). *Surgery.* 2014;155(6):977–988.

8. Tran KT, Smeenk HG, van Eijck CH, Kazemier G, Hop WC, Greve JW, et al. Pylorus preserving pancreaticoduodenectomy versus standard Whipple procedure: A prospective, randomized, multicenter analysis of 170 patients with pancreatic and periampullary tumors. *Ann Surg.* 2004;240(5):738–745.

9. Diener MK, Seiler CM, Rossion I, Kleeff J, Glanemann M, Butturini G, et al. Efficacy of stapler versus hand-sewn closure after distal pancreatectomy (DISPACT): A randomised, controlled multicentre trial. *Lancet.* 2011;377(9776):1514–1522.

10. Yeo CJ, Cameron JL, Lillemoe KD, Sauter PK, Coleman J, Sohn TA, et al. Does prophylactic octreotide decrease the rates of pancreatic fistula and other complications after pancreaticoduodenectomy? Results of a prospective randomized placebo-controlled trial. *Ann Surg.* 2000;232(3):419–429.

11. Lowy AM, Lee JE, Pisters PW, Davidson BS, Fenoglio CJ, Stanford P, et al. Prospective, randomized trial of octreotide to prevent pancreatic fistula after pancreaticoduodenectomy for malignant disease. *Ann Surg.* 1997;226(5):632–641.

12. Von Hoff DD, Ervin T, Arena FP, Chiorean EG, Infante J, Moore M, et al. Increased survival in pancreatic cancer with nab-paclitaxel plus gemcitabine. *NEJM.* 2013;369(18):1691–1703.

13. Tanaka M, Fernandez-del Castillo C, Adsay V, Chari S, Falconi M, Jang JY, et al. International consensus guidelines 2012 for the management of IPMN and MCN of the pancreas. *Pancreatology.* 2012;12(3):183–197.

14. Bakker OJ, van Brunschot S, van Santvoort HC, Besselink MG, Bollen TL, Boermeester MA, et al. Early versus on-demand nasoenteric tube feeding in acute pancreatitis. *NEJM.* 2014;371(21):1983–1993.

15. van Santvoort HC, Besselink MG, de Vries AC, Boermeester MA, Fischer K, Bollen TL, et al. Early endoscopic retrograde cholangiopancreatography in predicted severe acute biliary pancreatitis: A prospective multicenter study. *Ann Surg.* 2009;250(1):68–75.

16. van Santvoort HC, Besselink MG, Bakker OJ, Hofker HS, Boermeester MA, Dejong CH, et al. A step-up approach or open necrosectomy for necrotizing pancreatitis. *NEJM.* 2010;362(16):1491–1502.

17. Parikh P, Shiloach M, Cohen ME, Bilimoria KY, Ko CY, Hall BL, et al. Pancreatectomy risk calculator: An ACS-NSQIP resource. *HPB.* 2010;12(7):488–497.

18. Bassi C, Dervenis C, Butturini G, Fingerhut A, Yeo C, Izbicki J, et al. Postoperative pancreatic fistula: An international study group (ISGPF) definition. *Surgery*. 2005;138(1):8–13.

19. Wente MN, Bassi C, Dervenis C, Fingerhut A, Gouma DJ, Izbicki JR, et al. Delayed gastric emptying (DGE) after pancreatic surgery: A suggested definition by the International Study Group of Pancreatic Surgery (ISGPS). *Surgery*. 2007;142(5):761–768.

20. Andreou A, Vauthey JN, Cherqui D, Zimmitti G, Ribero D, Truty MJ, et al. Improved long-term survival after major resection for hepatocellular carcinoma: A multicenter analysis based on a new definition of major hepatectomy. *J Gastrointest Surg*. 2013;17(1):66–77.

21. Yu W, Wang W, Rong W, Wang L, Xu Q, Wu F, et al. Adjuvant radiotherapy in centrally located hepatocellular carcinomas after hepatectomy with narrow margin (<1 cm): A prospective randomized study. *J Am Coll Surg*. 2014;218(3):381–392.

22. Llovet JM, Ricci S, Mazzaferro V, Hilgard P, Gane E, Blanc JF, et al. Sorafenib in advanced hepatocellular carcinoma. *NEJM*. 2008;359(4):378–390.

23. Nordlinger B, Sorbye H, Glimelius B, Poston GJ, Schlag PM, Rougier P, et al. Perioperative FOLFOX4 chemotherapy and surgery versus surgery alone for resectable liver metastases from colorectal cancer (EORTC 40983): Long-term results of a randomised, controlled, phase 3 trial. *Lancet Oncol*. 2013;14(12):120–185.

24. Schadde E, Schnitzbauer AA, Tschuor C, Raptis DA, Bechstein WO, Clavien PA. Systematic review and meta-analysis of feasibility, safety, and efficacy of a novel procedure: Associating liver partition and portal vein ligation for staged hepatectomy. *Ann Surg Oncol*. 2015; 22(9):3109–3120.

25. Pitt HA, Kilbane M, Strasberg SM, Pawlik TM, Dixon E, Zyromski NJ, et al. ACS-NSQIP has the potential to create an HPB-NSQIP option. *HPB*. 2009;11(5):405–413.

26. Skandalakis JE, Weidman TA, Foster RS Jr, Kingsworth AS, Skandalakis LS, Skandalakis PN, Mirilas PS. *Skandalakis' Surgical Anatomy: The Embryologic and Anatomic Basis of Modern Surgery*. Athens, Greece: PMP; 2004.

27. Steinberg WM. A step-up approach, or open necrosectomy for necrotizing pancreatitis (comment on). *NEJM*. 2010;363(13):1286–1287.

28. De Waele JJ. A step-up approach, or open necrosectomy for necrotizing pancreatitis (comment on). *NEJM*. 2010;363(13):1286.

29. Warshaw AL. Improving the treatment of necrotizing pancreatitis–A step up. *NEJM*. 2010;362(16):1535–1537.

30. Beard RE, Hanto DW, Gautam S, Miksad RA. A comparison of surgical outcomes for noncirrhotic and cirrhotic hepatocellular carcinoma patients in a Western institution. *Surgery*. 2013;154(3):545–555.

31. Zheng Z, Liang W, Milgrom DP, Zheng Z, Schroder PM, Kong NS, et al. Liver transplantation versus liver resection in the treatment of hepatocellular carcinoma: A meta-analysis of observational studies. *Transplantation.* 2014;97(2):227–234.

32. Fisher WE, Jordan GL. Reply to letter: "A randomized prospective multicenter trial of pancreaticoduodenectomy with and without routine intraperitoneal drainage." *Ann Surg.* 2015;262(6):e107–108.

33. Bohara T. A randomized prospective multicenter trial of pancreaticoduodenectomy with and without routine intraperitoneal drainage [letter]. *Ann Surg.* 2016;263(2):e20.

34. Al-Omran M, Albalawi ZH, Tashkandi MF, Al-Ansary LA. Enteral versus parenteral nutrition for acute pancreatitis. *Cochrane Database Systematic Rev.* 2010(1):CD002837.

35. Li JY, Yu T, Chen GC, Yuan YH, Zhong W, Zhao LN, et al. Enteral nutrition within 48 hours of admission improves clinical outcomes of acute pancreatitis by reducing complications: A meta-analysis. *PloS ONE.* 2013;8(6):e64926.

36. Wereszczynska-Siemiatkowska U, Swidnicka-Siergiejko A, Siemiatkowski A, Dabrowski A. Early enteral nutrition is superior to delayed enteral nutrition for the prevention of infected necrosis and mortality in acute pancreatitis. *Pancreas.* 2013;42(4):640–646.

37. Italian Association for the Study of the Pancreas, Pezzilli R, Zerbi A, Campra D, Capurso G, Golfieri R, et al. Consensus guidelines on severe acute pancreatitis. *Digest Liver Disease.* 2015;47(7):532–543.

38. Guenter P, Boullata JI, Ayers P, Gervasio J, Malone A, Raymond E, et al. Standardized competencies for parenteral nutrition prescribing: The American Society for Parenteral and Enteral Nutrition Model. *Nutr Clin Practice.* 2015;30(4):570–576.

8

Colorectal Surgery

Blake Read • Raja Narayan • Cindy Kin

INTRODUCTION

Historically, investigation in colorectal surgery has focused on small, single-center series investigating optimal surgical techniques. Examples of such papers include reports on the "holy plane" in total mesorectal excision (see **b**, below), the Nigro protocol for squamous cell carcinoma of the anus (see **a**), and papers describing outcomes with various surgical techniques for inflammatory bowel disease. During the last decade, in an attempt to reduce postoperative length of stay, the research focus has shifted to the safety and outcomes of minimally invasive techniques in colorectal surgery. Results of these trials acknowledge the acceptability of laparoscopic-assisted resection for benign disease and for colon cancer, but potentially *worse* oncologic outcomes with this approach in cases of rectal cancer.

The last decade has also seen a growing movement to treat early rectal cancers with radiation and/or local excision, as an alternative to radical resection. Traditional proctectomy for the treatment of rectal cancer continues to generate controversy, given variable outcomes depending on surgeon experience and technique. Surgical treatment of diverticulitis continues to evolve, with management increasingly determined on a case-by-case basis. There are a multitude of clinical questions that remain to be answered, including the role of robotic surgery in colorectal operations, how we might improve rectal cancer outcomes, and whether radiation and/or local excision can safely replace radical resection for early rectal cancers. The following articles represent the best available data to inform current practice; however, any practitioner of colorectal surgery must review the literature frequently to keep abreast of this rapidly changing field.

a. Nigro Protocol

An evaluation of combined therapy for squamous cell cancer of the anal canal.

Nigro ND

Diseases Colon Rectum. 1984;27(12):763–766.

SYNOPSIS

Takeaway Point: Chemoradiation therapy is the treatment of choice for squamous cell cancer of the anal canal, with abdomino-perineal resection (APR) reserved for patients with persistent or recurrent disease.

Commentary: Prior to this trial, APR was the traditionally accepted management strategy for squamous cell carcinoma of the anal canal, with a 10-year survival rate of 52%. In the post–World War I era, British physicians began using radiation therapy as an alternative treatment, but the practice was discontinued because of toxicity. In the intervening years, radiation techniques advanced, and Dr. Nigro reports on the results of 104 patients who underwent combined chemotherapy and radiation for anal squamous cell carcinoma. He demonstrates complete clinical and pathologic response in most patients, with a low rate of severe toxicity. Largely as a result of this study, the standard of care for squamous cell carcinoma of the anal canal is now fluorouracil (5-FU), mitomycin, and radiation, often referred to as the "Nigro protocol," with abdominoperineal resection undertaken only for residual or recurrent disease, or for palliation.

ANALYSIS

Introduction: When this article was published, the standard of care for anal squamous cell cancer was abdominoperineal resection. Radiation as primary therapy was known to be effective, but had unacceptable complications. Advancements in more targeted techniques and concomitant chemotherapy with lower radiation doses reopened the door for nonoperative primary therapy.

Objectives: To evaluate the effects of radiation and chemotherapy in patients with squamous cell carcinoma of the anal canal.

Methods

Trial Design: Multicenter, nonrandomized, prospective case series.

Participants

Inclusion Criteria: Patients presenting to the author's institution with anal canal squamous cell carcinoma, as well as additional patients from other institutions via questionnaires.

Exclusion Criteria: Distant metastases at diagnosis, patients already included in other publications.

Intervention: External irradiation of 30 Gy to the primary tumor, pelvic and inguinal nodes over 21 days. Mitomycin C bolus (15 mg/m^2) on day 1, then 5-fluorouracil (1000 mg/m^2) continuously over days 1–4 and 28–31. Initial protocol included APR at 6 weeks after therapy, but after five of the first six patients were found to have no tumor in the operative specimen, the protocol was changed and abdominoperineal resection was not performed unless there was residual tumor.

Endpoints

Primary Endpoint: Presence of tumor following chemoradiation.

Secondary Endpoints: Survival, toxicity from chemoradiation.

Sample Size: From 1972 to 1982, 104 patients were included, 44 from the author's institution and 60 from other institutions.

Statistical Analysis: None (only raw data presented).

Results:

Baseline Data: 76 women and 28 men were included, with age ranging from 32 to 80 years. Initial tumor size ranged from 2 to 8 cm. Four had inguinal node metastases at diagnosis.

Outcomes: There was no residual gross tumor after chemoradiation in 97 of 104 patients; the seven with gross tumor still present all had initial tumors ≥5 cm. A total of 31 patients underwent abdominoperineal resection. Of the 24 without gross tumor who still underwent APR, only two specimens had microscopic disease. An additional seven patients underwent abdominoperineal resection for recurrent disease in the 3–12 months after chemoradiation. At follow-up of 2–11 years, 82 patients were disease-free; 60 of these patients had undergone only chemoradiation. Of the 20 deaths, 13 were attributable to disease progression. Five patients experienced severe adverse effects of chemoradiation requiring hospitalization.

Discussion

Conclusion: Chemoradiation alone is safe and effective for anal squamous cell cancer. Abdominoperineal resection should be performed for those with residual or recurrent disease.

Limitations: This is a small single-arm series with variable treatment protocols. No comparison group is presented, and only raw data are reported. The majority of patients were treated at outside centers and data was obtained by questionnaire only.

b. TME

Recurrence and survival after total mesorectal excision for rectal cancer.

Heald RJ, Ryall RD

Lancet 1986;1(8496):1479–1482.

SYNOPSIS

Takeaway Point: Low anterior resection for distal and midrectal adenocarcinomas has low rates of local recurrence when paired with complete excision of the mesorectum.

Commentary: Total mesorectal excision (TME) was first described in the 1930s, but Heald is responsible for promoting it as the standard surgical technique for proctectomy for rectal cancer. Noting the unsettling wide variations in local recurrence for rectal cancer, Heald surmised that a potential risk factor is failure to dissect within the avascular plane between the fascia propria of the rectum and the presacral fascia, thus maintaining the integrity of the mesorectal envelope. In this article, he describes excellent oncologic outcomes with few local recurrences in his personal series of 115 rectal cancer patients undergoing low anterior resection. He demonstrates that a wide mural margin does not provide additional oncologic benefit; hence, abdominoperineal excision with permanent end colostomy is not mandatory for low rectal cancers that are amenable to restorative proctectomy. The significance of this work is twofold; it emphasized the importance of sharp dissection within the presacral plane during proctectomy, and it demonstrated that restorative proctectomy for low rectal cancer is oncologically sound. These tenets have led to great advances in the surgical care of rectal cancer patients, reducing both local recurrence and permanent colostomy.

ANALYSIS

Introduction: The introduction of new stapling devices in the 1980s allowed for more distal colorectal anastomoses after proctectomy, but a distal mural margin of at least 5 cm was still considered oncologically necessary. However, extrarectal tumor spread was hypothesized to occur first within the mesorectum, raising the possibility that a smaller mural margin with total excision of the mesorectum might decrease the need for abdominoperineal excision.

Objectives: To examine the local control of rectal cancer using the surgical technique of total mesorectal excision with a reduction of the bowel wall margin.

Methods
Trial Design: Prospective consecutive single-surgeon series.
Participants
Inclusion Criteria: Patients with rectal or anal adenocarcinoma with the distal edge ≤15 cm from the anal verge undergoing curative anterior resections, with anus not palpably invaded by tumor where a clamp can be placed across the bowel distal to the tumor.

Exclusion Criteria: Patients with malignant polyps, carcinomas associated with polyposis or colitis, or undergoing palliative resection.

Intervention: Anterior resection of the rectum using a standard surgical technique consisting of proximal ligation of the inferior mesenteric vessels, sharp dissection under direct vision in the avascular plane between the visceral mesorectum and the somatic structures (autonomic nerve plexuses), widely placed peritoneal incisions to include the entire peritoneal reflection, and division of the middle rectal vessels far from the carcinoma. This allows the surgeon to free the rectum and mesorectum from the levators, thus preserving a small rectal reservoir devoid of visceral tissue that can be used for colorectal anastomosis.

Endpoints: 5-year overall and disease-free survival.

Sample Size: 115 rectal cancer patients referred for curative anterior resection at a single hospital with a policy of referring all rectal carcinomas to a single surgical firm from July 1978 to January 1986.

Statistical Analysis: Kaplan–Meier survival analysis, with corrected cumulative probability incorporating a predictive factor for patients followed for <5 years, and comparison of life tables by the log-rank test.

Results
Baseline Data: Of the 188 patients referred, 11% underwent abdominoperineal excision with end colostomy and 19% underwent palliative operations. Of the 115 patients undergoing curative restorative proctectomy, over 85% had mural resection margins <5 cm.

Outcomes: 30-day mortality was 2.6%. There were three pelvic recurrences and no staple line recurrences. The cumulative risk of local recurrence on the life table was 3.7%. The corrected cumulative survival probability at 5 years was 87.5%, overall tumor-free survival at 5 years was 81.7%, and the tumor-free survival by Dukes stage was: A 94%; B 87%; and C 58%. The height of anastomosis and length of mural margin did not influence survival.

Discussion

Conclusion: Total mesorectal excision during proctectomy for rectal cancers not only eliminates the difference in prognosis between proximal and distal rectal cancers and improves local recurrence rates but also allows for reduced mural margins and thus greater rates of sphincter preservation.

Limitations: The lack of a control group precludes comparison, and the use of a single surgeon's case series leads to lack of generalizability. The rates of survival and recurrence are a combination of actual and projected data. All analyses were univariate, and do not control for patient factors.

---

c. FAP-QOL

Quality of life after total colectomy with ileorectal anastomosis or proctocolectomy and ileal pouch–anal anastomosis for familial adenomatous polyposis.

Van Duijvendijk P, Slors JF, Taat CW, Oosterveld P, Sprangers MA, Obertop H, Vasen HF

Br J Surg. 2000;87(5):590–596.

SYNOPSIS

Takeaway Point: Patients with familial adenomatous polyposis who undergo total colectomy with ileorectal anastomosis versus total proctocolectomy with ileal pouch–anal anastomosis have largely comparable quality-of-life scores.

Commentary: The two surgical options for the treatment of familial adenomatous polyposis (FAP) are total colectomy with ileorectal anastomosis (IRA) and total proctocolectomy with ileal pouch-anal anastomosis (IPAA). A common assumption is that quality of life (QOL) outcomes with IPAA are much worse than with IRA. This may cause patients and physicians to choose IRA over IPAA, despite the fact that half of patients who undergo IRA will eventually require completion proctectomy due to rectal polyposis or cancer. This study sought to compare the QOL outcomes of FAP patients who have undergone IRA and IPAA. The authors found that the two groups were similar in all subscales of a generic QOL questionnaire, and all subscales of a disease-specific QOL scale, with the exception of worse defecation problems in the IPAA group. The demonstration of largely equivalent QOL outcomes between these two procedures is an important consideration in the process of shared decision-making for surgical intervention in patients with FAP.

ANALYSIS

Introduction: FAP patients develop hundreds of colon polyps, and colorectal cancer by age 40 if left untreated. Half of patients who undergo total colectomy with ileorectal anastomosis (IRA) will later require completion proctectomy for rectal polyps or cancer. Thus, more patients are choosing the more definitive, although technically more complex, total proctocolectomy with ileal pouch–anal anastomosis (IPAA) to remove all at-risk colorectal mucosa. Postoperative QOL is an important consideration for patients with FAP faced with this decision.

Objectives: To compare the QOL between FAP patients with an ileorectal anastomosis and an ileal pouch–anal anastomosis.

Methods

Trial Design: Cross-sectional study with age- and sex-matched controls.

Participants

Inclusion Criteria: Patients with FAP in a registry established by the Netherlands Foundation for the Detection of Hereditary Tumors, and a randomly selected group of age- and sex-matched normal controls.

Exclusion Criteria: Questionnaire nonresponders.

Intervention: Patients who underwent IRA or IPAA for FAP received the generic Short Form-36 Health Survey (SF-36) and the disease-specific European Organization for Research and Treatment of Cancer Colorectal Quality of Life Questionnaire (EORTC QLQ-CR38).

Endpoints: Generic and disease-specific QOL.

Sample Size: Of 323 eligible FAP registry patients, 279 (86%) responded; 183 patients who underwent IRA between 1961–1996 and 140 patients who underwent IPAA between 1984–1996. A control group of 279 of healthy volunteers completed the SF-36.

Statistical Analysis: The surgical groups were compared with the control group using univariate and multivariate analysis of variance, including the effect of sex, comorbidity, conversion from IRA to IPAA, age at survey, age at operation, length of follow-up, and IPAA anastomotic technique.

Results:

Baseline Data: IRA patients were older (mean age 41 vs. 37) and had a longer follow-up period (12 vs. 6.8 years).

Outcomes: There were no differences between the IRA and IPAA patients for all subscales of the generic QOL questionnaire, and both FAP groups had significantly poorer scores on all subscales than did the general population control group. The disease-specific QOL questionnaire showed more defecation problems in the IPAA group, but otherwise no difference in domains of body image, sexual function, gastrointestinal tract problems, micturition, and future perspective. Controlling for sex, comorbidities, conversion of IRA to IPAA, current age, and age at time of operation did not change the results.

Discussion

Conclusion: In most QOL domains, FAP patients who undergo IRA vs IPAA do not differ, except that the latter group reported more defecation problems. Both FAP groups have significantly lower QOL outcomes than age-matched controls in the general population.

Limitations: Limitations are inherent to a cross-sectional study capturing patients at different time points from surgery.

---

d. Dutch Trial

(1) Preoperative radiotherapy combined with total mesorectal excision for resectable rectal cancer.

Kapiteijn E, Marijnen CA, Nagtegaal ID, Putter H, Steup WH, Wiggers T, Rutten HJ, Pahlman L, Glimelius B, van Krieken JH, Leer JW, van de Velde CJ, Dutch Colorectal Cancer Group

NEJM. 2001;345(9):638–646.

(2) Preoperative radiotherapy combined with total mesorectal excision for resectable rectal cancer: 12-year follow-up of the multicentre, randomised controlled TME trial.

van Gijn W, Marijnen CA, Nagtegaal ID, Kranenbarg EM, Putter H, Wiggers T, Rutten HJ, Påhlman L, Glimelius B, van de Velde CJ, Dutch Colorectal Cancer Group

Lancet Oncol. 2011;12(6):575–582.

SYNOPSIS

Takeaway Point: A short course of preoperative radiation therapy prior to total mesorectal excision improves the local recurrence rate, but not overall survival, in patients with rectal adenocarcinoma.

Commentary: This trial was conducted to determine whether preoperative radiation therapy improved oncologic outcomes in patients with rectal cancer. The authors found that short-term pre-operative radiation therapy improves local control of rectal cancer compared to total mesorectal excision (TME) alone. The long-term outcomes demonstrate that 10-year local recurrence is reduced by over 50% in patients who undergo preoperative short-term radiotherapy compared to those who do not. These papers definitively established the standard of care for nonmetastatic rectal cancer: preoperative radiotherapy followed by TME. This trial followed strict quality control guidelines for radiation therapy, surgical technique, and detection of recurrence. Such results may not be representative of other centers with more variation in the delivery of radiation and in surgical technique and experience. This trial used short-course radiotherapy (5 Gy daily for 5 days) followed by TME. More common in the United States is long-course chemoradiotherapy (28 sessions over 5½ weeks for a total of 54 Gy), then TME 6–12 weeks later. Long-course chemoradiotherapy may be of particular benefit for shrinking large distal rectal tumors to make a sphincter-saving operation feasible, and short-course chemoradiotherapy is well suited to patients with metastatic disease who have already undergone upfront systemic chemotherapy, but thus far no trial has compared the two options directly.

ANALYSIS

Introduction: Preoperative radiotherapy and total mesorectal excision have both been shown to improve local recurrence rates of rectal cancer, but prior studies have not standardized a combination surgical and radiotherapy regimen.

Objectives: To investigate the efficacy of preoperative radiotherapy in combination with standardized total mesorectal excision in patients with rectal cancer.

Methods

Trial Design: Multicenter, randomized, prospective trial.

Participants

Inclusion Criteria: Patients with histologically confirmed rectal adenocarcinoma, with the distal tumor margin within 15 cm from the anal verge and below S1–2.

Exclusion Criteria: Distant metastases, fixed tumors, tumors treated by transanal excision, coexisting or prior history of cancer, prior chemotherapy or pelvic radiotherapy, prior colon surgery.

Intervention: The intervention group underwent radiotherapy to the primary tumor (5 Gy for 5 days), followed by total mesorectal excision, while the control group underwent surgery alone. Follow-up occurred every 3 months for 1 year, then annually for at least 2 years, with annual endoscopy and liver imaging. Participating surgeons were proctored for standard surgical technique. Pathologists used a uniform protocol, and a panel reviewed the specimens.

Endpoints

Primary Endpoint: Survival.

Secondary Endpoints: Local recurrence (tumor in the lesser pelvis or perineal wound), distant recurrence (tumor in any other area).

Sample Size: From January 1996 to December 1999, 1805 patients were enrolled from 84 Dutch, 13 Swedish, and 11 other European and Canadian institutions; 924 radiotherapy plus surgery and 937 surgery alone.

Statistical Analysis: χ^2 tests to compare proportions, Mann–Whitney tests to compare quantitative and ordinal variables, Kaplan–Meier method to measure survival, log-rank test to evaluate differences between the two groups, Cox proportional-hazards model to determine hazard ratios in the univariate and multivariate analyses.

Results

Baseline Data: Of the 1805 patients, 1653 had a curative resection, 57 did not have a macroscopically complete local resection, and 95 were found to have distant metastases intraoperatively. There was no tumor present in 28 specimens. The two groups were similar in age, gender, tumor location, operation type, and stage.

Outcomes: Survival at 2 years was comparable between the intervention and control arms (82% vs. 81.8%). Local recurrence rate at 2 years was lower in the intervention group [2.4% vs. 8.2%, hazard ratio (HR) 3.42]. Independent predictors of local recurrence were lack of preoperative radiotherapy, distance of the tumor from the anal verge, and TNM stage. Univariate subgroup analysis demonstrated that preoperative radiotherapy reduced local recurrence risk if the inferior margin was ≤ 10 cm from the anal verge, and for stage 2 and 3 disease, although this was not seen in the multivariate analysis. There was no difference in the risk of distant or overall recurrence. The intervention group had greater intraoperative blood loss (1000 vs. 900 mL), and those undergoing abdominoperineal resection after radiotherapy had more perineal wound complications (26% vs. 18%).

Discussion

Conclusion: Radiotherapy before total mesorectal excision improves local control of rectal cancer compared to surgical resection alone, but does not improve overall survival.

Limitations: Relatively short follow-up to adequately determine overall survival.

---

e. Fast Track

'Fast track' postoperative management protocol for patients with high comorbidity undergoing complex abdominal and pelvic colorectal surgery.

Delaney CP, Fazio VW, Senagore AJ, Robinson B, Halverson AL, Remzi FH

Br J Surg. 2001;88(11):1533–1538.

SYNOPSIS

Takeaway Point: A "fast track" recovery protocol can shorten hospital length of stay after major abdominal or pelvic surgery, even for patients with comorbidities.

Commentary: "Fast track" protocols to enhance postoperative recovery have been widely studied, but had previously focused on uncomplicated operations in relatively healthy patients. This study examines the use of a multimodal care plan to enhance recovery after complex colorectal operations in patients with and without comorbidities. During a 6-week time period, consecutive patients on one of several colorectal services at a single institution were assigned to this "fast track" pathway. The authors demonstrated that this group had a shorter length of stay than patients on other colorectal services during the same time period, at the same institution. Patients with comorbidities stayed a day longer than those without.

The readmission rate remained low. This article demonstrates that enhanced postoperative recovery pathways can be safely applied to more complicated patients without incurring harm or higher readmission rates.

ANALYSIS

Introduction: The median length of stay after major gastrointestinal surgery is 7 days. Better understanding of postoperative physiology as well as the adoption of laparoscopic surgery has enabled shorter lengths of stay. Multimodal fast-track protocols have been developed, but because of high readmission rates, they have not yet been studied in patients with comorbidities or those undergoing rectal or reoperative surgery.

Objectives: To determine whether a multimodal postoperative fast track with early discharge can be applied to patients with significant comorbidities undergoing major abdominal and pelvic colorectal surgery without increase in morbidity or readmission.

Methods
Trial Design: Prospective, unblinded, single-institution, stratified, controlled trial.

Participants
Inclusion Criteria: Consecutive patients undergoing elective laparotomy and intestinal resection over a 6-week period.

Exclusion Criteria: Smaller procedures (ventral hernia repair, loop ileostomy closure), cases requiring a planned second stage during the same hospitalization, and patients known to require postoperative parenteral nutrition.

Intervention: The fast-track protocol was explained preoperatively to patients. Epidurals and nasogastric tubes were not used. Postoperatively, patient-controlled analgesia (PCA) was used for pain control, with intravenous ketorolac as needed. Patients were allowed to walk on postoperative day 0, and offered liquids. On postoperative day 1, patients were encouraged to walk and sit in a chair, use the incentive spirometer, and offered solid food if able to tolerate liquids. On postoperative day 2, the urinary catheter was removed, and if oral intake was tolerated, the PCA was replaced with oral analgesia. Once patients passed either flatus or stool, were able to tolerate solid food, and were comfortable on oral analgesia, they were discharged.

Endpoints: Complications, length of stay, and readmission rates.

Sample Size: 58 of 60 consecutive patients at a single colorectal unit in the United States over a 6-week period in 2000.

Statistical Analysis: Study arms were compared using an independent-samples t-test for continuous variables with normal distribution. Mann–Whitney U-test was employed for nonparametric data. A χ^2 test was used for nonparametric discrete variables. Data analyzed on an intention-to-treat basis.

Results

Baseline Data: Mean age was 44.4, 38% were female, 59% had undergone at least one prior major laparotomy, and 62% had other comorbidities.

Outcomes: Patients with comorbidities had a longer length of stay (4.6 days) than did those without comorbidities (3.5 days, p 0.01), and patients with poor compliance to the protocol stayed longer than those with good compliance. The 30-day readmission rate was 7%. Patients on the fast-track service continued to have a shorter length of stay than did patients receiving standard care on other colorectal services in the 4 months after initiation of the protocol (mean stay 4.7 days vs. 7.7, p <0.001).

Discussion

Conclusion: Fast-track postoperative recovery protocols employing a multimodal approach can be successfully applied to patients undergoing major abdominal or pelvic surgery, even in the presence of comorbidities.

Limitations: This article reflects the experience of one colorectal service with a small sample size, and is subject to surgeon bias.

---

f. Non-op Rectal Cancer

Operative versus nonoperative treatment for stage 0 distal rectal cancer following chemoradiation therapy: Long-term results.

Habr-Gama A, Perez RO, Nadalin W, Sabbaga J, Ribeiro U Jr, Silva e Sousa AH Jr, Campos FG, Kiss DR, Gama-Rodrigues J

Ann Surg. 2004;240(4):711–717.

SYNOPSIS

Takeaway Point: Chemoradiation therapy for distal rectal adeno-carcinoma can result in complete clinical or pathologic response in a significant subset of patients, and this group may be safely managed with close follow-up rather than surgical resection.

Commentary: The traditional treatment strategy for distal rectal adenocarcinoma consists of neoadjuvant chemoradiation, surgical resection, and adjuvant radiation. In up to one-third of patients, chemoradiation results in a complete pathologic or clinical response. This study examines the outcomes of nonoperative versus operative treatment for patients who have complete clinical or pathologic response to chemoradiation. Complete responders were assigned to observation only, and incomplete responders underwent proctectomy. In the surgical group, 22 patients were found to have no disease in the surgical specimen. These pathologic complete responders who underwent surgery had worse overall survival and similar disease-free survival than did complete responders without surgery. This work is significant as it advocates for a major paradigm shift in rectal cancer treatment, from one that mandates resection for all patients to one that is tailored to response to chemoradiation. While standard practice in the United States largely still consists of radical resection after chemoradiation, there is increasing interest in local excision or observation strategies in patients who are complete responders. Multicenter trials comparing observation to resection after upfront chemoradiation are necessary.

ANALYSIS

Introduction: Distal rectal adenocarcinoma is traditionally treated with chemoradiation, radical resection, and systemic chemotherapy. Upfront chemoradiation may result in complete clinical or pathologic response in 10–30% of patients. Proctectomy causes significant morbidity, including high rates of permanent ostomy, and it is unclear whether it offers a survival benefit in the complete responders to chemoradiation.

Objectives: To report long-term oncologic outcomes in patients with distal rectal cancer with complete response to chemoradiation undergoing resection versus observation.

Methods
Trial Design: Nonrandomized parallel-group trial.
Participants
Inclusion Criteria: Patients with resectable distal rectal adenocarcinoma, located 0–7 cm from the anal verge.
Exclusion Criteria: Synchronous distant metastases.

Intervention: All patients underwent chemoradiation consisting of 5040 cGy over 6 weeks with concurrent 5-fluorouracil and folinic acid. Patients with complete response at 8 weeks underwent observation with monthly physical and digital rectal examination, proctoscopy, biopsy, serum carcinoembryonic antigen (CEA) levels, biannual abdominopelvic CT scans, and chest radiographs for year 1; examination every 2 months during year 2; and biannual examination thereafter. Patients with incomplete clinical response underwent immediate radical surgery.

Endpoints

Primary Endpoint: Clinical and pathologic response to chemoradiation.

Secondary Endpoints: Recurrence, overall and disease-free survival.

Sample Size: 265 patients enrolled at a single center in Brazil between 1991 and 2002; 71 (26.8%) had complete response to chemoradiation and were assigned to the observation group, and 194 had incomplete response and were assigned to the resection group. 22 in the resection group had complete pathologic response (pT0N0, stage p0) and made up resection group R.

Statistical Analysis: Analysis was performed with χ^2, Student's *t*-test, and Kaplan–Meier curves for survival analysis.

Results

Baseline Data: The observation group and resection group R (stage p0) were similar in gender, age, and prechemoradiation tumor characteristics, including size, distance from anal verge, and T and N stages.

Outcomes: Overall recurrence rate was 7% in the observation group, compared with 13.6% in resection group R. 5-year overall and disease-free survival rates were 100% and 92% in the observation Group, and 88 and 83% for resection group R. In all 93 patients considered to have either clinical ($n = 71$) or pathological ($n = 22$) stage 0 disease after CRT, 6.4% developed systemic recurrence, 2.2% died of disease progression, and 2.2% had endoluminal recurrence, for a 10-year survival of 97.7% and 10-year disease-free survival of 84%.

Discussion

Conclusion: First-line chemoradiation for distal rectal adenocarcinoma can offer complete response in a significant proportion of patients, in whom radical resection offers no survival or oncologic benefit. Close observation is an alternative strategy for this group.

Limitations: As this study is single-center, results may not be generalizable. This study was not randomized, and the study size was small. All analyses were univariate and did not control for patient or tumor characteristics.

---

g. Ventral Rectopexy

Long-term outcome of laparoscopic ventral rectopexy for total rectal prolapse.

D'Hoore A, Cadoni R, Penninckx F

Br J Surg. 2004;91(11):1500–1505.

SYNOPSIS

Takeaway Point: Laparoscopic ventral rectopexy is an effective intervention to correct rectal prolapse with excellent long-term outcomes, and does not worsen postoperative constipation.

Commentary: Traditional surgical interventions for rectal prolapse include perineal proctectomy, a shortened rectal reservoir that carries a high recurrence rate and poor bowel function, and abdominal rectopexy, complete rectal mobilization that is associated with increased constipation. Laparoscopic ventral rectopexy has been introduced as an alternative surgical technique, which involves no posterolateral mobilization of the rectum and uses mesh to close the rectovaginal septum. This study reports on a cohort of patients with rectal prolapse treated with laparoscopic ventral rectopexy. The authors report minimal postoperative complications, a low long-term recurrence rate, and improved bowel function with regard to constipation and continence. This article introduces a novel technique for rectal prolapse with excellent long-term results. This is a highly specialized surgical technique that has the potential to replace rectopexy and perineal proctectomy as the preferred treatment for rectal prolapse.

ANALYSIS

Introduction: Rectal prolapse can lead to progressive anal sphincter damage and fecal incontinence, and surgical correction aims to correct the prolapse, and protect or restore continence. Postoperative constipation is the most common side effect, occurring in up to half of patients, presumably due to autonomic denervation of the rectum. A laparoscopic nerve-sparing approach that avoids mobilization of the rectum has been developed.

Objectives:

The aim of this study was to assess the long-term outcome of patients who underwent a novel, autonomic nerve-sparing, laparoscopic technique for rectal prolapse.

Methods

Trial Design: Prospective cohort study.

Participants

Inclusion Criteria: All patients requiring surgery for full-thickness rectal prolapse.

Exclusion Criteria: Crohn's disease requiring ileocecal resection.

Intervention: The laparoscopic ventral rectopexy involves a peritoneal incision along the right side of the sacral promontory and the deepest part of the pouch of Douglas, incision of Denonvillier's fascia, and opening of the rectovaginal septum. There is no rectal mobilization or lateral dissection, so the rectum remains in the sacrococcygeal hollow. Mesh is sutured to the ventral aspect of the distal rectum and fixed to the sacral promontory, and the posterior vaginal fornix is brought up and sutured to the anterior side of the mesh in order to close the rectovaginal septum. The mesh is then covered with peritoneum by bringing the lateral borders of the incised peritoneum over the mesh. Follow-up occurred in person at 6 and 12 weeks, and by phone at a mean of 61 months postoperatively.

Endpoints: Intraoperative complications, early postoperative course, and long-term outcomes with regard to recurrence, continence, constipation, and sexual function.

Sample Size: 42 patients in one hospital in Belgium between March 1995 and December 1999.

Statistical Analysis: Descriptive statistics, Wilcoxon signed rank test for nonparametric paired data, and t-test for paired and unpaired samples.

Results

Baseline Data: Mean age was 49.7, 90% female. All except two cases were performed laparoscopically.

Outcomes: Mean postoperative stay was 5.8 days; this decreased from a mean of 7 days for the first 20 patients to a mean of 4.6 days for the next 22 patients ($p < 0.001$). Two patients developed a recurrence at 54 and 91 months' follow-up; both had previously failed a Delorme procedure. The majority of patients with preoperative incontinence had significant improvement (28 out of 31), and the majority of patients with preoperative constipation also saw improvement. Constipation did not worsen in any patients, and no new severe constipation developed. No sexual dysfunction was noted.

Discussion

Conclusion: Laparoscopic ventral rectopexy without posterolateral mobilization is effective in correcting rectal prolapse, and does not worsen bowel function.

Limitations: This was a small cohort study with no comparison group. The improvement in hospital length of stay over the course of the study, and the fact that both recurrences also occurred early in the study, imply a learning curve for a new surgical technique.

---

h. CLASICC Trial

(1) Short-term endpoints of conventional versus laparoscopic-assisted surgery in patients with colorectal surgery (MRC-CLASICC trial): Multicentre, randomised controlled trial.

Guillou PJ, Quirke P, Thorpe H, Walker J, Jayne DG, Smith AM, Heath RM, Brown JM, MRC CLASICC trial group

Lancet. 2005;365(9472):1718–1726.

(2) Five-year follow-up of the Medical Research Council CLASICC trial of laparoscopically assisted versus open surgery for colorectal cancer.

Jayne DG, Thorpe HC, Copeland J, Quirke P, Brown JM, Guillou PJ

Br J Surg. 2010;97(11):1638–1645.

SYNOPSIS

Takeaway Point: Laparoscopically assisted and open resection for colon cancer have comparable short-term and pathologic outcomes.

Commentary: The laparoscopic approach for colon cancer resection was rapidly adopted in the early 2000s without robust data compared to open resection. The CLASICC trial group sought to answer this question in a large multicenter randomized controlled trial. Short-term outcomes demonstrated that laparoscopic colorectal cancer resection offered similar intraoperative and postoperative complication and in-hospital mortality rates compared to open resection. Patients requiring conversion to open procedures had higher rates of intraoperative complications and postoperative transfusion. Pathologic specimens from laparoscopic resection had similar lymph node harvest and circumferential and longitudinal resection margins as open specimens. Laparoscopic anterior resection for rectal cancer, however, had a nonsignificant increased rate of circumferential resection margin positivity. This difference raises enough concern to warrant further trials to settle the question of the oncologic safety of the minimally invasive approach for rectal cancer. Five-year results reported in 2010 demonstrated no difference in overall or disease-free survival, and local and distant recurrence. The significance of this article is twofold: reassurance that laparoscopic colon cancer resection is oncologically and clinically safe compared to open resection, and strong motivation for future studies examining the outcomes of laparoscopic rectal cancer resection.

ANALYSIS

Introduction: The wide adoption of laparoscopic-assisted resection for colorectal cancer has occurred despite lack of evidence from large randomized trials showing its equivalence to open resection.

Objectives:
To compare short-term outcomes of open and laparoscopically assisted resection for colorectal cancer.

Methods
Trial Design: Pragmatic multicenter, randomized, controlled, open, parallel-group trial.

Participants

Inclusion Criteria: Patients with colorectal cancer amenable to right, left, or sigmoid colectomy, anterior resection, or abdominoperineal resection.

Exclusion Criteria: Patients with transverse colon adenocarcinoma, cardiopulmonary contraindications to pneumoperitoneum, acute bowel obstruction, other malignant disease in the past 5 years or synchronous adenocarcinomas, pregnancy, and associated gastrointestinal disease needing surgical intervention.

Intervention: Patients were randomized to laparoscopic-assisted or open surgery; resection was performed according to each surgeon's preferences. Laparoscopic surgeons had completed a minimum of 20 laparoscopic-assisted resections prior to entering the trial.

Endpoints

Primary Endpoints: Longitudinal and circumferential resection margins, proportion of Dukes C2 tumors (pathological analysis shows tumor going through the bowel wall with apical nodal metastases), and in-hospital mortality.

Secondary Endpoints: Intraoperative and postoperative complications at 30 and 90 days, quality of life (QOL) at 2 weeks and 3 months, and transfusion requirements.

Sample Size: 794 patients from 27 UK centers from July 1996 to 2002, randomized to open (268) and laparoscopic (526) surgery.

Statistical Analysis: Primary endpoints were compared with Pearson's χ^2 or Fisher's exact test, following an intention-to-treat and actual treatment group analysis. Sample size calculation estimated 1000 patients to obtain a confidence interval of 10%, although insufficient to detect true equivalency.

Results

Baseline Data: After excluding patients with missing data or who did not undergo resection, there were 253 open and 484 laparoscopic resections, 29% of whom required conversion. The groups were similar in baseline characteristics and staging, and most resections were undertaken with curative intent.

Outcomes: Positive circumferential and longitudinal resection margin rates did not differ between the groups, nor did the proportion of Dukes C2 tumors and lymph node harvest. In-hospital mortality rates were comparable (5% after open vs. 4% after laparoscopy, p 0.57). Intraoperative complications such as hemorrhage and cardiac events were similar between the treatment arms, but were higher in rectal resections, converted cases, and actual open cases (when the groups were defined by surgery received, rather than an intention-to-treat analysis). Transfusion requirement in the first week were the same between the treatment arms, but also higher in converted cases. Postoperative complications at 30 and 90 days were similar between the treatment arms, as was QOL. Median hospital stay was 2 days longer for open surgery, and duration of operation was longer in laparoscopic surgery (135 vs. 180 minutes). For cancers of the rectum, patients undergoing laparoscopic surgery had a trend toward higher rates of positive circumferential resection margin (CRM) (14% vs. 16%, p 0.8), higher intraoperative complication rates, and higher postoperative complication rates.

Discussion

Conclusion: Laparoscopic colon cancer resection has equivalent short-term clinical and pathologic outcomes, although the higher (albeit not statistically significant) CRM positivity rate in laparoscopic anterior resection raises concern for the minimally invasive approach for rectal cancer. Open surgery also carries a longer hospital stay and a higher rate of intraoperative complications.

Limitations: The surgeons' learning curve for laparoscopic resections (20 cases) was an underestimate as the conversion rate decreased each year of the study. Increased complication rates in converted cases may be skewed by relative inexperience at the beginning of the study period. Determination of the sample size was based on practical challenges with obtaining sufficient laparoscopic surgeons and loss of funding, and may have lacked statistical power.

---

i. COST Trial

Laparoscopic colectomy for cancer is not inferior to open surgery based on 5-year data from the COST Study Group trial.

Fleshman J, Sargent DJ, Green E, Anvari M, Stryker SJ, Beart RW Jr, Hellinger M, Flanagan R Jr, Peters W, Nelson H, Clinical Outcomes of Surgical Therapy Study Group

Ann Surg. 2007;246(4):655–666.

SYNOPSIS

Takeaway Point: Oncologic outcomes for colon cancer after laparoscopic colectomy are not inferior to open colectomy.

Commentary: Prospective randomized trials on short-term recovery and quality-of-life outcomes established the benefits of laparoscopic colectomy over open colectomy. However, because of reports of abdominal wall recurrences at laparoscopic port and extraction sites, the American Society of Colon and Rectal Surgeons and Society of American Gastrointestinal Endoscopic Surgeons restricted the use of laparoscopic colectomy for cancer. This multicenter trial of 872 patients with colon cancer randomized to laparoscopic versus open colectomy demonstrated a benefit in short-term recovery and quality of life in its initial publication, and found no difference in 3-year recurrence and overall survival rates between the two groups. This article reports 5-year oncologic outcomes, demonstrating no difference between the laparoscopic and open groups in overall and disease-free survival, recurrence rates, and sites of first recurrence for stage 1, 2, and 3 disease. This study definitively lifted the restriction on laparoscopic colectomy for colon cancer, allowing colon cancer patients to reap the quality-of-life and short-term recovery benefits of minimally invasive surgery. This article also highlighted the importance of standard surgical techniques to maximize oncologic outcomes.

ANALYSIS

Introduction: Because of concern over the oncologic safety of laparoscopic colectomy for cancer, the Clinical Outcomes of Surgical Therapy (COST) Study Group established a multicenter randomized controlled trial of laparoscopic versus open colectomy for colon cancer in 1994. The group had previously reported improved short-term recovery outcomes. This article reports on 5-year oncologic outcomes.

Objectives: To determine whether disease-free and overall survival are equivalent in patients with colon cancer undergoing laparoscopic versus open colectomy.

Methods

Trial Design: Noninferiority multicenter randomized trial.

Participants

Inclusion Criteria: Patients ≥18 years of age with left, right, or sigmoid colon adenocarcinoma.

Exclusion Criteria: Locally advanced (T4) or metastatic disease, emergent surgical indications, severe medical illness, inflammatory bowel disease, polyposis, pregnancy, or diffuse abdominal adhesions.

Intervention: Open or laparoscopically assisted colectomy for colon cancer, followed by surveillance with physical exam and CEA testing every 3 months for year 1, then every 6 months through year 5; chest x-ray every 6 months for 2 years and then annually; and colonoscopy every 3 years. The 66 included surgeons were credentialed to perform the operations based on oncologic principles.

Endpoints

Primary Endpoint: Time to tumor recurrence, defined as time from randomization to the first confirmed recurrence.

Secondary Endpoints: Disease-free survival, overall survival, complications, recovery parameters, and quality-of-life measures.

Sample Size: 872 patients with curable colon cancer, randomized to laparoscopic (435) and open (428) colectomy at 48 institutions in the United States between 1994 and 2001.

Statistical Analysis: One-sided log-rank test comparing time to recurrence; secondary endpoints were analyzed using two-sample t-test for continuous and χ^2 test for categorical variables. Cumulative incidence methods, log-rank test, Cox proportional-hazards regression, and Kaplan–Meier curves. Following the intention-to-treat principle, converted cases were analyzed in the laparoscopic group.

Results:

Baseline Data: 852 patients were included in the 5-year follow-up. In the laparoscopic arm, 21% required conversion. There was no difference in margins and lymph node harvest (median=12).

Outcomes: After a mean of 7 years' follow-up, 170 patients had experienced recurrences and 252 had died. Overall and disease-free survival, recurrence rates, and sites of first recurrence were similar in the two groups. The one-sided p value for time to recurrence in favor of the open procedure was 0.75, satisfying criteria to declare laparoscopic colectomy noninferior to open colectomy.

Discussion

Conclusion: Laparoscopic colon resection for curable colon cancer is not inferior to the open approach, with similar recurrence rates, overall and disease-free survival.

Limitations: The original accrual goal of 1200 patients in order to power the study was not met, although the authors used their prespecified modified statistical plan, which preserved adequate statistical power.

---

j. Sigma Trial

Laparoscopic sigmoid resection for diverticulitis decreases major morbidity rates: A randomized controlled trial: Short-term results of the Sigma Trial.

Klarenbeek BR, Veenhof AA, Bergamaschi R, van der Peet DL, van den Broek WT, de Lange ES, Bemelman WA, Heres P, Lacy AM, Engel AF, Cuesta MA

Ann Surg. 2009;249(1):39–44.

SYNOPSIS

Takeaway Point: Elective sigmoid resection for symptomatic sigmoid diverticulitis, when safe and feasible, should be done with a laparoscopic approach to minimize the risk of complications, reduce pain levels and narcotic use, shorten hospital stay, and improve quality of life.

Commentary: The Sigma Trial is a multicenter randomized controlled trial comparing postoperative outcomes in laparoscopic or open elective sigmoid resection for diverticular disease. This double-blinded trial used the same large dressing on all patients so that neither patients nor physicians conducting the postoperative evaluations and making discharge decisions were aware of the operative approach. Participating surgeons had prior experience of at least 15 laparoscopic and 15 open sigmoid resections. The authors found that while laparoscopic sigmoid resections took longer than open resections by almost an additional hour, they were associated with lower blood loss, less pain, shorter duration of systemic analgesia, shorter hospital stay, and lower rate of major complications. Quality-of-life measures at 6 weeks after surgery noted better outcomes in the laparoscopic group in the domains of pain, social functioning, and role limitations. This trial demonstrates that the laparoscopic approach toward elective sigmoid resection for diverticulitis is not only feasible but is also associated with improved perioperative outcomes. Most colon resections in the United States are done in an open fashion, so this represents an opportunity for improvement as more surgeons are trained in minimally invasive techniques.

ANALYSIS

Introduction: Open sigmoid resection for diverticulitis has been associated with high postoperative complication and mortality rates. Retrospective comparison studies suggest that the laparoscopic approach might offer improved outcomes.

Objectives: To determine whether laparoscopic sigmoid resection is associated with decreased postoperative complication rates compared to open sigmoid resection for symptomatic diverticulitis.

Methods
Trial Design: Prospective, multicenter, double-blind, parallel-arm, randomized controlled trial.

Participants
Inclusion Criteria: Patients with symptomatic sigmoid diverticulitis (diagnosed by CT scan or barium enema, and colonoscopy) defined as recurrent Hinchey 1 or 2a, Hinchey 2b, stricture, or recurrent bleeding requiring transfusions, and undergoing

operation at least three months from the last diverticulitis episode.

Exclusion Criteria: Failure to consent, prior colorectal resection or laparotomy for non–ob/gyn operations, and Hinchey III or IV diverticulitis.

Intervention: Open or laparoscopic sigmoid resection performed by surgeons with prior experience of at least 15 open and 15 laparoscopic sigmoid resections. Operations were conducted in a standardized fashion using a double-stapled anastomotic technique. Patients received standardized postoperative management with early mobilization and feeding, and were discharged if they were able to walk, managing with oral pain medication, and had a bowel movement. Patients, hospital staff, and postoperative care teams making discharge decisions were blinded to allocation as all patients had the same large abdominal dressing.

Endpoints

Primary Endpoints: All-cause 30-day mortality, major postoperative complications (anastomotic leak or other reoperation indication, intraabdominal abscess, postoperative bleeding requiring transfusion).

Secondary Endpoints: Minor complications (pneumonia, urinary tract infection, wound infection), pain scores, duration of systemic analgesia, length of stay, and quality-of-life measures at 6 weeks.

Sample Size: 104 patients, randomized into two arms of 52 each, from five tertiary care centers from 2002 to 2006.

Statistical Analysis: Independent-samples t-test for continuous variables with normal distribution, Wilcoxon W-test for nonparametric data, and Pearson χ^2 test for discrete variables. Intention-to-treat principle was used so converted cases remained in the laparoscopic arm.

Results

Baseline Data: Laparoscopic and open groups were similar in gender, age, BMI, ASA classification, comorbidities, previous abdominal surgery, surgical indication, and prior abscess drainage.

Outcomes: The laparoscopic group had a longer median operating time (183 vs. 127 minutes, p 0.0001) and lower intraoperative blood loss (100 vs. 200 mL, p 0.033). Laparoscopic patients had lower pain scores by 1.6 points and shorter lengths of hospital stay by 2 days (p 0.046) than did the open group. They also had fewer major complications than did the open group (9.6% vs. 25%, p 0.038), and at 6 weeks after surgery they had better scores on quality-of-life domains of pain, social functioning, and role limitations due to emotional or physical health.

Discussion

Conclusion: Patients undergoing laparoscopic sigmoid resection for symptomatic sigmoid diverticulitis had lower major postoperative complication rates, less pain, shorter hospital stay, and improved quality of life compared to patients undergoing open resection.

Limitations: The power calculation was based on a 23% reduction in postoperative complication rates with laparoscopic resection, but this hypothesis was not proved.

---

k. SNS for Fecal Incontinence

Sacral nerve stimulation for fecal incontinence: Results of a 120-patient prospective multicenter study.

Wexner SD, Coller JA, Devroede G, Hull T, McCallum R, Chan M, Ayscue JM, Shobeiri AS, Margolin D, England M, Kaufman H, Snape WJ, Mutlu E, Chua H, Pettit P, Nagle D, Madoff RD, Lerew DR, Mellgren A

Ann Surg. 2010;251(3):441–449.

SYNOPSIS

Takeaway Point: Sacral nerve stimulation is a safe and efficacious treatment for chronic fecal incontinence.

Commentary: Fecal incontinence (FI) refractory to dietary modification, biofeedback, and antidiarrheal medications often warrants more aggressive management. However, overlapping sphincteroplasty, while addressing the underlying mechanical defect, has not shown durability. Artificial bowel sphincter and dynamic graciloplasty are complex procedures with high complication rates. Sacral nerve stimulation (SNS) has been approved for urinary incontinence in the United States since the late 1990s, and for both urinary and fecal incontinence in Europe since 1994. As it had not yet been approved for fecal incontinence in the United States, this FDA-approved investigation sought to demonstrate its efficacy. SNS was found to result in therapeutic success defined as ≥50% reduction in weekly incontinent episodes in 83% of patients at one year, with 41% achieving perfect continence. This article is significant because it demonstrated that SNS is a safe and effective therapy with minimal morbidity for patients with fecal incontinence, and led to the 2011 FDA approval of the InterStim device for fecal incontinence. As a result, patients with FI in the United States now have the option of undergoing treatment with SNS.

ANALYSIS

Introduction: Fecal incontinence (FI) occurs in 1–2% of the population, and has a significant impact on quality-of-life (QOL) and healthcare costs. Existing treatment options are mediocre at best. Several small studies of sacral nerve stimulation (SNS) have demonstrated high success rates with low morbidity.

Objectives: To determine the safety and efficacy of SNS in a large population using an unbiased and rigorous FDA-approved investigational protocol.

Methods
Trial Design: Multicenter prospective nonrandomized trial.
Participants

Inclusion Criteria: Patients with >6 months (or >12 months after vaginal childbirth) of FI defined as two or more incontinent episodes per week, with failure or unsuitability of nonoperative treatment (dietary modification, antidiarrheals, biofeedback), age≥18 years.

Exclusion Criteria: Symptoms within 12 months of vaginal childbirth, congenital anorectal malformation, rectal surgery within 12 months (24 months if cancer), inflammatory bowel disease, pelvic radiation, active abscesses or fistulae, neurologic disease, complete spinal cord injury, anatomic limitations preventing electrode placement, pregnancy, medically refractory chronic diarrhea.

Intervention: A temporary electrode was placed in the S2, S3, or S4 foramen. Patients experiencing a reduction of ≥50% in the number of incontinent episodes or days per week in the 2-week test period underwent implantation of a permanent neurostimulation device. Patients completed a bowel diary at baseline, during the test period, at 3, 6, and 12 months, and annually.

Endpoints

Primary Endpoint: To demonstrate that ≥50% of patients would achieve therapeutic success, defined as ≥50% reduction in number of weekly incontinent episodes at 12 months

Secondary Endpoints: To demonstrate that ≥50% of patients at 12 months postimplant would achieve ≥50% reduction in number of incontinent days and urgent incontinent episodes per week, QOL scores.

Sample Size: 129 patients from 16 centers in North America and Australia between 2002 and 2008.

Statistical Analysis: Exact binomial test for a one-sample proportion, paired t–tests, or Wilcoxon signed-rank test.

Results

Baseline Data: Of the 129 who underwent the 2-week test stimulation, 120 demonstrated therapeutic success and underwent permanent implantation. Mean age was 60.5 years, 92% female, and mean FI duration of 6.8 years, most commonly due to obstetric trauma (46%) or postsurgical complications (21%).

Outcomes: Therapeutic success ($\geq 50\%$ reduction in number of incontinent episodes per week) was seen in 83% at 12 months (40% achieving perfect continence), 85% at 2 years, and 87% at 3 years. Weekly frequency of incontinent episodes decreased from 9.4 at baseline to 1.9 at 12 months, 2.7 at 2 years, and 1.4 at 3 years. Logistic regression analysis demonstrated that internal anal sphincter defects decreased the success rate (65% vs. 87%, p 0.025). Patients had improvement on all four QOL domains. Serious adverse events occurred in 26 patients, due primarily to implant site pain or infection, and infection led to device explant in 4% of patients.

Discussion

Conclusion: Sacral nerve stimulation results in greater than 50% improvement in FI in 83% of patients, with minimal morbidity.

Limitations: There was no control group, and the median length of follow-up was a little over 2 years, so long-term durability is unknown.

I. IPAA-QOL

Ileal pouch anal anastomosis: Analysis of outcome and quality of life in 3707 patients.

Faziom VW, Kiran RP, Remzi FH, Coffey JC, Heneghan HM, Kiratm HT, Manilich E, Shen B, Martin ST

Ann Surg. 2013;257(4):679–685.

SYNOPSIS

Takeaway Point: Restorative proctocolectomy with ileal pouch anal anastomosis offers excellent quality-of-life (QOL) and functional outcomes for patients with medically refractory ulcerative colitis, indeterminate colitis, and familial adenomatous polyposis.

Commentary: This retrospective analysis of over 4000 patients from the Cleveland Clinic in Ohio is the largest series of restorative proctocolectomy with ileal pouch anal anastomosis (IPAA) reported in the literature, with a considerable length of follow-up. Although the operation comes with a high morbidity rate, with over a third of patients having early postoperative complications, over a third developing pouchitis, and 5% having pouch failure, QOL and functional outcomes are excellent. The double-stapled method is associated with fewer complications and better function compared to the hand-sewn method. Patients with Crohn's disease were much more likely to develop pouch failure, so IPAA for known Crohn's disease should be reserved for highly selected patients.

ANALYSIS

Introduction: Restorative proctocolectomy with ileal pouch–anal anastomosis (IPAA) was first described in 1978 and has become the surgery of choice in medically refractory ulcerative colitis (UC), indeterminate colitis, familial adenomatous polyposis (FAP), and a highly selected subset of patients with Crohn's disease. The standard technique is the double-stapled ileal J pouch, using two loops of ileum for the reservoir. It is a technically complicated procedure with high risk of complications, which may affect functional outcomes and QOL.

Objectives: To report functional outcomes, complications, and QOL in the largest published series of IPAA.

Methods

Trial Design: Retrospective review of a prospectively maintained database.

Participants

Inclusion Criteria: Patients who underwent IPAA.

Exclusion Criteria: Patients who underwent redo IPAA.

Intervention: IPAA performed by 16 surgeons at one institution.

Endpoints: Early and late postoperative complications, functional outcomes, and quality of life.

Sample Size: 3707 patients at the Cleveland Clinic (Ohio) between 1984 and 2010.

Statistical Analysis: Student's t-test for two-sample comparisons and analysis of variance, followed by the Tukey honest significant differences (HSD) post hoc test where appropriate, χ^2 test for proportions and categorical variables.

Results

Baseline Data: Of the 3707 patients undergoing primary restorative proctocolectomy and IPAA, 79.7% had UC, 6% FAP, 4% Crohn's disease (most diagnosed postoperatively), 2.6% cancer/dysplasia, and 1.7% indeterminate colitis. The J configuration, fecal diversion, and double-stapled technique were predominant. Mean age was 38 years, and median follow-up was 84 months.

Outcomes: The 30-day mortality rate was 0.1%. Overall, 34.4% required readmission, and 14.9% required laparotomy for complications such as small-bowel obstruction (SBO). Early complications included wound infection in 7.4%, pelvic sepsis in 6.4%, and SBO in 5%. Late complications included pouchitis in 33.9%, chronic pouchitis in 15.9%, and SBO in 12.9%. Early and late anastomotic leaks occurred in 4.8% and 1.7%, early and late anastomotic strictures occurred in 5.2% and 11.2%, with Crohn's and UC patients more likely to develop an early stricture. Pouch failure occurred in 5.3% at a median of 30 months, treated with pouch excision, redo IPAA, or fecal diversion. At 10 years, 95% of patients with UC had an intact functioning pouch. Independent predictors of pouch failure include Crohn's disease, age >70 at surgery, completion proctectomy or mucosectomy at the time of IPAA, and postoperative anastomotic leak, pelvic sepsis, and pouch fistula. Anastomotic leak and stricture, postoperative hemorrhage, pouch fistula, obstruction, and pouch failure were more common with the hand-sewn technique.

On a 10-point scale at 1, 5, and 10 years, patients reported good to excellent quality of life (8–9), quality of health (8–9), energy level (7–8), and happiness with their current medical situation (9–10). Less than half reported dietary restrictions, and even less reported restrictions in social, work, and sexual domains.

Discussion

Conclusion: IPAA, despite high complication rates, offers excellent functional outcomes and quality of life for patients who require total proctocolectomy.

Limitations: Single-center retrospective study with heterogeneous operative technique (hand-sewn vs. stapled), may not be generalizable.

m. ACOSOG Z6051

Effect of laparoscopic-assisted resection vs open resection of Stage II or III rectal cancer on pathologic outcomes: The ACOSOG Z6051 randomized clinical trial.

Fleshman J, Branda M, Sargent DJ, Boller AM, George V, Abbas M, Peters WR Jr, Maun D, Chang G, Herline A, Fichera A, Mutch M, Wexner S, Whiteford M, Marks J, Birnbaum E, Margolin D, Larson D, Marcello P, Posner M, Read T, Monson J, Wren SM, Pisters PW, Nelson H

JAMA 2015;314(13):1346–1355.

SYNOPSIS

Takeaway Point: For patients with stage II or III rectal cancer, laparoscopic resection fails to meet noninferiority criteria and may provide a worse oncologic outcome than open resection.

Commentary: This multicenter, randomized clinical trial was undertaken to determine whether laparoscopic-assisted resection was noninferior to open resection for stage II or III rectal cancer with regard to pathologic outcomes. The results demonstrated that laparoscopic proctectomy failed to meet the noninferiority criteria, and thus, the authors conclude that laparoscopic proctectomy for rectal cancer may lead to poorer oncologic outcomes. It is unclear why laparoscopic proctectomy had worse pathologic outcomes; it does not appear to be surgeon-related as all participants were credentialed in proper standard surgical technique. This study calls into question the movement toward minimally invasive proctectomy at a time when new technologies such as robotic surgery and transanal single-port total mesorectal excision are being developed and adopted in centers throughout the world. Rectal cancer outcomes in the United States lag behind outcomes achieved in Europe, potentially as a result of inadequate surgical resection. The OSTRiCH (Optimizing the Surgical Treatment of Rectal Cancer) Consortium has recently been established to improve the quality of rectal cancer care in the United States.

ANALYSIS

Introduction: The completeness of a total mesorectal excision for rectal cancer predicts the likelihood of local recurrence. No multicenter study has demonstrated oncologic equivalency for laparoscopic versus open resection for locally advanced disease.

Objectives: To determine whether laparoscopic resection for stage II and III rectal cancer is noninferior to open resection, based on gross pathologic and histologic specimen evaluation.

Methods

Trial Design: Multicenter noninferiority randomized (and balanced) nonblinded trial.

Participants

Inclusion Criteria: Age ≥18 years; BMI ≤34; ECOG score <3; histologically proven rectal adenocarcinoma ≤12 cm from the anal verge; clinical stage II, IIIA, IIIB (no T4) determined by MRI or transrectal ultrasound; operation within 4–12 weeks of completion of neoadjuvant therapy with fluorouracil-based chemoradiation or radiation alone.

Exclusion Criteria: Invasive pelvic malignancy within 5 years, psychiatric disorder affecting compliance, ASA IV or V, systemic disease or other condition precluding laparoscopic approach.

Intervention: Laparoscopic or open resection performed by credentialed surgeons, with standard technique including proximal ligation of feeding vessels, splenic flexure mobilization, and sharp or energy dissection outside the visceral fascia of the mesorectum. The hand-assisted hybrid approach wherein the upper abdominal dissection is performed laparoscopically and the pelvic dissection is performed open was included in the open arm.

Endpoints

Primary Endpoint: Successful resection (defined as distal margin ≥1 mm, circumferential radial margin >1 mm, and completeness of total mesorectal excision).

Secondary Endpoints: Disease-free survival, rate of local recurrence, quality of life, blood loss, length of stay, pain medication use.

Sample Size: Of 486 enrolled from 2008 to 2013 from 35 North American institutions, 462 were analyzed (240 laparoscopic, 222 open).

Statistical Analysis: Assuming 90% oncologic success in open resections, 240 per arm provides 80% power to detect noninferiority if laparoscopic oncologic success were 84%. Categorical variables were analyzed with χ^2 test, continuous variables with Wilcoxon rank sum test. Modified intent-to-treat analysis was performed.

Results

Baseline Data: The two groups were similar in gender, age, race, BMI, operation type, tumor location and size, ECOG score, clinical stage, and neoadjuvant therapy. Low anterior resection (LAR) was performed in 77% and abdominoperineal resection (APR) in 23%. Mesorectal excision was complete in 77% of the specimens and nearly complete in 16.5%.

Outcomes: Successful resection (the primary composite outcome) was 86.9% in the open arm and 81.7% in the laparoscopic arm (p for noninferiority = 0.41) and thus did not support noninferiority. In the laparoscopic group, conversion to open resection occurred in 11.3% and 2.7% required conversion from low anterior resection to abdominoperineal resection, compared with none in the open group. Operative time was longer in the laparoscopic group, whereas length of specimen, length of stay, readmission rate, and complication rate did not differ.

Discussion

Conclusion: Laparoscopic resection for stage II or III rectal cancer failed to meet the criterion of noninferiority for pathologic outcomes, and thus may be oncologically inferior to open resection.

Limitations: The analysis uses a novel composite pathologic outcome, which is likely to correlate with long-term oncologic outcomes but has not yet been validated.

9

Hernia Surgery

Jared Forrester • Christina Vargas • James Lau

INTRODUCTION

Hernias are so ubiquitous that even in this era of superspecialization, hernia repairs belong to the general surgeon. The history of hernia repairs reflects the evolution of surgery itself. Over the centuries, thanks to the ingenuity of some of the greatest names in surgical history, hernia repair has matured from a reckless effort with near 100% recurrence, to its current position as routine standard of care. Today, the maturation of young surgeons can be marked by their ability to repair these defects.

Inguinal hernias and their attempted repairs can be traced to ancient times, when the Egyptians and Greeks experimented with external trusses or transscrotal high ligation of hernia sacs.[1] Open repairs have undergone numerous iterations, from ligation to orchiectomy, eventually progressing to tissue repairs as understanding of the anatomy improved. Published accounts of early hernia repairs started with Ambroise Paré in the late 1500s.[2] As the antiseptic, then aseptic, technique joined with the anesthetic revolution, hernia surgery became safer and more formalized in the mid-1800s.[3] Since then, there have been numerous evolutions and revolutions in technique.

A myriad of approaches to hernia repair persist because no technique has eliminated the two looming problems associated with repair: pain and recurrence. Three key advancements, however, have substantially decreased the incidence of these complications. The tissue repair developed by Eduardo Bassini in 1888 and the tension-free repair with onlay mesh developed by Irving Lichtenstein in 1984 both dramatically reduced recurrence rates compared with historic methods. The third advancement, the introduction of the laparoscopic hernia repair, as reported by Ger, Shultz, and Corbitt in 1990, has improved the incidence of chronic pain.

Inguinal anatomy is complicated, and the price for a poor understanding of its complexity is chronic pain and recurrence for the patient. Laparoscopy has flipped the lens with which we approach the inguinal hernia from the anterior abdominal wall to the retroperitoneal arena, adding to the intricate anatomical knowledge required for a successful procedure. The mastery of this approach requires more mentored practice than open techniques, but ultimately decreases chronic neurologic pain while preserving the low recurrence rate associated with the tension-free repair. While open inguinal hernia repair is the quintessential intern case, the laparoscopic approach is appropriately allocated to the senior surgical resident.

The articles that follow chronicle the journey that surgeons have taken throughout history to repair these abdominal wall defects. When reviewing these seminal works, make note of the struggles, limitations, nuances, and especially the remaining challenges with regard to hernia repair. When performing these operations, you may hear, "I thought it would be a routine hernia." Those who accept the challenge of building a practice around hernia repairs, however, will tell you, "There is no routine hernia." Inguinal hernias are ubiquitous, technically demanding to repair, and worthy of scientific and surgical rigor. It is one of the most important problems surgeons address, and the hernia surgeon is the quiet champion of many grateful patients who enjoy an improved quality of life as the result of our efforts.

---

a. Halsted Repair

The radical cure of inguinal hernia in the male.

Halsted WS

Ann Surg. 1893;17(5):542–556.

SYNOPSIS

Takeaway Point: The Halsted hernia repair has mortality and recurrence rates low enough to recommend routine surgical repair of inguinal hernias.

Commentary: In this article, Dr. Halsted presents his method for primary inguinal hernia repair, accompanied by his initial 3-year experience at Johns Hopkins Hospital. At the time of publication, operative repair for groin hernias was associated with high morbidity and very high recurrence rates. Dr. Halsted argues in this article that his technique carries low mortality and recurrence rates and thus routine surgical repair should be attempted for all hernias. In addition to the description of the Halsted technique, it is interesting to note several of the details surrounding the procedure in the 1890s: standard postoperative bed rest of 21 days, Dr. Halsted's assessments of the stages of wound healing and strength, and his avoidance of "tissue constriction" as part of aseptic technique. Scientific reporting has evolved considerably since this report was published, and the details of the series are not always clear. Although the Halsted technique is not standard today (see **c**, below), his procedure represents a major advancement in hernia repair. His recommendation that all hernias should be repaired is no longer standard of care (see **g**, below); however, his report demonstrated for the first time the safety and potential utility of herniorraphy.

ANALYSIS

Introduction: At the time of this publication, most surgeons would operate for "radical cure" of inguinal hernia only in situations of strangulation or inability to retain the hernia with a truss. The ability to operatively repair hernia defects with an acceptable long-term success rate had not been previously established, and most operations involved only ligation of the sac.

Objectives: Dr. Halsted, prior to this article, had published a description of his new technique for recreating the inguinal canal. Dr. Bassini of Padua had published a very similar technique during the same year. In this article, Dr. Halsted compares the two techniques, presents his outcomes, and makes recommendations for the routine operative repair of groin hernias.

Methods

Trial Design: Prospective single-institution case series.

Participants: All patients undergoing herniorraphy at a single institution.

Intervention: Groin hernia repair using the Halsted or McBurney method. In comparison to the Bassini repair which always brings the cord through the internal ring, Halsted places the cord structures above the external oblique. Postoperatively patients were kept on bed rest for 21 days.

Endpoints

Primary Endpoint: Hernia recurrence.

Secondary Endpoints: Wound infection, death.

Sample Size: 82 patients from one institution, enrolled between 1889 and 1893.

Statistical Analysis: Descriptive.

Results

Baseline Data: 82 total patients: 5 femoral hernias, 76 inguinal hernias, 1 umbilical hernia. 64 males, 18 females. Five patients underwent McBurney repair, and 58 underwent Halsted repair. Age ranged from 14 months to 58 years. Follow up was variable, ranging from <1 month to 3 years.

Outcomes: Two out of the five hernias treated with McBurney repair recurred. There were no recurrences in the 58 cases of Halsted repair, which healed "per primum," but six recurrences occurred in cases complicated by wound infection or noncompliance.

Discussion

Conclusion: Routine repair of inguinal hernia can be performed with low risk of mortality and a low rate of recurrence.

Limitations: Single-institution case series only. Limited baseline data and variable follow-up. Patient population was not homogenous: pediatric and adult patients; inguinal, femoral, and umbilical hernias were included. No statistical analysis was performed.

---

b. Shouldice Repair

Short-stay surgery (Shouldice technique) for repair of inguinal hernia.

Glassow F

Ann R Coll Surg Engl. 1976;58(2):133–139.

SYNOPSIS

Takeaway Point: The Shouldice technique allows for successful repair of groin hernias with immediate postoperative ambulation and short hospital stay.

Commentary: There are several components to the Shouldice technique for inguinal hernia repair, including local anesthetic, extensive dissection of the internal ring, early ambulation, and early return to work. This is a very large single-surgeon series of this technique with low recurrence rates. The author argues that this technique will result in significant decreases in healthcare and lost wage costs from groin hernias. Of note, Dr. Glassow evaluated recurrence as his only outcome measure in making his case for the adoption of these changes. It is worth noting that although mesh repairs are now the most common technique for repair of inguinal hernias, the Shouldice Hospital in Toronto continues to perform only the repair described in this study for over 7000 hernias per year, with results similar to those seen in this series.

ANALYSIS

Introduction: When this study was published, the average length of stay following groin hernia repair in the United States was 5.7 days, and was associated with significant hospital and loss of wage costs. A few small case series had appeared indicating that early postoperative ambulation and shorter length of hospital stay were associated with fewer complications, including recurrence, but the practice had not been clearly established.

Objectives: The intention of this article is to demonstrate that, using a standardized technique for the repair, a short hospital stay and an early return to normal activity are compatible with a low recurrence rate.

Methods
Trial Design: Retrospective single-surgeon case series.
Participants
Inclusion Criteria: All groin hernia repairs performed by a single surgeon at Shouldice Hospital in Toronto.

Exclusion Criteria: Combined inguinal and femoral hernias.

Intervention: The Shouldice technique consists of local anesthesia, complete dissection around the internal ring to identify secondary defects, tissue reconstruction of the posterior inguinal canal, immediate ambulation after repair, and discharge after 72 hours with skin staples removed and without a dressing on the surgical site. Patients whose occupations do not require heavy activity return to work the following week; laborers return to work within 4 weeks.

Endpoints: None (retrospective case series).

Sample Size: 14,982 total repairs by a single surgeon from 1945 to 1973 at the Shouldice Hospital in Toronto.

Statistical Analysis: Descriptive.

Results

Baseline Data: 14,982 herniorrhaphies performed; 123 ipsilateral combined inguinal and femoral hernias excluded. 13,108 primary herniorrhaphies, 1874 recurrences. 7863 primary indirect repairs, 3814 primary direct repairs, 798 combined indirect and direct, and 633 primary sliding hernias. Of recurrent hernia repairs, there were 627 indirect, 927 direct, 249 combined indirect and direct, and 71 sliding hernias.

Outcomes: Overall recurrence rate for primary hernia repair was 0.6% (73 of 13,108) with annual follow-up from 1 to 21 years in more than 95% of the sample. 18 of 1874 patients (1%) who underwent repair of recurrent hernia experienced additional recurrence.

Discussion

Conclusion: Repair of groin hernias may be successfully performed using local anesthesia with early ambulation and short stay without an increase in recurrence. Long-term follow-up in a large single-surgeon series suggests that inguinal and femoral recurrence rates may decrease with increasing surgeon experience.

Limitations: Single-institution and single-surgeon data; large variability in length of follow-up. Retrospective report without secondary outcome data (death, wound infection, length of stay). No comparison group.

---

c. Lichtenstein Repair

The tension-free hernioplasty.

Lichtenstein IL, Shulman AG, Amid PK, Montllor MM

Am J Surg. 1989;157(2):188–193.

SYNOPSIS

Takeaway Point: The Lichtenstein tension-free repair demonstrated no recurrences in 1000 consecutive repairs with follow-up ranging from 1 to 5 years.

Commentary: Dr. Lichtenstein and colleagues present a review of the factors that contribute to hernia recurrence: suture line tension, iatrogenic apposition of nonanatomic structures, and inherent weakness of the aponeurotic tissue in which medial and lateral sutures are placed. He then presents a description of his tension-free repair with polypropylene mesh under local anesthesia. This article is primarily the description of a new technique. He does present a results section, where he states that after 1000 consecutive cases, followed for 1–5 years, there have been no recurrences. He does not give any information about his patients or any specific follow-up data. Despite the lack of outcomes data in this preliminary descriptive paper, the technique he describes has replaced primary tissue repair to become the mainstay of herniorraphy.

ANALYSIS

Introduction: At the time of publication, previous large studies had demonstrated a recurrence rate of at least 10% following primary repair of inguinal hernias using the techniques of Bassini, Halsted, Shouldice, and McVay. Lack of adequate follow-up in most reports led to extreme variability in outcomes. Lichtenstein proposes that the cause of recurrent hernia is the tension created by approximating normally unopposed tissues.

Objectives: To demonstrate the results of a new tension-free hernia repair "without distortion of the normal anatomy and without any suture line tension."

Methods
Trial Design: Single-center, prospective cohort study.

Participants: Not defined. Inclusion/exclusion criteria: not defined.

Intervention: Tension-free inguinal hernia repair with mesh. All wounds were sprinkled with an antibiotic powder (polymyxin and bacitracin); no systemic antibiotics were given.

Endpoints
Primary Endpoint: Hernia recurrence.

Secondary Endpoints: Infection, hematoma, time until return to normal activity.

Sample Size: 1000 patients.

Statistical Analysis: Descriptive.

Results
Baseline Data: 1000 consecutive hernia repairs were performed using the tension-free technique with polypropylene mesh.

Outcomes: Follow-up ranged from 1 to 5 years. No recurrences or infections were seen. Two hematomas resolved spontaneously. Patients resumed work within an average of 2–3 postoperative days.

Discussion
Conclusion: Tension-free hernia repair with mesh offers a dramatically lower rate of recurrence, and local anesthesia enables same-day discharge and prompt return to normal activity.

Limitations: Descriptive study with no detailed reporting of patient characteristics or outcomes, limited follow-up. No comparison group.

---

d. Open versus Laparoscopic Repair (Liem)
Comparison of conventional anterior surgery and laparoscopic surgery for inguinal-hernia repair.

Liem MS, van der Graaf Y, van Steensel CJ, Boelhouwer RU, Clevers GJ, Meijer WS, Stassen LP, Vente JP, Weidema WF, Schrijvers AJ, van Vroonhoven TJ

NEJM. 1997;336(22):1541–1547.

SYNOPSIS

Takeway Point: Laparoscopic inguinal hernia repair results in faster recovery and fewer recurrences than open repair.

Commentary: This multicenter randomized trial compares laparoscopic extraperitoneal repair with an open approach, and demonstrates faster return to work, less postoperative pain, and fewer recurrences in the laparoscopic group. The authors achieved excellent (97%) follow-up, and the study included teaching and nonteaching hospitals and surgeons with a range of experience levels. However, it is worth noting that the authors compared laparoscopic mesh repair to an open repair without mesh. Moreover, there is no discussion of potentially different open techniques amongst surgeons. This may account for the higher rate of late recurrences in the open group, given prior studies demonstrating reduced recurrence with a tension-free prosthetic mesh repair (see **c**, above). Additionally, all patients undergoing open repair were required to have general anesthesia, despite the feasibility of local anesthesia for open repair (see **b**, above). This eliminates one potential benefit of an open operation, and could contribute to the longer recovery time. Although these limitations lessen the generalizability of the results, this trial demonstrates the superiority of laparoscopic repair specifically for decreasing rates of postoperative pain.

ANALYSIS

Introduction: Previous small trials suggest that laparoscopic repair of inguinal hernia is associated with improved postoperative pain and faster recovery in comparison with open approach. These benefits have not been established in a large, multicenter trial.

Objectives: To compare conventional anterior repair with extra-peritoneal laparoscopic repair in terms of postoperative recovery, complications, and recurrence rates in patients with primary or first recurrent unilateral hernias.

Methods

Trial Design: Prospective, randomized, unblinded multicenter trial.

Participants

Inclusion Criteria: Patients over age 20 diagnosed with primary or first-recurrent unilateral inguinal hernia, planning to undergo surgical repair with general anesthesia.

Exclusion Criteria: Concurrent surgical procedure, prior extensive lower abdominal surgery, severe local inflammation or radiation, pregnancy >12 weeks, mentally incompetent patients, inability to speak Dutch.

Intervention: Open inguinal hernia repair without mesh or laparo-scopic extraperitoneal repair with polypropylene mesh.

Endpoints

Primary Endpoint: Hernia recurrence.

Secondary Endpoints: Time to resume normal activities, death, score on activities of daily living questionnaire, postoperative pain, complications.

Sample Size: 1051 patients enrolled between February 1994 and June 1995, with 994 analyzed (487 laparoscopic and 507 open repair).

Statistical Analysis: Intention-to-treat analysis, two-tailed t-test, χ^2 test, Fisher's exact test, ANOVA, Kaplan–Meier survival curves, log-rank test.

Results

Baseline Data: Baseline characteristics were well balanced between the two groups. Overall mean age was 55, and 95% of patients were male.

Outcomes: 6% of patients who underwent open repair experienced hernia recurrence compared with 3% of those who had laparoscopic repair (p 0.05) in a median follow-up period of 607 days. Median operative time was 5 minutes shorter in the open repair group ($p < 0.001$). There were six patients with postoperative wound abscess in the open surgery group and none in the laparoscopic group (p 0.03). 14% of patients who had open repair reported chronic pain compared with 2% of those who had laparoscopic repair ($p < 0.001$). Postoperative visual analog pain scores were lower in the laparoscopic group ($p < 0.001$). Median time to resume usual activity was 10 days in the open group and six in the laparoscopic group ($p < 0.001$). 82% of hernia recurrences after laparoscopic repair were diagnosed in the first year; 10 of the 17 laparoscopic recurrences were from surgeons with limited laparoscopic experience.

Discussion

Conclusion: Patients with inguinal hernias who undergo extraperitoneal laparoscopic repair return to their usual activities more quickly with less pain and fewer recurrences than do those who undergo open repair.

Limitations: A moderate number of patients were excluded or crossed over after randomization. Exclusion criteria included inability to speak Dutch and prior extensive lower abdominal surgery, potentially limiting generalizability. No details given regarding differences in open surgical techniques.

---

e. Tension-Free Mesh versus Shouldice

Randomized trial of Lichtenstein versus Shouldice hernia repair in general surgical practice.

Nordin P, Bartelmess P, Jansson C, Svensson C, Edlund G

Br J Surg. 2002;89(1):45–49.

SYNOPSIS

Takeaway Point: Lichtenstein tension-free mesh repair for open inguinal hernias is a technically easier procedure and results in shorter operative time and decreased rates of recurrence compared to the Shouldice repair.

Commentary: This randomized clinical trial comparing Lichtenstein tension-free mesh repairs versus Shouldice repairs for open inguinal hernias demonstrated an increased rate of recurrence in the Shouldice group at 3 years (4.7% vs. 0.7%). Additionally, the Lichtenstein repair had a shorter mean operative time (54 vs. 61 minutes), which the authors argue is due to the shorter learning curve for the mesh repair. There were no significant differences seen with respect to hospital stay, return to normal activity, or pain. Although there were no statistically significant differences in postoperative complications, the only two cases of testicular atrophy occurred in the Lichtenstein group.

The authors conclude that the Lichtenstein repair allows the surgeon to acquire a high technical standard relatively quickly, and decreases the rate of hernia recurrence. Notably, a recent Cochrane meta-analysis of 16 randomized controlled trials concurred that Shouldice repairs have a higher recurrence rate than mesh repairs (OR 3.80, 95% CI 1.99–7.26), although the quality of data on most of the trials is somewhat poor.[5] In summary, this single-center randomized trial addresses the safety, efficacy, and ease of learning of tension-free mesh repair for open inguinal hernias.

ANALYSIS

Introduction: Recurrence rates after open inguinal hernia repair can vary widely with quotes of 0.1–20% after 5 years. The lowest recurrence rates are reported from specialized hernia centers (0.1% for Lichtenstein and <1% for Shouldice). Few surgeons have been able to reproduce these results with most randomized trials reporting around a 5% recurrence rate.

Objectives: The aim was to compare the Shouldice procedure and Lichtenstein hernia repair with respect to recurrence rate, technical difficulty, convalescence and chronic pain.

Methods

Trial Design: Single-center randomized control trial.

Participants

Inclusion Criteria: Men, 25–75 years old with unilateral, primary inguinal hernia.

Exclusion Criteria: Irreducibility, femoral hernia, coagulation abnormalities, anticoagulation treatment, and patients determined to be unsuitable for general anesthesia.

Intervention: Patients were randomized to either Shouldice repair or Lichtenstein tension-free mesh repair. The five participating surgeons underwent a pretrial training program during which both techniques were taught and performed in a standard fashion.

Endpoints

Primary Endpoint: Hernia recurrence, operative time, complete recovery time, severity of pain using visual analog scale (VAS), and testicular atrophy with follow-up at 8 weeks, 1 year, and 3 years.

Secondary Endpoints: Postoperative surgical complications including hematoma, infection, seroma, swelling, and urinary complaints.

Sample Size: 297 patients from one center between 1994 and 1998, with 148 randomized to Shouldice repair and 149 randomized to Lichtenstein tension-free mesh repair.

Statistical Analysis: Mann–Whitney U-test, sample size estimation of 152 patients per arm with an assumed difference in recurrence rate of at least 5%, power of 80, and $\alpha = 0.05$.

Results

Baseline Data: 300 patients eligible, 3 excluded, 297 randomized. Baseline patient characteristics were balanced between the Shouldice and Lichtenstein groups (age, type of work, and type of hernia).

Outcomes: There was significantly longer mean operating time with all five surgeons using the Shouldice repair (61 vs. 54 minutes, $p < 0.01$). There were no statistically significant differences in postoperative complications between the two groups; however, the only two cases of testicular atrophy occurred in the Lichtenstein group (one due to deep scrotal infection, another due to postoperative orchitis). There were no statistically significant differences in pain between the two groups at any time. Shouldice repair had a higher recurrence rate [4.7%; 95% CI (1.3–8.1)] versus the Lichtenstein repair [0.7%; 95% CI (0.0–2.0)] after 3 years. There was no association between individual surgeon and recurrence rate.

Discussion

Conclusion: Lichtenstein tension-free mesh repair for inguinal hernias is a method that is relatively easy to learn, allows for shorter operative times, and results in consistently lower recurrence rates than the Shouldice repair at nonspecialized hernia centers.

Limitations: For the power of the study to reach 80% with $\alpha = 0.05$, each group required 152 patients. The study was minimally underpowered. Although statistically significant, the clinical significance of a 7-minute difference in operative time is not clear. No cost-benefit analysis was performed.

---

f. Open versus Laparoscopic Repair (Neumayer)

Open mesh versus laparoscopic mesh repair of inguinal hernia.

Neumayer L, Giobbie-Hurder A, Jonasson O, Fitzgibbons R Jr, Dunlop D, Gibbs J, Reda D, Henderson W, Veterans Affairs Cooperative Studies Program

NEJM. 2004;350(18):1819–1827.

SYNOPSIS

Takeaway Point: Open-mesh hernia repair is superior to laparoscopic mesh repair of primary inguinal hernias.

Commentary: This multicenter randomized trial follows 2000 veterans undergoing repair of both primary and recurrent inguinal hernias. The authors found that recurrence and complication rates after laparoscopic repair of primary inguinal hernias were significantly higher than after open repair. Recurrence rates after either type of repair for recurrent hernias were similar. This contradicts the earlier Liem study (see **d**, above), which showed significantly higher recurrence rates after open repair. This well-designed study offers evidence in support of open-mesh repair over laparoscopic repair, although it has important limitations. Two years may be insufficient follow-up to judge a difference in recurrence rates, and the difference between primary and recurrent hernia outcomes indicates the need for subgroup analyses that are not adequately powered in this study. It is also interesting to note the authors' evaluation of surgeon experience. In contrast with prior studies, the rate of recurrence after laparoscopic repair became comparable to open repair for surgeons who have performed more than 250 procedures.

ANALYSIS

Introduction: Open tension-free herniorrhaphy is associated with recurrence rates of <5%, with minimal morbidity and mortality. The laparoscopic tension-free repair has been reported to have lower recurrence rates, and is associated with substantially less pain in the postoperative period. However, the laparoscopic approach requires general anesthesia, and has the potential for more serious intraoperative complications.

Objectives: To compare recurrence rates and complication rates after open repair with mesh and laparoscopic repair with mesh.

Methods
Trial Design: Prospective, randomized, unblinded, multicenter trial.

Participants
Inclusion Criteria: Men aged 18 or older with inguinal hernia.

Exclusion Criteria: ASA class IV or V; contraindication to general anesthesia; bowel obstruction, strangulation, or perforation; local or systemic infection; contraindication to laparoscopy; previous mesh repair; life expectancy <2 years.

Intervention: Lichtenstein open-mesh repair or laparoscopic mesh repair (either transabdominal or totally extraperitoneal approach).

Endpoints

Primary Endpoint: Hernia recurrence within 2 years.

Secondary Endpoints: Complications, death, pain, functional status, and activity level.

Sample Size: 2164 patients block-randomized and stratified by type of hernia (primary or recurrent), unilateral/bilateral, and study site. 1087 randomized to open repair and 1077 to laparoscopic repair at 14 Veterans Affairs hospitals between 1999 and 2001.

Statistical Analysis: Intention-to-treat analysis, logistic regression analysis, adjusted odds ratios, Cox regression analysis.

Results

Baseline Data: 93 patients in the open repair arm and 88 in the laparoscopic repair arm did not undergo intervention. 97 patients assigned to laparoscopic repair underwent open repair, and 16 assigned to open repair underwent laparoscopic repair. The two groups were balanced in terms of ASA classification and baseline characteristics. In the laparoscopic group, 90% underwent totally extraperitoneal repair and 10% underwent transabdominal repair.

Outcomes: The rate of recurrence at 2 years in the laparoscopic group was 10.1% compared with 4.9% in the open group. In subgroup analyses, laparoscopic repair of primary hernias produced a higher recurrence rate (10.1%) compared with 4% in the open repair group. For patients with recurrent hernias, 10% had recurrence after laparoscopic repair and 14.1% had recurrence after open repair (not statistically significant).

Ancillary Data: 39% of patients who underwent laparoscopic repair had a complication, compared with 33.4% who underwent open repair. Intraoperative, immediate postoperative, and life-threatening complications occurred significantly more frequently in the laparoscopic repair group. Those who underwent open repair reported significantly higher pain immediately postoperatively and at 2 weeks, but the two groups were similar in overall pain assessments by three months postoperatively. Time to resume activity was significantly shorter following laparoscopic repair (4 days) relative to open repair (5 days).

Post hoc evaluation of surgeon experience found that recurrence rate after laparoscopic repair for surgeons who had performed 250 or fewer laparoscopic repairs was >10% compared with <5% for surgeons who had performed more than 250.

Discussion

Conclusion: For repair of primary inguinal hernias, the tension-free open-mesh repair technique has a lower recurrence rate and lower complication rate than laparoscopic mesh repair.

Limitations: Limited to veteran population (all male, older age than the general population), 2-year follow-up. Moderate amount of crossover after randomization. Not adequately powered for subgroup analyses.

---

g. Watchful Waiting

(1) Watchful waiting vs repair of inguinal hernia in minimally symptomatic men: a randomized clinical trial.

Fitzgibbons RJ Jr, Giobbie-Hurder A, Gibbs JO, Dunlop DD, Reda DJ, McCarthy M Jr, Neumayer LA, Barkun JS, Hoehn JL, Murphy JT, Sarosi GA Jr, Syme WC, Thompson JS, Wang J, Jonasson O

JAMA. 2006;295(3):285–292.

(2) Long-term results of a randomized controlled trial of a nonoperative strategy (watchful waiting) for men with minimally symptomatic inguinal hernias.

Fitzgibbons RJ Jr, Ramanan B, Arya S, Turner SA, Li X, Gibbs JO, Reda DJ, Investigators of the Original Trial

Ann Surg. 2013;258(3):508–515.

SYNOPSIS

Takeaway Point: At 2 years, watchful waiting is an acceptable option for men with minimally symptomatic inguinal hernias. After 10 years, most will require surgery for increasing symptoms.

Commentary: This randomized, prospective comparison of watchful waiting versus surgical repair in minimally symptomatic patients with inguinal hernias demonstrated no difference in patient-reported pain or physical component score at 2 years. They conclude that watchful waiting is an acceptable alternative to surgical repair in this population. It is possible that the median follow-up of 3.2 years may be too short to appreciate the full impact of the watchful waiting strategy, and the authors do not address the potential for increasing operative risk as patients age during a watchful waiting approach. Regardless, this is a large, well-designed randomized trial that provides invaluable information regarding the natural history of asymptomatic or minimally symptomatic inguinal hernias. The follow-up study by the same authors followed those in the watchful waiting group an additional seven years, to address some of the concerns raised in the first study. The rate of crossover in the original study doubled when followed out to 10 years, although less than half of patients had complete follow-up data. Although watchful waiting is a safe strategy, most patients will proceed to eventual surgery for increasing symptomatology.

ANALYSIS

Introduction: Watchful waiting as an alternative to repair of inguinal hernias in adult men has not been previously substantiated in the literature. Patients are typically referred for repair of inguinal hernias in order to prevent acute incarceration or strangulation, but the actual incidence of these events in patients with minimally symptomatic hernias is unknown.

Objectives: To compare pain and the physical component score (PCS) of the SF-36 at 2 years in men with minimally symptomatic inguinal hernias treated with watchful waiting or surgical repair.

To assess the long-term crossover (CO) rate in men undergoing watchful waiting (WW) as a primary treatment strategy for their asymptomatic or minimally symptomatic inguinal hernias.

Methods

Trial Design: Prospective, randomized multi-institution trial.

Participants

Inclusion Criteria: Male patients over age 18 with asymptomatic or minimally symptomatic inguinal hernia (no hernia pain or difficulty in reducing the hernia within 6 weeks).

Exclusion Criteria: Undetectable hernia, local or systemic infection, ASA >3.

Intervention: Watchful waiting patients were screened at 6 months and annually for hernia symptoms but received no intervention. Patients randomized to surgical repair underwent standard, open, tension-free repair with follow-up at 3 and 6 months, then annually.

Endpoints

Primary Endpoint: Pain and discomfort interfering with daily life at 2 years, and change in PCS at 2 years.

Secondary Endpoints: Complications, patient-reported pain, functional status, activity level, satisfaction, crossover rate.

Sample Size: 724 patients from five VA hospitals between 1999 and 2002, 366 randomized to watchful waiting and 358 to surgical repair. 254 of the original watchful waiting group at the end of the 2 years were followed for an additional 7 years.

Statistical Analysis: Intention to treat analysis, χ^2 test, Fisher exact test, t-test, ANOVA, O'Brien–Fleming sequential proportion tests, O'Brien–Fleming sequential z-test, Dunnett t-test.

Results

Baseline Data: 724 patients randomized, 4 excluded, 720 eligible. Most baseline patient characteristics were balanced between watchful waiting and surgical repair groups. The surgical repair cohort had significantly higher BMI, and more patients assigned to watchful waiting had enlargement of their hernia in the prior 6 weeks. Of the original 366 patients assigned to watchful waiting, 85 (23%) underwent surgical repair during the original 2-year follow-up period. 62 (17%) of patients assigned to surgery did not undergo repair. In the follow-up study, 254 patients in the watchful waiting arm consented to long-term follow-up, and 167 had complete follow-up data. These patients were followed for an additional 7 years, and a cumulative total of 141 patients crossed over to surgery.

Outcomes: Intention-to-treat analysis at 2 years revealed no significant difference in pain or PCS between groups. Both cohorts had less pain at 2 years than at baseline. The reduction in perception of pain was significantly greater for patients assigned to surgical repair (p 0.01); as-treated analysis produced similar results. >97% of patients in both groups were satisfied or very satisfied with their care. A total of three patients required emergency surgery but there was no mortality.

Ancillary Data: Acute incarceration occurred in one patient (0.3%) assigned to watchful waiting within 2-year follow up; one acute incarceration with bowel obstruction occurred at 4 years in the watchful waiting group. The acute hernia complication rate was found to be 0.0018 events per patient-year.

Discussion

Conclusion: The watchful waiting strategy for men with asymptomatic or minimally symptomatic inguinal hernias is an acceptable alternative to repair. Acute hernia complications occurred at a rate of 1.8 per 1000 patient-years. Over time, symptoms are more likely to require operative therapy.

Limitations: The influence of significant differences in baseline patient characteristics is unclear. Follow-up for primary endpoints ended at 2 years. The follow-on study tracked some of the watchful waiting group to 7 years, but median follow-up was still only 3.2 years. Significant loss to follow-up during the second study.

REFERENCES

1. Patino JF. A history of the treatment of hernia. In: Nyhus LM, Condon RE, eds. *Hernia.* 4th ed. Philadelphia: Lippincott; 1995:3–15.

2. Pare A. In: Keynes G, ed. *The Apologie and Treatise.* London: Falcon Educational Books; 1951.

3. Marcy HO. A new use of carbolized cat gut ligatures. *Boston Med Surg J.* 1871;85:315–316.

4. Edwadia TE. Inguinal hernia repair: The total picture. *J Minimal Access Surg.* 2006;2(3):144–146.

5. Amato B, Moja L, Panico S, Persico G, Rispoli C, Rocco N, Moschetti I. Shouldice technique versus other open techniques for inguinal hernia repair [review]. *Cochrane Database Syst. Rev.* April 18, 2012;4:CD001543.

10

Stomach Surgery

Rima Ahmad • John Mullen

The stomach is host to a variety of benign and malignant conditions that may present acutely, as in the case of a bleeding or a perforated peptic ulcer, or indolently, as is often the case with gastric cancer.

Peptic ulcer disease is among the most common benign conditions, and its natural course has evolved significantly over the years. While antrectomies, vagotomies, and other acid-reducing procedures were common several decades ago, the introduction of acid-suppressing medications and the discovery (and eradication) of *Helicobacter pylori* have virtually eliminated such operations.[1–4] Nonetheless, gastric and duodenal perforations due to complicated peptic ulcer disease remain a frequent cause for presentation to the emergency room and account for nearly 10% of hospital admissions related to peptic ulcer disease.[1] As critical care and supportive treatments have improved, nonoperative approaches can be considered in subsets of patients with high operative risk due to medical comorbidities, or whose perforations appear to be self-contained.[5] Similarly, the availability of acid-suppressing medications and therapies eradicating *H. pylori* have made less radical and less invasive surgical approaches, such as laparoscopic primary and/or omental patch repair, more common.

Acute upper GI hemorrhage is the most common presentation of peptic ulcer disease, although it may represent other etiologies, including Mallory–Weiss tears or varices. A certain proportion of patients will have self-limited episodes of bleeding, but ongoing bleeding requires upper GI endoscopy. There are a number of advanced endoscopic techniques to stop active bleeding, including cauterization, injection sclerotherapy with epinephrine, and clip application.[6] As these techniques have evolved, so has the debate as to which endoscopic therapies are most effective, which we will examine in the chapter that follows. Surgical intervention is now reserved for the rare circumstances in which the patient is in shock or in which endoscopic therapies have failed.

Esophageal and gastric varices are a manifestation of an underlying disease process, most commonly cirrhosis. Spontaneous bleeding occurs at a rate of 5–15% per year,[7] and studies have shown that variceal size and degree of decompensated cirrhosis (as graded by Child's score) are strong predictors of bleeding.[8] Gastric varices are associated with higher rates of bleeding and are commonly due to splenic vein thrombosis.[7] Endoscopy is recommended for screening and monitoring of patients who are likely to develop bleeding varices,[7] and endoscopic ligation can be undertaken to either eradicate them or, at a minimum, to reduce their bleeding risk. Prophylactic treatment is often considered for those patients at the highest risk of bleeding.

Gastric adenocarcinoma is the most common malignancy of the stomach, and without endoscopic screening most patients in Western countries present with advanced disease. As a result, the average 5-year survival rate for patients undergoing surgery is less than 30%.[9] Comparatively, the incidence of gastric cancer is much higher in the East,[10] and routine endoscopic screening programs result in a much higher proportion of gastric cancers diagnosed at an early, curable stage.[11] Much of the evolution in the treatment of gastric cancer in the West has come about in the last 15–20 years, with a number of pioneering trials demonstrating improved survival rates with the use of multimodality therapy for adenocarcinomas of the distal esophagus, gastroesophageal (GE) junction, and stomach. Furthermore, there has been a great deal of debate about the optimal surgical management of gastric cancer, including the appropriate extent of gastric resection (subtotal vs. total gastrectomy) and of regional lymph node dissection (D1 vs. D2 lymphadenectomy). We will review several of these important trials in this chapter.

As the practice of surgery has become more focused on minimally invasive techniques, surgery on the stomach has followed the same trend. Laparoscopic and endoscopic procedures are becoming more common, although open surgery continues to be the predominant mode for oncologic resections. As this balance changes, the debate regarding adequate lymph node dissection will undoubtedly be a key point of consideration. Underlying these issues are differences in the approach to gastric cancer and treatment outcomes between Eastern and Western centers, led by the possibility that the etiology of gastric cancer, and even the underlying biology of the disease, may be different between East and West. The extent of these differences and their clinical implications have yet to be effectively demonstrated and remain an area in need of further investigation.

---

a. D1 versus D2 Dissection: Dutch Trial
Extended lymph-node dissection for gastric cancer.

Bonenkamp JJ, Hermans J, Sasako M, van de Velde CJ, Welvaart K, Songun I, Meyer S, Plukker JT, Van Elk P, Obertop H, Gouma DJ, van Lanschot JJ, Taat CW, de Graaf PW, von Meyenfeldt MF, Tilanus H, Dutch Gastric Cancer Group

NEJM. 1999;340(12):908–914.

SYNOPSIS

Takeaway Point: Extended D2 lymph node dissection for gastric cancer results in higher morbidity and mortality and does not result in improved survival or locoregional tumor control when compared with D1 dissection.

Commentary: Eastern centers with high volumes of gastric cancer have long emphasized extensive lymph node dissections for adequate disease staging and improved locoregional tumor control. However, Western centers have not been able to replicate the same advantages with an extensive lymph node dissection. This multi-center trial was among the first large-scale efforts to investigate the use of D2 lymph node dissection in a Western population, and this publication serves as a report of long-term survival data at 5 years. Initial data from the Dutch study, published in 1995, demonstrated higher complication and mortality rates among the D2 group, despite active observation by master surgeons.[12] Patients underwent splenectomy and distal pancreatectomy as a routine part of their resection, and this was postulated to be the major cause of the increased morbidity of the procedure. The group concluded that splenectomy should not be an essential part of the procedure, and they could not recommend a D2 lymph node dissection as a routine procedure during the resection of gastric cancer. The MRC and Italian trials (see **b** and **m**, below) did not necessitate resection of the spleen and distal pancreas in their protocols. While some patients in the MRC trial did undergo this more aggressive resection, allowing for subset comparison, the Italian trial carried out only pancreas-preserving resections. These three trials represent a progressive tailoring of the D2 dissection technique for safe application among Western populations.

ANALYSIS

Introduction: D2 lymph node dissection has been performed with very low morbidity and has been shown to improve disease staging and lead to better locoregional tumor control in patients with gastric cancer in the East. However, the safety and the potential benefit of D2 lymph node dissection have not been demonstrated in a Western population.

Objectives: To examine the safety and long-term outcomes of D1 versus D2 lymph node dissection in patients undergoing surgery for gastric cancer.

Methods

Trial Design: Multicenter randomized controlled trial.

Participants

Inclusion Criteria: Age <85 years with histologically proven gastric cancer and no evidence of metastatic disease.

Exclusion Criteria: Prior gastric resection, other malignant disease.

Intervention: Resection with D1 lymph node dissection or D2 lymph node dissection, including splenectomy and distal pancreatectomy.

Endpoints

Primary Endpoint: Survival.

Secondary Endpoint: Risk of relapse.

Sample Size: 996 patients enrolled from August 1989 to July 1993 from 80 Dutch hospitals, with 380 in the D1 group and 331 in the D2 group.

Statistical Analysis: Kaplan–Meier survival curves with log-rank testing.

Results

Baseline Data: Median age 66 years; 57% male. No difference in T stage, extent of resection, rate of R0 resection, or lymph node involvement between the groups. Median follow-up time was 72 months.

Outcomes: In-hospital mortality occurred in 47 patients overall (7%). There was an overall complication rate of 25% with D1 dissection and 43% with D2 dissection (p <0.001), with in-hospital mortality at 4% and 10% for D1 and D2 groups, respectively (p 0.004). There was no difference in 5-year survival (45% and 47% for D1 and D2 dissections, HR = 1.0). Recurrence occurred in 43% versus 37% of the patients in the D1 and D2 groups, respectively (HR 0.84).

Discussion

Conclusion: The group could not recommend D2 dissection because of the higher morbidity and mortality of the procedure and no significant advantage in 5-year survival or locoregional control.

Limitations: Despite direct observation, there was a high noncompliance rate, resulting in inadequate dissection among 36% of the D1 group and 51% of the patients in the D2 group. The authors suggested that this rate was inflated as a result of poor separation of lymph nodes from the specimen, but it nevertheless remains quite significant.

---

b. D1 versus D2 Dissection: MRC Trial

Patient survival after D1 and D2 resections for gastric cancer: Long-term results of the MRC randomized surgical trial.

Cuschieri A, Weeden S, Fielding J, Bancewicz J, Craven J, Joypaul V, Sydes M, Fayers P, Surgical Co-operative Group

Br J Cancer. 1999;79(9–10):1522–1530.

SYNOPSIS

Takeaway Point: Extended D2 lymph node dissection does not provide improved survival among patients with gastric cancer and is highly morbid, due to pancreaticosplenic resection.

Commentary: This article was the culmination of long-term data from the Medical Research Council (MRC) trial, an early prospective study to look at the effects of D2 resection on outcomes for gastric cancer in Western centers, and an attempt to replicate its advantages as espoused by Eastern centers. Although they could not show any survival difference, the authors postulated that much of the early mortality in the D2 group may have been due to resection of the pancreas and spleen, once considered essential to achieve adequate lymph node clearance but no longer mandated according to the Japanese Gastric Cancer Association. Although a subset analysis of patients who did not undergo pancreaticosplenectomy showed improved survival among the D2 group, this could not be definitively attributed to the dissection. The authors recommend against removal of the spleen or pancreas unless tumor involvement necessitated it, thereby limiting the mortality of these resections. This conclusion, along with results from the Dutch trial (see **a**, above) set the stage for the newer Italian trial discussed next. Presenting the case that the increased morbidity of the D2 dissection may be countered by elimination of the pancreaticosplenectomy portion of the procedure, this trial also left open the possibility of improved survival among this subset.

ANALYSIS

Introduction: While an extended D2 lymph node dissection is the standard of care for gastric cancer in Eastern centers, early use by Western surgeons was associated with higher in-hospital morbidity and mortality, particularly related to the splenectomy and distal pancreatectomy.

Objectives: To examine the long-term outcomes of D1 versus D2 lymph node dissection for gastric cancer.

Methods
Trial Design: Multicenter randomized controlled trial.

Participants
Inclusion Criteria: Histologically proven gastric cancer, TNM stage I–III.

Exclusion Criteria: Age <20 years, prior gastric resection, other malignancy, comorbidity that would preclude D2 dissection.

Intervention: Randomization to D1 or D2 dissection that included pancreaticosplenectomy in patients without antral tumors.

Endpoints
Primary Endpoint: Overall survival.

Secondary Endpoints: Recurrence-free survival.

Sample Size: 400 patients from 80 centers primarily in the United Kingdom, enrolled between August 1989 and July 1993, were randomized into equal groups of 200 to undergo D1 or D2 dissection.

Statistical Analysis: Survival was calculated using Kaplan–Meier curves with log-rank testing and Cox proportional-hazards models, intention-to-treat analysis.

Results
Baseline Data: The cohort was 67% male, with 75% over the age of 60 and 40% over age 70.

Outcomes: Overall survival by intention to treat was equivalent in the two groups, at 35% and 33% for D1 and D2 groups, respectively (p 0.63). Recurrence-free survival was not significantly different. The spleen and pancreas were both resected in 56% of the D2 group and only 4% of the D1 group. Although significantly more lymph nodes were sampled in the D2 arm (median of 17 compared to 13 in the D1 arm), only 46 patients met the strict criteria of more than 26 lymph nodes considered adequate by the Japanese definition. When looking only at patients without pancreaticosplenectomy, those in the D2 arm had an improved survival compared to the D1 group, but they also had a higher proportion of antral tumors. In subgroup analyses, the D2 group with pancreaticosplenectomy had the poorest survival, and the D2 group with preservation of the pancreas and spleen had the best overall survival.

Discussion
Conclusion: There is no long-term survival difference between patients undergoing D1 and D2 lymph node dissection. Pancreaticosplenic resection drastically increases mortality and may obscure any survival advantage of the D2 dissection, and should therefore not be a part of the resection unless these organs are directly involved by tumor.

Limitations: Although it was clear that pancreaticosplenectomy caused higher mortality rates, improved survival for D2 dissection without it could be proved only on subset analysis. Multivariate analysis controlled for a number of confounding factors, but it is unclear whether the subgroup analysis was adequately powered. The majority of patients in the D2 group fell short of the strict definition by both lymph node group and number.

---

c. Subtotal versus Total Gastrectomy
Subtotal versus total gastrectomy for gastric cancer: Five-year survival rates in a multicenter randomized Italian trial.

Bozzetti F, Marubini E, Bonfanti G, Miceli R, Piano C, Gennari L, Italian Gastrointestinal Tumor Study Group

Ann Surg. 1999;230(2):170–178.

SYNOPSIS
Takeaway Point: Subtotal gastrectomy does not show a decreased survival when compared to total gastrectomy and should be the

preferred resection in patients with distal tumors where adequate margins can be obtained.

Commentary: While subtotal gastrectomy (SG) and total gastrectomy (TG) were both in use for resection of antral gastric tumors, there was a concern among proponents of TG that a subtotal resection resulted in poorer long-term outcomes. This trial provides evidence of equal survival between the two techniques and put forth the argument for preferentially performing SG in order to decrease rates of postoperative complications as well as long-term nutritional difficulties.

ANALYSIS

Introduction: Distal gastric tumors of the body and antrum have been cured with subtotal gastric resection or total gastrectomy. Total gastrectomy (TG) has a higher potential for complications and long-term nutritional difficulties among patients. There is concern, however, that subtotal gastrectomy (SG) may yield poorer long-term disease control.

Objectives: To examine survival outcomes with subtotal versus total gastrectomy for gastric cancer.

Methods

Trial Design: Multicenter randomized controlled trial.

Participants

Inclusion Criteria: Age >75 years with cancer of the distal stomach.

Exclusion Criteria: Previous gastric resection, other malignancy, previous chemotherapy, metastatic disease.

Intervention: Randomized to SG or TG.

Endpoints

Primary Endpoint: Mortality.

Secondary Endpoint: None.

Sample Size: 618 patients from 28 Italian centers between April 1982 and December 1993. The SG group contained 315 patients, and the TG group contained 303 patients.

Statistical Analysis: Kaplan–Meier survival with Cox proportional-hazards regression modeling.

Results

Baseline Data: The cohort was 58% male, 86% between stages T1b and T3, and 22% with tumors larger than 5 cm. Extension of resection to other structures outside of the stomach occurred in 18%. Splenectomy was performed significantly more often in the TG group (18% vs. 5%), but there were no other differences between the two groups.

Outcomes: Overall survival for patients undergoing SG was 36%, compared to 39% for those undergoing TG. The adjusted hazard ratio for survival was 1.01 between the groups. When analyzing for other prognostic factors, patients with tumors isolated to the antrum had worse prognosis than did those in the body of the stomach. As expected, other factors that decreased survival included T3 or T4 disease and involvement of the spleen or other extragastric structures.

Discussion
Conclusion: Subtotal gastrectomy has long-term survival outcomes similar to those of total gastrectomy and should be considered in all patients with anatomically eligible tumors.

Limitations: Although the authors suggested decreased operative and long-term complications with subtotal gastrectomy as compared to total gastrectomy, they did not seek to analyze these factors in this study. The total gastrectomy group had significantly more patients undergoing splenectomy.

---

d. *H. pylori* and Ulcer Healing
Eradication of *Helicobacter pylori* prevents recurrence of ulcer after simple closure of duodenal ulcer perforation: Randomized controlled trial.

Ng EK, Lam YH, Sung JJ, Yung MY, To KF, Chan AC, Lee DW, Law BK, Lau JY, Ling TK, Lau WY, Chung SC

Ann Surg. 2000;231(2):153–158.

SYNOPSIS

Takeaway Point: *H. pylori* eradication results in lower peptic ulcer recurrence rates among high-risk patients.

Commentary: This single-center study examined *H. pylori* as a risk factor for peptic ulcer recurrence in patients who previously presented with an episode of perforation and documented *H. pylori* infection. A simple patch repair, as is commonly performed for perforated peptic ulcer, carries a high risk of recurrent symptomatic disease. Participants in this trial were randomized to either a proton pump inhibitor (PPI) alone or *H. pylori* eradication therapy along with a PPI. Although both groups were documented as having experienced complete healing of their initial ulceration, those with eradication of their infection had a much lower rate of ulcer recurrence at one-year follow up. This article forms part of the literature that supports symptomatic peptic ulcer disease as an indication for treatment of *H. pylori* infection with antibiotic eradication therapy.[13,14]

ANALYSIS

Introduction: Uncomplicated peptic ulcer disease is treated with *H. pylori* eradication; however, perforated duodenal ulcers represent advanced disease with a high risk of ulcer relapse. It is unclear whether eradication of the bacteria prevents the need for additional acid suppression surgery.

Objectives: To determine whether eradication of *H. pylori* could lead to sustained ulcer remission in patients who underwent only simple repair for duodenal ulcer perforation.

Methods

Trial Design: Randomized controlled trial.

Participants

Inclusion Criteria: Patients with perforated duodenal ulcers requiring emergent omental patch repair who were proven to have *H. pylori* by positive biopsy culture or positive rapid urease test along with identification of helical organisms by Gram stain or histology.

Exclusion Criteria: Age <16 or >75 years, previous gastrectomy or vagotomy, pregnancy, use of antibiotics or acid suppressants within 4 weeks, actively undergoing treatment for another illness, or perforation larger than 1 cm not amenable to patch repair.

Intervention: Treatment with *H. pylori* eradication therapy (bismuth, tetracycline, metronidazole, and omeprazole) compared to treatment with just omeprazole.

Endpoints

Primary Endpoint: Healing of ulceration.

Secondary Endpoints: *H. pylori* eradication, recurrent ulceration.

Sample Size: 99 patients from a single center between September 1994 and January 1997, with 51 randomized to eradication therapy and 48 to omeprazole alone.

Statistical Analysis: χ^2 test and Student's t-test.

Results

Baseline Data: Mean age among patients was 44 years, and 85% were male. Of the cohort, 20% underwent laparoscopic repair of their perforation. Baseline characteristics were similar between the two groups.

Outcomes: There was an initial dropout of 9 patients from both groups, leaving 44 patients in the treatment arm and 46 in the control arm. At initial follow-up endoscopy, 8 weeks from initiation of therapy, *H. pylori* had been eradicated in 84% of the treatment group and 17% of the control group. Ulcers had completely healed in 82% and 88% of patients in the therapy and control groups, respectively (*p* 0.58). The remaining patients' ulcers did not heal despite continued omeprazole therapy, so they were deemed as having failed treatment and were excluded from further analysis. Among the 78 patients that followed up at 1 year, 18 had ulcer recurrence, 5% in the treatment group, and 38% in the omeprazole-only control group (*p* <0.01). On testing, patients were found to be *H. pylori*–positive in 1 of 2 recurrences in the treatment arm and 14 of 16 in the control arm.

Discussion

Conclusion: There was no difference in the rates of ulcer healing between those receiving treatment for *H. pylori* and those receiving only omeprazole. Treatment for *H. pylori* decreased the recurrence of both occult and symptomatic peptic ulcer disease compared with omeprazole alone.

Limitations: Cross contamination of groups, with patients in the control group receiving antibiotic courses for other indications in the postoperative period that may have treated their *H. pylori*. Further, the treatment group did not all achieve eradication of their organism. The follow-up period of 1 year is relatively short for this disease process.

---

e. SWOG Gastric Cancer Trial

Chemoradiotherapy after surgery compared with surgery alone for adenocarcinoma of the stomach or gastroesophageal junction.

Macdonald JS, Smalley SR, Benedetti J, Hundahl SA, Estes NC, Stemmermann GN, Haller DG, Ajani JA, Gunderson LL, Jessup JM, Martenson JA

NEJM. 2001;345(10):725–730.

SYNOPSIS

Takeaway Point: Postoperative chemoradiation after R0 resection for gastric cancer improves survival and reduces disease recurrence.

Commentary: This trial by the Southwest Oncology Group (SWOG) sought to establish a precedent for adjuvant therapy in the treatment of gastric cancer in order to improve on the high recurrence rates after surgical resection. The group compared patients who received only surgery (the standard of care at the time) with those undergoing postoperative chemoradiation therapy and found a survival advantage of 9 months and an increased recurrence-free survival of 17% with adjuvant therapy. This trial definitively established a role for adjuvant therapy in gastric cancer and resulted in a new standard of care, and it paved the way for further investigation into the routine use of chemotherapy and radiotherapy for this disease, including the MAGIC and CROSS trials discussed later in this chapter (see **j** and **k** below).

ANALYSIS

Introduction: Gastric cancer in the West is often diagnosed at an advanced stage and thus carries a poor prognosis even after complete surgical resection. The high rate of relapse makes it important to consider multimodality therapy, but adjuvant chemotherapy has not provided a significant survival advantage over surgery alone. Most relapses occur within the region of the resection bed, making postoperative radiation an attractive possibility.

Objectives: To compare surgery followed by chemoradiation therapy to surgery alone in the treatment of gastric cancer.

Methods
Trial Design: Randomized controlled trial.
Participants

Inclusion Criteria: Patients with histologically confirmed gastric or GE junction adenocarcinoma and stage IB–IV disease who underwent R0 resection. World Health Organization (WHO) performance status <2, adequate nutritional support throughout the study, and able to start therapy 20–41 days postoperatively.

Exclusion Criteria: Metastatic disease, significant hepatic or renal dysfunction.

Intervention: Surgery followed by chemoradiation using fluoro-uracil and leucovorin, given with radiation therapy in 25 fractions to a total of 45 Gy, compared to surgical resection alone.

Endpoints

Primary Endpoint: Overall survival.

Secondary Endpoints: Relapse-free survival, local and distant recurrence.

Sample Size: Single-center trial from August 1991 to July 1998 with 556 patients, 275 randomized to postoperative chemoradiation and 281 to surgery alone.

Statistical Analysis: Survival analysis was carried out with Cox regression models using an intention-to-treat analysis. Patients were stratified by T and N stage for the analysis. Power calculation estimated that 550 patients would provide 90% power to detect a 40% survival difference.

Results

Baseline Data: Of the cohort, 72% were male. Tumors were anatomically located as follows: 54% antrum, 24% body, 20% GE junction, and 2% multicentric. Nodal involvement was present in 85% of patients. There was no difference in any factors between the two groups.

Outcomes: In the 281 patients assigned adjuvant chemoradiation, 64% completed the prescribed course. Toxic effects were severe enough to cause cessation of therapy in 17% of patients. Survival at 3 years was 41% in the surgery-alone group and 50% in the adjuvant chemoradiation group, with median survival of 27 and 36 months, respectively (p 0.005). Hazard ratio for death in the surgery alone group was 1.35. Three-year relapse-free survival was 31% in the surgery-alone group compared with 48% in the chemoradiation group, with a median of 19 months and 30 months, respectively (p <0.001). Local recurrence decreased from 29% to 19% with adjuvant therapy, and regional recurrence decreased from 72% to 65%. Hazard ratio for relapse was 1.52 in the surgery-only group.

Discussion

Conclusion: Adjuvant chemoradiation in gastric cancer can prolong survival and reduce the rate of locoregional recurrence.

Limitations: Only 64% of patients completed all of the prescribed therapy, and a high proportion of patients experienced side effects severe enough to withdraw from therapy. Although patients were stratified by N stage, 54% of patients only had a D0 lymph node dissection and thus were likely understaged.

f. Laparoscopic Ulcer Repair

Laparoscopic repair for perforated peptic ulcer: A randomized controlled trial.

Siu WT, Leong HT, Law BK, Chau CH, Li AC, Fung KH, Tai YP, Li MK

Ann Surg. 2002;235(3):313–319.

SYNOPSIS

Takeaway Point: Laparoscopic repair of a perforated peptic ulcer is a safe alternative to open surgery and results in less postoperative pain and a faster recovery.

Commentary: This single-center, prospective, randomized controlled trial sought to establish laparoscopic omental patch repair as a viable alternative to open surgery among patients undergoing emergent repair of a perforated peptic ulcer. Theorizing that the advantages of laparoscopic surgery in other fields would be equally applicable in this circumstance, the authors were able to demonstrate reduced postoperative pain and quicker return to activity, without any additional risks. Laparoscopic omental patch repair is now widely used in the treatment of patients who present acutely with perforated peptic ulcers.

ANALYSIS

Introduction: Laparoscopic surgery is gaining greater application in acute care surgery. Patients for whom a simple omental patch repair is to be performed may benefit from the advantages of laparoscopic surgery, but this had not previously been studied.

Objectives: To compare the outcome of laparoscopic and open omental patch repair for perforated peptic ulcers.

Methods

Trial Design: Randomized controlled trial.

Participants

Inclusion Criteria: Age >16 years with clinical peritonitis and perforated peptic ulcer on exploratory surgery.

Exclusion Criteria: Bleeding from the ulcer, history of prior abdominal surgery, gastric outlet obstruction, ulcer in location other than pylorus or duodenum.

Intervention: Patients randomized to laparoscopic or open omental patch repair, randomization occurred after decision was made for surgery.

Endpoints

Primary Endpoint: Postoperative use of IV analgesia.

Secondary Endpoints: Operative time, hospital admission length, postoperative pain score, complications, mortality, return to daily activities.

Sample Size: 121 patients from a single center, enrolled between January 1994 and June 1997. 63 patients randomized to laparoscopic repair and 58 to open repair.

Statistical Analysis: Factors compared using Student's t-test, χ^2 test, and Mann–Whitney test.

Results

Baseline Data: Mean age of the cohort was 55 years, 81% male patients. Most patients fell into ASA classes I and II (82%). Ulcers were found to be in the stomach in 23% of cases and the duodenum in 77%, with a mean size of 5.2 mm in the laparoscopic group and 4.7 mm in the open group. The two groups showed no statistically significant baseline differences.

Outcomes: Laparoscopic repair could be completed in all except nine assigned cases (13%). Operative times were shorter for laparoscopic repair, but this was not clinically significant. Postoperative pain was reduced in patients undergoing laparoscopic repair, as judged by use of postoperative IV medication and visual analog pain scores on postoperative days 1 and 3. There was no difference in postoperative ileus or time to resume a regular diet. The open group had seven cases of pneumonia, versus none in the laparoscopic group (p 0.05). Perioperative mortality, postoperative leak, and wound complications were equivalent between the two groups. Patients who underwent laparoscopic repair returned to daily activity in a mean of 10 days compared to 26 days in the open group (p 0.01).

Discussion

Conclusion: Laparoscopic omental patch repair for a perforated ulcer can be performed safely, with less postoperative pain and faster recovery. Apart from a reduced incidence of postoperative pneumonia, there is no other difference in short- or long-term complications when compared to open repair.

Limitations: The mean age of the cohort was 55 years, and over 80% of patients were ASA class I or II, a healthier population than the elderly patients with multiple comorbidities who often present with a perforated ulcer. Gastric body ulcers were determined to harbor too high a risk for malignancy and are not represented in this study.

g. Prophylaxis of Variceal Rebleeding

Variceal ligation plus nadolol compared with ligation for prophylaxis of variceal rebleeding: A multicenter trial.

de la Peña J, Brullet E, Sanchez-Hernández E, Rivero M, Vergara M, Martin-Lorente JL, Garcia Suárez C

Hepatology. 2005;41(3):572–578.

SYNOPSIS

Takeaway Point: Combination therapy with endoscopic variceal ligation and β-blockade is the most effective approach to secondary prophylaxis for esophageal varices.

Commentary: Patients with varices who experience an episode of UGI bleeding are at high risk for recurrent bleeds. Secondary prophylaxis is imperative in these patients and can be accomplished by medical therapy with β-blockers or endoscopic variceal ligation (EVL). This study demonstrates a greater risk reduction with the use of combination therapy, with EVL and nadolol, justifying a more aggressive regimen in the treatment of these high-risk patients. The authors demonstrate not only a reduced occurrence of rebleeding, but also a lower rate of forming recurrent varices. Although a major hindrance to β-blockade is patient tolerance, the therapy was relatively well tolerated among the patients in this study, with only 7% stopping treatment because of side effects. The combination therapy was so effective at the planned interim analysis that the study was stopped early, leading to a smaller sample size. Despite the small size, the results have proved to be important in establishing the multimodal aggressive approach recommended by the American College of Gastroenterology for secondary prophylaxis of esophageal varices.

ANALYSIS

Introduction: Patients who survive an initial episode of variceal bleeding have a high risk of rebleeding. Secondary prophylaxis of varices may be carried out with endoscopic or medical therapy, but neither therapy reaches the underlying goal of optimal control. As these therapies act through different mechanisms, it is possible that combination therapy may yield improved results.

Objectives: To assess the efficacy of a combination therapy between a portal hypotensive agent such as nadolol and EVL versus EVL alone for the secondary prophylaxis of variceal bleeding.

Methods

Trial Design: Randomized controlled trial.

Participants

Inclusion Criteria: Age 18–75 years with a diagnosis of cirrhosis, presenting with acute UGI bleeding from esophageal or gastro-esophageal varices.

Exclusion Criteria: Bleeding fundal varices, hepatocellular carcinoma (HCC), portal vein thrombosis, portosystemic shunt, prior endoscopic ligation or sclerotherapy, pregnancy, refractory ascites, ASA class IV or V, or medical contraindication to receiving β-blockers.

Intervention: After resolution of acute bleed, treatment with EVL until variceal elimination, either alone or in combination with nadolol, titrated to reduction of resting heart rate by 25%. EVL was performed for new varices as discovered on regular follow-up.

Endpoints

Primary Endpoint: Rebleeding of varices.

Secondary Endpoints: Mortality, complications of treatment, eradication of varices, recurrence of varices, treatment failure resulting in uncontrolled bleeding, repeated rebleeding within 3 months, need for other therapies such as transjugular intrahepatic portosystemic shunt (TIPS), or complications leading to death.

Sample Size: 80 patients were enrolled from four hospitals in Spain from June 1999 to October 2003; 43 were randomized to EVL and nadolol together, and 37 to EVL alone.

Statistical Analysis: Student's t-test, Mann–Whitney test, χ^2 test, and Kaplan–Meier analysis with log-rank testing; sample size calculation required 85 patients per group to detect a risk reduction of 16%.

Results

Baseline Data: Mean age of the cohort was 60 years, with a 75% male predominance. Cirrhosis was most commonly alcoholic (66%), with 25% viral and 9% other causes. 15% of patients were Child's A, 56% Child's B, and 29% Child's C. There were no baseline differences between groups.

Outcomes: Eradication of varices was accomplished in all enrolled patients, with no significant difference in number of treatments required between groups. Recurrent bleeding occurred in 38% of patients treated with EVL alone compared to 14% in the combined therapy group (p 0.006). The probability of recurrence at one year was higher in the EVL-alone group (77% vs. 54% in the combined group, *p* 0.06). This difference was maintained at 2-year follow-up, with recurrence rates of 97% and 68% for the EVL-alone and combined groups, respectively (*p* 0.06). A total of 3% of patients suffered adverse effects in the EVL-alone group compared to 33% in the combined group, with three patients in this group withdrawing from the study due to adverse effects from nadolol. Treatment failure rate was 29% in the EVL-alone group and 5% in the EVL+ nadolol group (*p* <0.05). Mortality was similar between groups.

Discussion

Conclusion: Combination therapy with EVL and nadolol reduces risk of recurrent bleeding from esophageal varices, although it does not improve mortality.

Limitations: The study was terminated early because of the demonstrated difference between groups, and thus calculations of power are inaccurate. Application is limited to patients without a contraindication to β-blockers, which may be a significant proportion of patients with varices.

---

h. EVL in Primary Prophylaxis of Varices

Endoscopic variceal ligation versus propranolol in prophylaxis of first variceal bleeding in patients with cirrhosis.

Lay CS, Tsai YT, Lee FY, Lai YL, Yu CJ, Chen CB, Peng CY

J Gast Hep. 2006;21(2):413–419.

SYNOPSIS

Takeaway Point: Endoscopic ligation and propranolol therapy have equal efficacy as primary prophylaxis for esophageal varices in patients with cirrhosis.

Commentary: This single-center randomized controlled trial remains one of the most compelling studies to advocate for primary prophylaxis of esophageal varices with endoscopic ligation. It demonstrates not only that there is no difference in bleeding or long term mortality with endoscopic variceal ligation (EVL) versus medical therapy but also higher compliance and tolerance with EVL than propranolol. This study is among the references cited by the American College of Gastroenterology in their guidelines to treat esophageal varices. These guidelines recommend variceal ligation therapy as an effective and preferred method of primary prophylaxis against bleeding.

ANALYSIS

Introduction: Patients with advanced cirrhosis and esophageal varices are at risk for upper gastrointestinal (UGI) bleeding, which may be life-threatening in patients with depressed physiologic reserve. The Japanese Research Society for Portal Hypertension has been able to delineate characteristics that identify varices at high risk of bleeding, and it is in this patient population that it becomes prudent to provide primary prophylaxis against bleeding episodes.

Objectives: To determine, in a controlled and prospective manner, whether EVL or propranolol therapy of high-risk varices affects the risk of first variceal bleeding and improves the chances of survival of cirrhotic patients with no previous bleeding from the upper gastrointestinal tract.

Methods
Trial Design: Randomized controlled trial.

Participants

Inclusion Criteria: Patients with high-risk varices on endoscopy, as defined by the Japanese Research Society for Portal Hypertension, with cirrhosis from any cause.

Exclusion Criteria: Presence of gastric or other ectopic varices, history of prior UGI bleed, other life-limiting comorbidity.

Intervention: Randomization to either EVL, which consisted of repeated sessions of endoscopic band ligation until eradication, or until varices became too small to ligate; or to propranolol therapy, titrated to reduction of the resting heart rate by 20%, or highest tolerated dose.

Endpoints

Primary Endpoint: Occurrence of UGI bleeding, all-cause mortality.

Secondary Endpoints: Compliance with therapy.

Sample Size: Single-center trial, enrolling a cohort of 100 patients with cirrhosis between January 1998 and December 2002, with 50 randomized to EVL and 50 to propranolol therapy.

Statistical Analysis: Univariate analysis was carried out using the χ^2 and Student's t-test, as well as Kaplan–Meier life tables with log-rank analysis. Cox proportional-hazards models were used for multivariate analysis.

Results

Baseline Data: Mean age of 56 years, 78% male, all with cirrhosis (70% viral causes, 21% alcoholic, 9% other). The severity of cirrhosis by Child–Pugh class was 45% A, 39% B, and 16% C. There were no differences between the randomized groups.

Outcomes: There was no difference between patients treated with EVL and propranolol therapy with regard to the occurrence of bleeding (22% vs. 24%, p 0.68), death from bleeding (10% vs. 8%, p 0.72), or all-cause mortality at 2 years (28% vs. 24%, p 0.34). Eradication of varices was achieved in 90% of patients who underwent EVL, in a mean of 5.2 sessions per patient. The remaining 10% of patients ($n = 5$) were noncompliant or lost to follow-up. Target therapy of 20% reduction in resting heart rate was achieved in 75% of the patients treated with propranolol therapy. Side effects were experienced in 50% of patients on propranolol, and caused 20% ($n = 10$) to discontinue therapy. Two of these patients later had variceal bleeding.

Discussion

Conclusion: Bleeding rates from esophageal varices and subsequent mortality are equal when comparing EVL to propranolol prophylaxis. However, treatment with EVL may result in fewer adverse effects and enhanced treatment compliance.

Limitations: Although of very sound methodology, this study's impact is somewhat limited by its small sample size garnered from a single Eastern center. Furthermore, in a high proportion of cases cirrhosis was due to viral hepatitis disease, reflective of the typical etiology among this population. The natural course of the disease may be different among other populations where alcohol abuse and steatohepatitis account for a higher incidence of disease.

---

i. Hemostatic Efficacy in High-Risk Bleeding Ulcers
Comparison of hemostatic efficacy for epinephrine injection alone and injection combined with hemoclip therapy in treating high-risk bleeding ulcers.

Lo CC, Hsu PI, Lo GH, Lin CK, Chan HH, Tsai WL, Chen WC, Wu CJ, Yu HC, Cheng JS, Lai KH

Gastrointest Endosc. 2006;63(6):767–773.

SYNOPSIS

Takeaway Point: Combined endoscopic hemoclip and epinephrine injection therapy provides superior hemorrhage control to epinephrine injection therapy alone for both initial bleed and rebleed from UGI ulcers.

Commentary: Endoscopic control of bleeding ulcers is performed in a number of ways, usually per the endoscopist's preference. This study established that hemoclips as an adjunct to injection therapy results in more effective control of hemorrhage with a decreased likelihood of rebleeding. The authors encourage the use of combination therapy as primary treatment for clearly bleeding ulcers, rather than as a secondary adjunct after initial therapy has already failed. They also demonstrate that this approach results in lower rates of retreatment or progression to surgery, suggesting that a more aggressive approach is warranted during the first endoscopic treatment for bleeding ulcers. This is now the approach recommended by the American College of Gastroenterology (ACG) in their guideline for treatment of bleeding peptic ulcers.

ANALYSIS

Introduction: There are a number of endoscopic methods to control active hemorrhage, including injection therapy and endoclip ligation. While both have proven to be safe and efficacious in treating acute bleeding, the impact of treatment choice on rebleeding rates has not been established.

Objectives: To evaluate the impact of epinephrine injection alone versus epinephrine injection with hemoclip therapy for actively bleeding ulcers on reduction of recurrent bleeding rate, the need for surgery, and mortality.

Methods

Trial Design: Randomized controlled trial.

Participants

Inclusion Criteria: Patients with UGI bleed who were found to have a peptic ulcer on endoscopic examination with evidence of bleeding (defined as the presence of a visible vessel, whether actively bleeding at the time of examination or not, or adherent clot).

Exclusion Criteria: Other lesions that could be a source of the bleed, including malignancy; predisposition to bleeding [platelet count <50,000 mm^{-3}, prolonged prothrombin time (PT), or active therapeutic anticoagulation therapy]; presence of other acute clinical disease, including stroke and sepsis.

Intervention: Patients were randomized to combination endoclip therapy and epinephrine injection or epinephrine injection alone. Patients experiencing rebleeding after injection therapy alone were again randomized between the two treatments for their second therapy.

Endpoints

Primary Endpoint: Cessation of hemorrhage after first therapy, as visualized by endoscope for 5 minutes after administration of therapy.

Secondary Endpoints: Cessation of hemorrhage after therapy for rebleeding, need for surgical intervention, length of stay, 30-day mortality.

Sample Size: 105 patients enrolled at a single center in Taiwan from July 2003 to July 2004, with 53 patients randomized to epinephrine injection alone and 52 to combination therapy.

Statistical Analysis: Student's t-test, χ^2, and Fisher exact test.

Results

Baseline Data: The patients had a median age of 64 years, and 77% were men. Ulcers were found in the stomach (51%) and duodenum (49%). There were no baseline differences between the groups.

Outcomes: Patients achieved hemostasis in 98% and 92% of cases with combination versus injection therapy alone, respectively (p 0.18). Rebleeding was more likely in patients who underwent injection therapy alone (4% vs. 21%, p 0.08), as well as those who developed hypovolemic shock before therapy, had an actively bleeding ulcer, or an ulcer >2 cm. Patients who rebled after injection therapy alone and were randomized for further therapy achieved cessation of bleeding in 100% of cases with combination therapy, and 33% with injection therapy alone (p 0.02). A total of 9% of patients needed surgical intervention in the injection only arm, versus none in the combination therapy arm (p 0.02). There were no differences in hospital stay or 30-day mortality between the groups.

Discussion

Conclusion: Combination therapy with both endoclips and injection therapy reduces the occurrence of rebleeding from acutely hemorrhaging ulcers, when compared to injection alone. This remains true for secondary control after rebleeding.

Limitations: There was no control group that received endoclip therapy alone, so it remains unclear whether endoclips simply provide greater hemorrhage control regardless of the use of epinephrine.

j. MAGIC Trial

Perioperative chemotherapy versus surgery alone for resectable gastroesophageal cancer.

Cunningham D, Allum WH, Stenning SP, Thompson JN, Van de Velde CJ, Nicolson M, Scarffe JH, Lofts FJ, Falk SJ, Iveson TJ, Smith DB, Langley RE, Verma M, Weeden S, Chua YJ, MAGIC Trial Participants

NEJM. 2006;355(1):11–20.

SYNOPSIS

Takeaway Point: A combination of neoadjuvant and adjuvant chemotherapy provides a survival advantage over surgery alone for gastric cancer.

Commentary: This study established a new approach to the treatment of gastric cancer with the introduction of neoadjuvant therapy. During this large multicenter trial, patients were randomized to either (1) three cycles of neoadjuvant and three cycles of adjuvant chemotherapy or (2) surgical resection alone, which was the standard of care at the time when the study was initiated (this study enrolled patients concurrently with the SWOG study; see **e**, above). The treatment group had improved survival, decreased incidence of disease recurrence, smaller tumors at resection, and a greater proportion of early-stage disease. This trial introduced the possibility of downstaging with preoperative therapy, a circumstance that may improve chances for a complete resection. Although the proportion of patients who were able to receive the complete treatment protocol was low, the effects of the study were far-reaching, and this same treatment protocol has since become an established and validated standard therapy for gastric cancer.

ANALYSIS

Introduction: Surgical resection alone confers a poor prognosis and a high disease recurrence rate for patients with advanced gastric cancer. While a number of adjuvant chemotherapy regimens have been shown to improve survival, there is limited experience with neoadjuvant therapy in this setting.

Objectives: To determine whether a regimen of epirubicin + cisplatin + infused fluorouracil (ECF) given before and after radical surgery improves the outcomes of operable gastric cancer compared to surgery alone.

Methods

Trial Design: Randomized controlled trial.

Participants

Inclusion Criteria: Patients of all ages with histologically proven gastric or lower GE junction adenocarcinoma, clinically staged as T2 or higher.

Exclusion Criteria: Previous chemotherapy or radiotherapy, uncontrolled cardiac disease, creatinine clearance < 60 mL/min, or WHO performance status > 1.

Intervention: Chemotherapy with ECF, delivered as three cycles preoperatively and three cycles postoperatively, or surgical resection alone.

Endpoints

Primary Endpoint: Survival at 5 years.

Secondary Endpoints: Local recurrence and distant recurrence.

Sample Size: A cohort of 503 patients from 45 centers, mostly in the United Kingdom, between July 1994 and April 2002; 250 randomized to chemotherapy and 253 to surgery alone.

Statistical Analysis: An intention-to-treat analysis was performed using χ^2 and Mann–Whitney tests, as well as Kaplan–Meier analysis with log-rank testing for survival, and Cox proportional-hazards models to determine hazard ratios. Sample size calculations required 500 participants and 250 deaths to detect a 15% difference in survival.

Results

Baseline Data: The median age of the cohort was 62 years, and 79% of patients were male. Pretreatment characteristics were balanced between groups.

Outcomes: Of the 250 patients assigned to receive chemotherapy, 42% received all six cycles. In total, 92% of these patients eventually underwent surgery as compared to 96% in the surgery-alone group. Resection was curative in 69% of the patients in the chemotherapy group and 66% in the surgery-only group. There were a higher proportion of earlier stage tumors in the chemotherapy group, with 51% of tumors either T1 or T2, compared with 37%

in the surgery-alone group (p 0.002). Median tumor size was 3 cm, compared with 5 cm in the surgery-alone group (p <0.001), and nodal involvement was N0 or N1 among 84% of the ECF-treated patients versus 71% in the surgery-alone group. Five-year survival reached 36% in the chemotherapy group compared to 23% in the surgery-alone group (p 0.009). Overall recurrence was 39% compared to 57% in the surgery-alone group, and local and distant recurrences were 14% and 24% in the chemotherapy arm and 21% and 37% in the surgery-only arm, respectively (p <0.001).

Discussion

Conclusion: A combination regimen of preoperative and postoperative chemotherapy conferred an absolute 5-year survival benefit of 13% and a decreased recurrence rate of 18%. There was a high rate of treatment intolerance, resulting in only 42% of patients receiving the full six cycles.

Limitations: Treatment was poorly tolerated, with a high noncompletion rate. The overall 30-day mortality rate was high at 15%, and complication rates were 45%, although there were no differences between groups. Surgery alone was the standard of care when this trial was initiated, so there was no comparison with chemoradiation, which has since been demonstrated to improve survival.

---

k. CROSS Trial

Preoperative chemoradiotherapy for esophageal or junctional cancer.

van Hagen P, Hulshof MC, van Lanschot JJ, Steyerberg EW, van Berge Henegouwen MI, Wijnhoven BP, Richel DJ, Nieuwenhuijzen GA, Hospers GA, Bonenkamp JJ, Cuesta MA, Blaisse RJ, Busch OR, ten Kate FJ, Creemers GJ, Punt CJ, Plukker JT, Verheul HM, Spillenaar Bilgen EJ, van Dekken H, van der Sangen MJ, Rozema T, Biermann K, Beukema JC, Piet AH, van Rij CM, Reinders JG, Tilanus HW, van der Gaast A, CROSS Group

NEJM. 2012;366(22):2074–2084.

SYNOPSIS

Takeaway Point: Neoadjuvant chemoradiation for esophageal carcinoma is well tolerated and improves survival.

Commentary: This trial established a new standard of care with regard to preoperative therapy for esophageal carcinoma. Patients receiving preoperative chemoradiation have higher rates of

R0 resection compared to surgery alone. Median survival time doubled, and 29% of patients achieved a complete pathologic response. Although the benefits are less dramatic when examining individual histologies, there remains a demonstrable difference. At a time when there was no standard treatment regimen for esophageal cancer, this trial stands as one of the largest and most prominent to show a definite benefit of therapy. Using a combination of carboplatin and paclitaxel, the authors put forward an effective regimen that was well tolerated and has been widely adopted into practice.

ANALYSIS

Introduction: The use of neoadjuvant therapy in esophageal carcinoma is hindered by lack of a standardized regimen and concrete data demonstrating a definite survival benefit.

Objectives: To compare neoadjuvant chemoradiotherapy followed by surgery versus surgery alone in patients with potentially curable esophageal or esophagogastric junction carcinoma.

Methods

Trial Design: Randomized controlled trial.

Participants

Inclusion Criteria: Age 18–75 years with histologically confirmed squamous, undifferentiated, or adenocarcinoma of the esophagus or GE junction with WHO performance level ≤ 2 and T1–T3 tumors.

Exclusion Criteria: Tumor length > 8 cm and/or width > 5 cm; metastatic disease; history of previous chemotherapy or radiotherapy; other malignant disease; or failure of renal, hepatic, pulmonary, or hematopoietic system.

Intervention: Preoperative chemoradiation with carboplatin and paclitaxel delivered with 41.4 Gy of radiation in 23 fractions, or surgery alone.

Endpoints

Primary Endpoint: Overall survival.

Secondary Endpoints: Complete (R0) resection, treatment completion.

Sample Size: 366 patients enrolled from two Dutch centers between March 2004 and December 2008; 178 patients were randomized to chemoradiation and 188 to surgery alone.

Statistical Analysis: Survival examined with Kaplan–Meier analysis and log-rank testing, as well as Cox proportional-hazards model. Sample size calculations required 175 patients per group to detect an overall difference in median survival of 22 months.

Results

Baseline Data: Median age 60 years, 78% male. Tumors by histology were 75% adenocarcinoma, 23% squamous cell carcinoma, and 2% other. Median tumor size was 4 cm. Tumors were at the GE junction in 24%, distal third of esophagus in 58%, middle third in 13%, and proximal third in 2%. Baseline characteristics were balanced between the groups.

Outcomes: 91% of patients receiving neoadjuvant chemoradiation completed therapy. Of the patients going directly to surgery, 13% were found to be unresectable, versus 4% in the chemoradiation group (p 0.002). Complete (R0) resection was achieved in 92% of patients receiving chemoradiation, compared to 69% in the surgery-only group (p <0.001), and a pathologic complete response was noted in 29%. The incidence of positive lymph nodes was decreased in the neoadjuvant therapy group compared to the surgery-alone group (31% vs. 75%, p <0.001). There was no difference in postoperative complications. Five-year survival was 47% in the neoadjuvant group and 34% in the surgery-alone group, with median survivals of 49 and 24 months, respectively (p 0.003). Hazard ratio for death was 0.66 in the neoadjuvant group. The observed survival rates did not change when controlling for tumor histology.

Discussion

Conclusion: Preoperative chemoradiation with carboplatin and paclitaxel is well tolerated and results in prolonged survival among patients with esophageal or GE junction carcinoma.

Limitations: The cohort consisted largely of distal esophageal or GE junction tumors, and there was no separate analysis to determine whether these results were different by tumor location. Similarly, a proportionately small percentage of patients had squamous cell carcinoma, and patients were not analyzed separately by histology. Therefore, this study is of limited applicability for patients with proximal gastric tumors or with tumor histologies other than adenocarcinoma.

I. Transfusion Strategies for UGI Bleeding

Transfusion strategies for acute upper gastrointestinal bleeding.

Villanueva C, Colomo A, Bosch A, Concepción M, Hernandez-Gea V, Aracil C, Graupera I, Poca M, Alvarez-Urturi C, Gordillo J, Guarner-Argente C, Santaló M, Muñiz E, Guarner C

NEJM. 2013;368(1):11–21.

SYNOPSIS

Takeaway Point: A restrictive transfusion strategy (hemoglobin transfusion threshold 7 mg/dL) has improved mortality and complication rates in comparison with a liberal transfusion strategy in patients with active UGI bleeding.

Commentary: This single-center randomized controlled trial sought to determine whether a restrictive transfusion strategy as espoused by TRICC (see TRICC Trial, Chapter 4, article **b**) and other trials was applicable in the setting of active UGI bleeding. Prior trials, including TRICC, specifically excluded patients with active bleeding due to legitimate concerns that patient outcomes would suffer without an aggressive blood replacement strategy. In this study, the authors randomized patients with an UGI bleed to blood transfusion using a liberal hemoglobin threshold of 9 mg/dL, or a restrictive threshold of 7 mg/dL, and were able to establish that a restrictive strategy decreased mortality and the incidence of rebleeding. This trial confirmed that, similar to other critically ill patients, patients with UGI bleeds have better outcomes when their transfusions are limited to lower hemoglobin goals.

ANALYSIS

Introduction: Although the shift in paradigm toward a restrictive transfusion strategy in critical care was not extended to patients with active GI bleeds, it has been suggested that a higher intravascular volume (and, by association, a higher portal pressure) puts patients at risk for further bleeding, and thus actively bleeding patients may benefit from a similarly restrictive strategy.

Objectives: To determine whether a restrictive transfusion strategy confers better patient outcomes compared to a liberal transfusion strategy in the setting of acute UGI bleeding.

Methods

Trial Design: Randomized controlled trial.

Participants

Inclusion Criteria: Age >18 years, evidence of UGI bleed [eg, melena or bloody nasogastric tube (NGT) output].

Exclusion Criteria: Lower gastrointestinal (LGI) bleed, acute coronary or neurologic ischemia, recent transfusion or trauma, low risk of bleeding (determined by Rockall score), massive exsanguinating bleed, refusal by patient or attending physician to receive transfusions per protocol.

Intervention: Transfusion for patients dropping below hemoglobin of 7 mg/dL, with a target range of 7–9 mg/dL, compared with a control transfusion threshold of 9 mg/dL and target range of 9–11 mg/dL.

Endpoints

Primary Endpoint: All-cause mortality within 45 days.

Secondary Endpoints: Rebleeding requiring intervention, in-hospital complications requiring intervention.

Sample Size: A total cohort of 889 patients from a single center between June 2003 and December 2009, with 444 in the restrictive transfusion group and 445 in the liberal transfusion group.

Statistical Analysis: Kaplan–Meier analysis with log-rank testing, Cox proportional-hazards regression; sample size calculations estimating 430 patients per arm to detect a mortality difference of at least 5%.

Results

Baseline Data: The etiology of the bleed was ulceration in 49% and variceal in 21% of patients. Cirrhosis was present in 31% of the cohort. There were no differences between groups, including hemoglobin levels at admission.

Outcomes: Patients in the restrictive group received a mean of 1.5 units of blood, versus 3.7 units in the liberal group (p <0.001). In total, 51% in the restrictive arm and 14% in the liberal arm did not require transfusions (p <0.001). All-cause mortality for the restrictive group was 5% at 45 days, compared to 9% in the liberal group (p 0.02). This remained true when controlling for baseline disease and etiology of bleeding. Mortality due to bleeding was 0.7% in the restrictive group and 3.1% in the liberal group (p 0.01). Rebleeding occurred in 10% of the restrictive group and 16% of the liberal group (p 0.01), requiring surgical intervention in 2% and 6%, respectively (p 0.04). There was a higher incidence of overall complications in the liberal group (48% vs. 40%, p 0.02), and a higher incidence of cardiac events and pulmonary edema in particular.

Discussion

Conclusion: A restrictive transfusion protocol with a hemoglobin transfusion threshold of 7 mg/dL improves mortality and complication rates among patients with an active UGI bleed. Furthermore, there is a reduction in rebleeding and progression to surgical intervention with a restrictive transfusion strategy.

Limitations: The study's cohort excluded patients with massive exsanguinating bleeding, a qualifier that was not well defined. Violation of the protocol occurred in 9% of the patients in the restrictive strategy group.

---

m. D1 versus D2 Dissection: Italian Trial

Randomized clinical trial comparing survival after D1 or D2 gastrectomy for gastric cancer.

Degiuli M, Sasako M, Ponti A, Vendrame A, Tomatis M, Mazza C, Borasi A, Capussotti L, Fronda G, Morino M, Italian Gastric Cancer Study Group

Br J Surg. 2014;101(2):23–31.

SYNOPSIS

Takeaway Point: D2 lymph node dissection with a pancreas-preserving technique can be carried out for more accurate staging without increasing mortality, but it does not improve survival.

Commentary: Numerous groups have attempted to demonstrate the use of D2 lymph node dissection as defined by the Japanese Gastric Cancer Association (JGCA) in Western centers and found the technique limited by its high perioperative risk. This was ascribed mainly to the previously mandated splenectomy and distal pancreatectomy that was thought to be required for full lymph node clearance. The Italian Gastric Cancer Study Group (IGCSC) sought to evaluate the pancreas-preserving technique for D2 dissection, and found their mortality rate to meet that reported by Eastern centers. This trial reported on long-term survival and found that, although overall survival was no different between D1 and D2 groups, patients with T2-T4 stage cancers who underwent D2 dissection demonstrated a 21% disease-specific survival benefit at 5 years. After disappointing results from the Dutch and MRC trials (see **a** and **b**, above), this study ultimately demonstrated that D2 dissection can be carried out safely in the West with a low perioperative mortality rate and improved tumor staging. It is because of this increased staging accuracy that pancreas- and spleen-preserving D2 dissection has been the recommendation forwarded by the National Comprehensive Cancer Network (NCCN) for gastric cancer resections.[15] In practice, safe lymph node harvest that does not endanger surrounding organs often falls short of the strict definition of a D2 dissection but can still provide greater staging information than a simple D1, and has been termed a "D1+ dissection."

ANALYSIS

Introduction: The application of D2 dissection for gastric cancer has long been established as the standard of care in the East, but adoption has been limited in Western centers because of high morbidity and mortality, especially associated with pancreatic or splenic resection. This has prompted the elimination of routine pancreatic and splenic resection from the D2 dissection, but a clear survival benefit has not yet been demonstrated.

Objectives: To determine the influence of extended lymph node (LN) dissection without routine splenectomy or pancreatectomy on long-term survival in gastric cancer.

Methods

Trial Design: Randomized controlled parallel-group superiority trial.

Participants

Inclusion Criteria: Age < 80 years with histologically proven gastric cancer and no comorbidities that would preclude extensive surgical resection.

Exclusion Criteria: Prior gastric surgery, other malignant disease, resection under emergent circumstances, unresectable disease.

Intervention: D1 nodal dissection or D2 dissection as defined by the JGCA, with preservation of pancreas and allowance of one deficient group out of the D2 nodes.

Endpoints

Primary Endpoint: Overall survival.

Secondary Endpoint: Disease-specific survival.

Sample Size: Cohort of 267 patients from five Italian centers, enrolled between June 1998 and December 2006. The D1 group consisted of 133 patients, with 134 in the D2 group.

Statistical Analysis: Categorical data with χ^2 test, continuous data with t-test or Mann–Whitney test. Survival by Kaplan–Meier analysis with log-rank testing and Cox multivariate regression model. Sample size analysis calculated 160 patients needed in each arm to detect a 15% absolute increase in survival rate.

Results

Baseline Data: 30% of patients were over 70 years old, and 49% were male. Total gastrectomy was performed in 25% of patients and distal gastrectomy in 75% of patients. Splenectomy was performed in 8% of patients. Nodal metastases were found in 53% of patients. Baseline characteristics were well balanced between the groups, although the D1 group had significantly more low-grade (IA) tumors (30.8% vs. 18.7%, p 0.021).

Outcomes: Median number of harvested lymph nodes was 25 in the D1 group and 33 in the D2 group (p 0.015). Perioperative morbidity and mortality were equivalent. Those undergoing D1 dissection had a 67% overall survival rate and a 71% disease-specific survival (DSS) rate, not significantly different from 64% and 73% in the D2 group, respectively. Among T1 tumors, DSS was 98% in the D1 group versus 83% in the D2 group (p 0.015). However, in tumors staged T2–T4, DSS was 38% in the D1 group and 59% in the D2 group (p 0.055). Patients over 70 years of age undergoing D2 dissection had a DSS of 51%, compared to 75% in the D1 group (p 0.018).

Discussion

Conclusion: D2 dissection without pancreaticosplenic resection did not demonstrate an improved overall survival when compared to D1 dissection.

Subgroup analyses showed no survival benefit to D2 dissection among T1 cancers but did show a trend towards improved DSS among patients with T2–T4 stage cancers that approached significance.

Limitations: There was a significant rate of contamination for patients undergoing D1 dissection, yielding a higher than usual lymph node harvest for this group, as well as noncompliance with D2 dissection in 33% of patients assigned to that arm. There was also a higher distribution of early-stage tumors in the D1 group and later-stage tumors in the D2 group. Although subgroup analyses controlling for stage reached statistical significance, the study was not powered to look for these differences. Enrollment was significantly slower than anticipated, and so they did not reach their goal sample size for the overall trial.

REFERENCES

1. Wang YR, Richter JE, Dempsey DT. Trends and outcomes of hospitalizations for peptic ulcer disease in the United States, 1993 to 2006. *Ann Surg.* 2010;251(1):51–58.

2. Hermansson M, Ekedahl A, et al. Decreasing incidence of peptic ulcer complications after the introduction of the proton pump inhibitors, a study of the Swedish population from 1974–2002. *BMC Gastroenterol.* 2009;9:25.

3. Malfertheiner P, Chan FK, McColl KE. Peptic ulcer disease. *Lancet.* 2009;374(9699):1449–1461.

4. Papastergiou V, Georgopoulos SD, Karatapanis S. Treatment of *Helicobacter pylori* infection: Past, present and future. *World J Gastrointest Pathophysiol.* 2014;5(4):392–399.

5. Søreide K, Thorsen K, Søreide JA. Strategies to improve the outcome of emergency surgery for perforated peptic ulcer. *Br J Surg.* 2014;101(1):e51–e64.

6. Muguruma N, Kitamura S, et al. Endoscopic management of nonvariceal upper gastrointestinal bleeding: State of the art. *Clin Endosc.* 2015;48(2):96–101.

7. Garcia-Tsao G, Sanyal AJ, et al. Practice Guidelines Committee of the American Association for the Study of Liver Diseases; Practice Parameters Committee of the American College of Gastroenterology. Prevention and management of gastroesophageal varices and variceal hemorrhage in cirrhosis. *Hepatology.* 2007;46(3):922–938.

8. North Italian Endoscopic Club for the Study and Treatment of Esophageal Varices. Prediction of the first variceal hemorrhage in patients with cirrhosis of the liver and esophageal varices. A prospective multicenter study. *NEJM.* 1988;319(15):983–989.

9. SEER Statistics. *Stomach Cancer* (available at http://seer.cancer.gov/statfacts/html/stomach.html; accessed 4/15/15).

10. International Agency for Research on Cancer (IARC) Fact Sheet. *Stomach Cancer* (available at http://globocan.iarc.fr/Pages/fact_sheets_cancer.aspx; accessed 4/12/15).

11. Inoue M, Tsugane S. Epidemiology of gastric cancer in Japan. *Postgrad Med J.* 2005l;81(957):419–424.

12. Bonenkamp JJ, Songun I, Hermans J, Sasako M, Welvaart K, Plukker JT, et al. Randomised comparison of morbidity after D1 and D2 dissection for gastric cancer in 996 Dutch patients. *Lancet.* 1995;345(8952):745–748.

13. Wong CS, Chia CF, Lee HC, Wei PL, Ma HP, Tsai SH, et al. Eradication of *Helicobacter pylori* for prevention of ulcer recurrence after simple closure of perforated peptic ulcer: A meta-analysis of randomized controlled trials. *J Surg Res.* 2013;182(2):219–226.

14. Tomtitchong P, Siribumrungwong B, Vilaichone RK, Kasetsuwan P, Matsukura N, Chaiyakunapruk N. Systematic review and meta-analysis: *Helicobacter pylori* eradication therapy after simple closure of perforated duodenal ulcer. *Helicobacter.* 2012;17(2):148–152.

15. NCCN Clinical Practice Guidelines in Oncology. *Gastric Cancer*, Version 3. 2015 (available at http://www.nccn.org; accessed 7/30/15).

11

Small Bowel Surgery

Vicki Sein • Ara Feinstein

Surgery of the small bowel is a mainstay of practice for the general and acute care surgeon. Any abdominal operation must take into consideration the small bowel, both as a potential site of pathology or iatrogenic injury during the operation itself, and postoperatively, when ileus or adhesive small bowel obstruction may extend hospital length of stay. Despite the widespread importance of small bowel pathology to surgeons, the care of these patients relies on traditional surgical teaching. Evidence-based management in this area remains nascent, with few randomized controlled trials providing data to either support or refute dogma. Surgeons' reluctance to undertake a study that appears to deviate from standard care may contribute, in part, to the paucity of high-quality data.

Of the extant studies in the area, many focus on streamlining care for patients with postoperative ileus or adhesive small bowel obstruction. Nonpharmocologic methods such as gum chewing,[1] as well as newer pharmaceuticals such as Alvimopan,[2] have been studied in an attempt to reduce the incidence of postoperative ileus, and Gastrografin has been suggested to facilitate resolution of partial small bowel obstruction.[3] Surgical technique has also evolved over the years, with the development of new energy devices for mesenteric ligation and the linear cutting stapler for bowel anastomoses. It has now become common practice to use a variety of staplers for intestinal anastomoses, but controversy remains regarding the equivalency of hand-sewn and stapled anastomoses.

The topics presented in this review highlight recent developments and recommendations regarding the management of surgical issues of the small bowel. This discussion represents a sampling of the few high-quality studies in the area, and demonstrates the need for rigorous clinical trials to further inform surgical practice. Hopefully, further randomized controlled trials will clarify factors to improve outcomes in patients with small bowel disease, and ultimately guide standardization of care.

a. Gastrografin for Adhesive Small Bowel Obstruction
Randomized clinical study of Gastrografin administration in patients with adhesive small bowel obstruction.

Biondo S, Parés D, Mora L, Martí Ragué J, Kreisler E, Jaurrieta E

Br J Surg. 2003;90(5):542–546.

SYNOPSIS

Takeaway Point: The use of oral Gastrografin can help diagnose a complete small bowel obstruction, and hasten resolution of a partial small bowel obstruction.

Commentary: The authors present a randomized study of orally administered Gastrografin to identify patients who will need an operation for a small bowel obstruction, and to speed recovery of bowel function in patients with partial obstructions. They demonstrate an overall shorter hospital stay in patients receiving Gastrografin studies, both those requiring surgery, and those managed nonoperatively. Gastrografin has the potential to expedite identification of patients with complete small bowel obstruction who will require operation, and to hasten the resolution of partial obstructions that can be safely managed conservatively.

ANALYSIS

Introduction: Controversy continues to exist over the appropriate timing of operative intervention in adhesive small bowel obstruction (SBO). Determining whether the obstruction is complete or partial is an important decision point in the management of these patients. Oral administration of Gastrografin has been used to differentiate partial from complete obstructions, and may have a therapeutic effect in early adhesive SBO.

Objectives: To evaluate the ability of Gastrografin to resolve a partial SBO.

Methods
Trial Design: Single-center, prospective, randomized trial.

Participants

Inclusion Criteria: Any patient admitted with signs or symptoms of postoperative small bowel obstruction.

Exclusion Criteria: Age < 18 years, pregnancy, allergy to iodine, known nonspecific inflammatory bowel disease, symptoms suggestive of strangulating obstruction (fever, tachycardia, continuous pain with peritoneal irritation, metabolic acidosis), obstruction complicating an infective intraabdominal process such as diverticular disease, known abdominal cancer, prior abdominal radiotherapy, intestinal obstruction within the first 4 weeks after an abdominal operation, or known or suspected intestinal vascular disorder.

Intervention: 100 mL Gastrografin administered via nasogastric tube (NGT) after decompression in the emergency department. The NGT was then clamped for 3 hours, and serial abdominal radiographs were obtained. If the Gastrografin did not reach the colon in 24 hours, laparotomy was performed. If symptoms did not resolve by 4–5 days, laparotomy was performed.

Endpoints

Primary Endpoint: Success of nonoperative management and length of hospital stay.

Secondary Endpoints: Readmission, time between admissions, surgical operation, mortality.

Sample Size: 92 patients at one center in Spain between February 2000 and November 2001, making up 100 visits, were randomized; 10 episodes in 9 patients were later excluded because the final diagnosis was not SBO. Of the included patients, 44 episodes in 42 patients were randomized to Gastrografin and 46 episodes in 41 patients to the control group.

Statistical Analysis: ANOVA, χ^2 test, Student's t-test.

Results

Baseline Data: All groups had similar baseline characteristics. Overall, 85.6% of episodes resolved with conservative management.

Outcomes

Primary: In patients who were treated successfully with nonoperative management, hospital stay was significantly decreased in the Gastrografin group (2.8 days vs. 5.8 days, $p < 0.001$). All patients who had contrast in the colon at 24 hours were successfully treated nonoperatively.

Secondary: Patients in the Gastrografin group had a decreased total length of stay after surgical intervention.

Discussion

Conclusion: The use of oral Gastrografin early in the course of an adhesive small bowel obstruction may identify a complete obstruction and better stratify patients to operative intervention, and can shorten the time to resolution of partial obstructions.

Limitations: The diagnosis of bowel obstructions was based on plain radiographs, and in patients with CT scans the decision to go to the operating room may be based on different factors. The difference in total length of stay may represent earlier operation for the Gastrografin group (after 24 hours) rather than the 4–5 days of nonoperative management allowed for the control group.

---

b. Alvimopan and Postoperative Ileus

Alvimopan, a novel, peripherally acting μ opioid antagonist: Results of a multicenter, randomized, double-blind, placebo-controlled, phase III trial of major abdominal surgery and postoperative ileus.

Wolff BG, Michelassi F, Gerkin TM, Techner L, Gabriel K, Du W, Wallin BA, Alvimopan Postoperative Ileus Study Group

Ann Surg. 2004;240(4):728–734.

SYNOPSIS

Takeaway Point: In patients undergoing gastrointestinal (GI) surgery, the μ-opioid receptor antagonist alvimopan speeds recovery of GI tract function and reduces in-hospital stay.

Commentary: The authors present a large, multicenter, randomized controlled trial, comparing alvimopan at 6 and 12 mg doses to placebo for patients undergoing laparotomy with either bowel resection or radical hysterectomy. The patients receiving alvimopan had accelerated GI recovery and decreased time to discharge with equivalent opioid usage. The improved effect of the 12 mg dose has raised the question of whether even higher doses should be used. The effectiveness of the drug among patients undergoing laparoscopic surgery or epidural analgesia, techniques associated with both decreased incidence and duration of postoperative ileus, has not been studied, and therefore the effectiveness of alvimopan in such scenarios is uncertain.

ANALYSIS

Introduction: Multiple factors are thought to contribute to the pathogenesis of postoperative ileus (POI), one of which may be the action of opioid analgesics on μ-opioid receptors in the GI tract. Alvimopam is a peripherally acting antagonist of the μ receptor, and acts in the GI tract to attenuate the antimotility effects of opioid analgesics.

Objectives: The present study was performed to evaluate the efficacy and safety of alvimopan (6 or 12 mg) for the management of POI in patients undergoing partial bowel resection with primary anastomosis or radical hysterectomy.

Methods
Trial Design: Multicenter, randomized, placebo-controlled, double-blinded, parallel-group study.

Participants
Inclusion Criteria: ≥18 years of age, scheduled to undergo a partial small- or large-bowel resection with primary anastomosis or radical total abdominal hysterectomy (rTAH), scheduled to receive post-operative pain management with intravenous patient-controlled analgesia with opioids, and scheduled to have the nasogastric tube (NGT) removed at the end of surgery.

Exclusion Criteria: Epidural analgesia, NGT insertion after surgery, ileostomy or colostomy, surgical procedure not specified by the protocol, cancellation of surgery.

Intervention: Patients were randomized to receive an oral dose of alvimopan (6 or 12 mg) or identical placebo capsules at least 2 hours before surgery and then twice daily beginning on postoperative day (POD) 1 until hospital discharge, or for a maximum of 7 days of postoperative treatment.

Endpoints
Primary Endpoint: Time to recovery of gastrointestinal function, as defined by the latter of two events: time until patient tolerated solid food, or time until either flatus or bowel movement (BM).

Secondary Endpoints: Time (in hours) from the end of surgery to first flatus, first BM, tolerance of solid food, ready for hospital discharge (based solely on the recovery of GI function as defined by the surgeon), and time to discharge order written.

Sample Size: 510 patients from 34 North American centers were randomized, 165 to placebo, 169 to 6 mg alvimopan, and 176 to 12 mg alvimopan.

Statistical Analysis: Cox proportional-hazards model, Kaplan–Meier cumulative survival curve, modified intention-to-treat (MITT) analysis.

Results

Baseline Data: Baseline characteristics were similar between groups. Fewer patients underwent small bowel resection in the placebo group. Forty-one patients were excluded from analyses, 16 from the placebo group and 25 from the two treatment arms. The remaining 469 patients comprised the MITT population.

Outcomes

Primary: The time to recovery of GI function was significantly accelerated by alvimopan at 6 mg (105 vs. 120 hours, $p < 0.05$) and 12 mg doses (98 hours, $p < 0.001$).

Secondary: Time to hospital discharge was decreased in both alvimopan groups, by 13 hours for the 6-g group (p 0.070) and by 20 hours for the 12-mg group (p 0.003) compared with the placebo group. The average opioid consumption was similar between all groups.

Discussion

Conclusion: In patients undergoing open bowel resection or radical hysterectomy, alvimopan speeds recovery of GI function and time to hospital discharge.

Limitations: This study demonstrates an increased drug effect at the 12 mg dose, but it is unknown whether the incremental increase in effect would continue with higher medication doses. Additionally, this study does not address laparoscopic surgery, patients on chronic opioid therapy, or those with epidural analgesia. The study utilized a modified intent to treat analysis, which excluded from the outcome analysis those who did not have an efficacy evaluation and did not undergo the specified surgery. This resulted in a moderate number of randomized patients being excluded from the analysis.

---

c. Gum Chewing for Postoperative Ileus

Does gum chewing ameliorate postoperative ileus? Results of a prospective, randomized, placebo-controlled trial.

Matros E, Rocha F, Zinner M, Wang J, Ashley S, Breen E, Soybel D, Shoji B, Burgess A, Bleday R, Kuntz R, Whang E

J Am Coll Surg. 2006;202(5):773–778.

SYNOPSIS

Takeaway Point: Contrary to conclusions from previous studies, gum chewing may not reduce the duration of postcolectomy ileus.

Commentary: Postoperative ileus is a major determinant of length of hospital stay, and therefore cost, in patients undergoing colon surgery. Many methodologies have been tested to shorten the time to recovery of bowel function. This study aims to examine the effects of gum chewing on postoperative ileus after colon surgery. Using a three-group design with an acupressure bracelet as placebo, patients were studied for time to return to bowel function and readiness for discharge. The authors found no significant difference in the time to first postoperative flatus, time to first bowel movement, or time to readiness for discharge. This trial contradicts the results of prior studies, although all have had relatively small sample sizes and difficulty quantifying outcomes.[4] The variability between study outcomes highlights the difficulty associated with studying the duration and effect of postoperative ileus.

ANALYSIS

Introduction: Postoperative ileus is a major source of morbidity and prolonged hospital stay after abdominal operations. Previous studies have suggested that postoperative gum chewing is associated with an earlier return of bowel function.

Objectives: To determine whether gum chewing is more effective than a placebo in hastening bowel recovery and shortening hospitalization after open colectomy.

Methods
Trial Design: Single-center, prospective, randomized, placebo-controlled study.

Participants
Inclusion Criteria: Age 18–85 years, scheduled to undergo open segmental colonic resection, low anterior resection, abdominoperineal resection, hemicolectomy, or end colostomy reversal.

Exclusion Criteria: Metastatic disease, history of inflammatory bowel disease, prior abdominal radiation, mint allergy, dentures, concomitant resection of small intestine, nasogastric tube drainage beyond the first postoperative morning, diverting ileostomy, or more than one bowel anastomosis during the operation.

Intervention: Patients were randomized to one of three postoperative regimens: (1) standard of care, (2) acupressure bracelet worn in a sham location on the dorsum of the wrist (placebo), or (3) chewing gum. Subjects in the latter two groups were instructed to either wear the bracelet or chew gum for 45 minutes 3 times daily at 9 AM, 4 PM, and 8 PM.

Endpoints

Primary Endpoint: Time to passage of flatus.

Secondary Endpoints: Time to first postoperative bowel movement, time until patients were ready for discharge (defined as passing gas and tolerating two regular meals in the absence of complications), time until actual discharge, and complications at 30 days.

Sample Size: 66 patients at one institution between April 2003 and June 2004; 21 received standard of care, 22 received active therapy, 23 received the placebo bracelet.

Statistical Analysis: Log-rank test, Kaplan–Meier curves, ANOVA, and χ^2 test.

Results

Baseline Data: All three groups had similar baseline characteristics.

Outcomes

Primary: The median time to first flatus was not statistically significant between standard of care, placebo, and gum (67, 72, and 60 hours, p 0.384).

Secondary: There was no significant difference in the time to first bowel movement, time to readiness for discharge, or time until actual discharge.

Discussion

Conclusion: Postoperative gum chewing does not show a statistically significant effect in the reduction of postoperative ileus, as measured by the passage of first flatus.

Limitations: This is a small single-institution study. Patients included in the study all had laparotomies, and no arm of the study included laparoscopic surgery. Additionally, the majority of patients included in this study had epidural analgesia, thus making it difficult to generalize these findings to patients treated with oral or IV narcotic medications.

---

d. Lanreotide and Pancreatic and Enterocutaneous Fistulae

Randomized, placebo-controlled, double-blind study of the efficacy of lanreotide 30 mg PR in the treatment of pancreatic and enterocutaneous fistulae.

Gayral F, Campion JP, Regimbeau JM, Blumberg J, Maisonobe P, Topart P, Wind P, Lanreotide Digestive Fistula Study Group

Ann Surg. 2009;250(6):872–877.

SYNOPSIS

Takeaway Point: Administration of lanreotide, a long-acting somatostatin analog, can decrease enterocutaneous fistula output and shorten time to closure when compared to placebo.

Commentary: This is a randomized, double-blinded, placebo-controlled, multicenter trial, evaluating the efficacy of 30 mg of intramuscular lanreotide for reduction of enterocutaneous fistula output and time to fistula closure. Somatostatin is commonly used to decrease fistula output, and is dosed as a continuous infusion. This makes somatostatin a cumbersome treatment for patients with enterocutaneous or pancreatic fistulae, as it generally requires inpatient status and intravenous access. Unlike somatostatin, lanreotide is long-acting, requiring injections once every 10 days, making it a compelling alternative therapy. The drug gained FDA approval for treatment of neuroendocrine tumors in 2014.

This study had a three-phase design, in which nonresponders at 72 hours were unblinded, and if administered lanreotide, the medication was stopped. If they had been in the placebo group, lanreotide was administered. The study group demonstrated similar closure rates between placebo and lanreotide after the first injection, and the authors concluded that these fistulae would have likely resolved spontaneously. For patients requiring a second dose, lanreotide significantly decreased fistula output and improved time to closure.

ANALYSIS

Introduction: Enterocutaneous fistula formation is a serious complication of gastrointestinal and pancreatic surgery. Somatostatin, a naturally occurring hormone that inhibits gastrointestinal, biliary, and pancreatic exocrine secretion, has been used to decrease fistula output, but it requires continuous intravenous infusion due to a short half-life. Lanreotide is a synthetic analogue of somatostatin available in an intramuscular prolonged-release (PR) formulation.

Objectives: To assess the efficacy of lanreotide 30 mg PR to decrease the drainage volume of digestive fistulae, and its potential influence on spontaneous fistula closure.

Methods

Trial Design: Multicenter, randomized, placebo-controlled, double-blinded, three-phase trial.

Participants

Inclusion Criteria: Age 18–80 years, with simple externalized pancreatic, duodenal, or small intestine fistula. Pancreatic fistula drainage of at least 100 mL/24 hours over 2 days or 50 mL/24 hours for 3 consecutive days plus amylase concentration in fistula output of at least three times serum. Duodenal or small intestine fistula drainage of at least 100 mL/24 hours over 2 days.

Exclusion Criteria: Expected surgical treatment of fistula, uncontrolled intraabdominal sepsis, Crohn's disease, radiation-induced lesion, mesenteric vascular insufficiency, fistula in a cancer-infiltrated area, distal obstruction, exposed fistula of small intestine, intraabdominal foreign body, previous transplantation, long-term corticotherapy, previous curative treatment of the fistula with a somatostatin analog within the last month, contraindication to intramuscular injection, hypersensitivity to the test material, pregnancy or ongoing nursing, unlicensed drug received within the previous months.

Intervention: Intramuscular injection of either lanreotide 30 mg PR or placebo. 72 hours after the first injection, subjects showing a reduction of at least 50% of their fistula were kept on double-blind treatment and constituted group 1. Blinding was lifted for patients deemed nonresponders at 72 hours. If they had received placebo initially, they were subsequently treated with open-label lanreotide 30 mg PR (group 2); if they had initially received lanreotide, they were switched to an alternative treatment at the discretion of the investigator (group 3). All groups received a total of seven injections of drug or placebo.

Endpoints

Primary Endpoint: Rate of responders on double-blind treatment (group 1).

Secondary Endpoints: Closure time, defined as the interval between the day of first injection and the day of spontaneous fistula closure, rate of fistula closure at last visit, number of injections received by each patient, fistula recurrence rate, mortality.

Sample Size: 111 patients were randomized from two countries; four patients without primary efficacy data were removed from the intention-to-treat (ITT) population, which thus comprised 107 patients, of whom 54 were randomized to lanreotide and 53 to placebo.

Statistical Analysis: Logistic regression model, nonparametric analysis of covariance model, Kaplan–Meier curves.

Results

Baseline Data: Baseline characteristics including fistula location, drainage, and duration were similar between groups. There was a higher percentage of patients on total parenteral nutrition (TPN) in the placebo group, and conversely a higher percentage on enteral nutrition in the lanreotide group.

Outcomes

Primary: Lanreotide recipients had a 3.1 times higher likelihood of a 50% decrease of the fistula output after the first double-blinded dose (p 0.006). The likelihood of a response on lanreotide was higher among those patients with pancreatic fistula (p 0.014). For patients with small bowel fistula, there was a trend toward a higher responder rate for lanreotide, although the difference was not statistically significant (p 0.184).

Secondary: Ten patients (seven on lanreotide and three on placebo) were discontinued after the second dose due to death, adverse event, lack of efficacy, withdrawn consent, procedural errors, or loss to follow-up, or at the discrepancy of the investigator. Median fistula closure time for patients on lanreotide or placebo in the double-blind group 1 was 14 days and 17 days, respectively. In the entire ITT cohort, median time to fistula closure in the lanreotide group (n = 54) was 17 days, versus 26 days in the placebo group (n = 53). Fistula recurrence occurred in one patient on lanreotide. Overall closure rates were similar between the two groups.

Discussion

Conclusion: In patients with enterocutaneous fistulae, lanreotide administration decreased fistula output and shortened time to fistula closure by nine days, compared to placebo.

Limitations: Many fistulae resolved early with either placebo or lanreotide, which were likely fistulae that would have closed spontaneously. Lanreotide is a long-acting formulation, which may be unavailable or cost-prohibitive. The fistula output criteria for this study was relatively low, and high-output fistulas, which traditionally require surgery for closure, were not investigated.

---

e. Hand Suture versus Stapled Anastomosis

HAnd suture versus STApling for closure of loop ileostomy (HASTA trial): Results of a multicenter randomized trial. (DRKS00000040).

Löffler T, Rossion I, Bruckner T, Diener MK, Koch M, von Frankenberg M, Pochhammer J, Thomusch O, Kijak T, Simon T, Mihaljevic AL, Krüger M, Stein E, Prechtl G, Hodina R, Michal W, Strunk R, Henkel K, Bunse J, Jaschke G, Politt D, Heistermann HP, Fusser M, Lange C, Stamm A, Vosschulte A, Holzer R, Partecke LI, Burdzik E, Hug HM, Luntz SP, Kieser M, Büchler MW, Weitz J, HASTA Trial Group

Ann Surg. 2012;256(5):828–835.

SYNOPSIS

Takeaway Point: For takedown of a loop ileostomy, there is no difference in short-term outcomes, including rate of bowel obstruction, between stapled or hand-sewn small bowel anastomosis.

Commentary: There continues to be significant variability among surgeons with regard to technique for small bowel anastomoses. To address this issue, this multicenter trial compared hand suture versus stapling for small bowel anastomosis during closure of a loop ileostomy. All patients had a diverting ileostomy placed after low anterior resection (LAR) for rectal cancer. After closure of the ileostomy, there were no significant differences in the rates of postoperative ileus, postoperative bowel obstruction, or anastomotic leak between the two groups. The stapled closure led to a statistically significant reduction in operative time, although this mean difference was only 15 minutes, and the two techniques were equivalent in terms of outcomes at 30 days. This study supports surgeon preference and experience as a valid determinant for the method used for performing a small bowel anastomosis.

ANALYSIS

Introduction: Bowel obstruction is the main complication encountered after closure of an ileostomy. Previous studies comparing rates of bowel obstruction after hand-sewn versus stapled techniques for loop ileostomy closure have been small and single-center.

Objectives: The objective of the HASTA trial was to compare hand suture versus stapled loop ileostomy closure in a randomized controlled trial.

Methods
Trial Design: Multicenter pragmatic randomized controlled parallel-group superiority trial.

Participants
Inclusion Criteria: Patients ≥18 years of age, scheduled for elective ileostomy closure with history of LAR and creation of a protective loop ileostomy for rectal cancer.

Exclusion Criteria: Pathologic findings in routine preoperative diagnostic tests (eg, anastomotic leakage) that prevent ileostomy closure; participation in another intervention trial.

Intervention: The stapler group underwent side-to-side anastomosis with an Ethicon linear cutter-and-stapler (TLC 75), with loop apex and spout cross-stapled with the TLC and then oversewn with 5-0 polydioxanone equivalent suture. The hand suture technique was left to the discretion of each surgeon. A surgical workshop was carried out during the first investigators' meeting before the start of the trial, and skills (number of ileostomy closures, board certification) of all participating surgeons were recorded to correlate with the primary endpoint.

Endpoints

Primary Endpoint: Rate of bowel obstruction within 30 days of ileostomy closure.

Secondary Endpoints: Operative time, rate of wound infection, rate of reoperation due to anastomotic leakage of ileostomy closure, time to first tolerance of solid food and first bowel movement, length of postoperative hospital stay, mortality, and costs of surgical procedure.

Sample Size: 337 patients from 27 centers in Germany were randomized to stapled or hand-sewn ileostomy closure, 168 to stapler and 166 to hand-sewn.

Statistical Analysis: Sample size calculations, logistic regression model. Secondary variables were analyzed descriptively by tabulation of appropriate measures.

Results

Baseline Data: The groups were similar for patient and procedure characteristics. Mean time between LAR and ileostomy closure was 6 months, and 41% of ileostomy closures were performed as teaching procedures. Six of the hand-sewn group crossed over; 10 of the stapler group had hand-sewn closures.

Outcomes

Primary: The rate of bowel obstruction after one month did not differ significantly between the stapled and hand-sewn groups (10.3% vs. 16.6%, p 0.10). Technique of hand-sewn anastomosis (side-to-side vs. end-to-end) also had equivalent rates of bowel obstruction (p 0.76).

Secondary: Operative time was shorter in the stapled group, by a mean of 15 minutes ($p < 0.001$). There was no significant difference in rates of anastomotic leak between the two groups. Infection rate, time to food tolerance or bowel movement, and the mean duration of hospital stay were similar between the two groups.

Discussion

Conclusion: In patients undergoing takedown of a loop ileostomy, there is no difference in bowel obstruction, leak, or time to return of bowel function when comparing stapled to hand-sewn anastomoses.

Limitations: All patients in this study had their initial surgery performed for rectal cancer with placement of a loop ileostomy, and thus it is difficult to generalize these findings to patients having a small bowel anastomosis for another purpose. Additionally, this study had relatively short-term (30-day) follow-up.

---

f. Nonoperative Management in Adhesive Small Bowel Obstruction

Trials of nonoperative management exceeding 3 days are associated with increased morbidity in patients undergoing surgery for uncomplicated adhesive small bowel obstruction.

Keenan JE, Turley RS, McCoy CC, Migaly M, Shapiro ML, Scarborough JE

J Trauma Acute Care Surg. 2014;76(6):1367–1372.

SYNOPSIS

Takeaway Point: Nonoperative management of small bowel obstruction exceeding 3 days is associated with increased morbidity and postoperative length of hospitalization.

Commentary: This is a review of ACS-NSQIP data from 2005 to 2010. The authors reviewed patients who were admitted for adhesive small bowel obstructions and underwent surgery. They determined that trials of nonoperative management exceeding 3 days were associated with higher rates of postoperative infection, deep-space infection, urinary tract infection, and DVT. On the basis of these findings, the authors conclude that in general, trials of nonoperative management for adhesive small bowel obstruction should not exceed 3 days. It is worth noting that this is a retrospective database study, and does not include any small bowel obstructions that were successfully managed nonoperatively.

ANALYSIS

Introduction: The management of adhesive small bowel obstruction (ASBO) is a common but controversial topic in general surgery. In the absence of signs of intestinal compromise or complete obstruction, trials of nonoperative management are generally undertaken, but the optimal length of this trial is still a topic of debate.

Objectives: To determine the potential impact of incremental delays in the surgical management of patients with uncomplicated ASBO in whom an initial trial of nonoperative management has been attempted.

Methods

Trial Design: Retrospective review of ACS-NSQIP database.

Participants

Inclusion Criteria: Any patient who underwent a surgical procedure for treatment of an adhesive small bowel obstruction.

Exclusion Criteria: Operation on the first day of hospitalization, evidence of sepsis, operation more than 10 days after admission, previous operation within 30 days of the index operation, transfer from another facility, index operation by a non-general surgeon, outpatient classification, ASA 5 status, pregnancy.

Intervention: None.

Endpoints

Primary Endpoint: 30-day morbidity and mortality, length of hospitalization.

Secondary Endpoints: Specific complications (including surgical site infection, wound dehiscence, pneumonia, pulmonary embolism, major bleeding, systemic sepsis).

Sample Size: 9297 patients from the 2005–2010 ACS-NSQIP Participant User Files.

Statistical Analysis: ANOVA, Kruskal–Wallis test, nonparsimonious multivariate logistic or linear regression, and χ^2 test.

Results

Baseline Data: Overall, 34% of patients received operation after 1 day of hospitalization; 20% after 2 days; 14% after 3 days. Patients who received operations later in the course of their hospital stay were more likely to have concomitant diagnoses, and were less likely to have signs of SIRS preoperatively.

Outcomes: The overall rate of postoperative mortality was 4.4%, and the morbidity rate was 29.6%. Overall morbidity was increased in patients who had a preoperative stay of 3 days or greater, with an increase in surgical site infection (SSI), organ/deep-space SSI, urinary tract infection (UTI), and DVT. Overall 30-day mortality was not associated with preoperative length of hospitalization.

Discussion

Conclusion: Nonoperative management for adhesive small bowel obstruction exceeding 3 days is associated with higher postoperative morbidity and increased length of stay.

Limitations: This study was a retrospective review of the ACS-NSQIP database. The database does not include data on patients who had bowel obstructions that resolved without operative management, and thus it is difficult to generalize the results as the percentage of patients who would recover nonoperatively after 3 days is unknown. In addition, there were no data regarding imaging studies or physical exams, which would typically influence the decision to operate in the setting of ASBO. Patients who had delayed operations also had higher rates of comorbid conditions, which raises the possibility that the delay was due to higher operative risk.

REFERENCES

1. Matros E et al. Does gum chewing ameliorate postoperative ileus? Results of a prospective, randomized, placebo-controlled trial. *J Am Coll Surg.* 2006;202(5):773–778.

2. Wolff B et al. Alvimopan, a novel, peripherally acting mu opioid antagonist: Results of a multicenter, randomized, double-blind, placebo-controlled, phase III trial of major abdominal surgery and postoperative ileus. *Ann Surg.* 2004;240(4):728–734; discussion 734–735.

3. Biando S et al. Randomized clinical study of Gastrografin administration in patients with adhesive small bowel obstruction. *Br J Surg.* 2003;90(5):542–546.

4. Asao T et al. Gum chewing enhances early recovery from postoperative ileus after laparoscopic colectomy. *J Am Coll Surg.* 2002;195:30–32.

12

Appendix Surgery

Dre Irizarry • Stephen Odom

INTRODUCTION

Into the 18th century, descriptions of inflammatory diseases of the appendix appeared only as solitary case reports with conflicting nomenclature and an unclear natural history.[1] Only in the mid-19th century, when nitrous oxide and chloroform anesthesia granted a degree of safety to laparotomy, did early operation for appendicitis gain favor.[1] In contrast to these humble beginnings, appendectomy is now the most common emergency operation in the United States, with more than 300,000 appendectomies performed annually.[2]

Acute appendicitis arises from luminal obstruction by external compression (eg, lymphadenopathy) or internal obstruction by fecalith, tumor, ingested debris, or more rarely, parasites. If untreated, mucosal and serosal ischemia develops, followed by perforation with resultant peritoneal contamination and sepsis. The rise of antibiotics as a complement to surgical management has markedly decreased the septic consequences and mortality associated with this disease.

The diagnosis and management of appendicitis have changed in recent decades. Perhaps most significant is the acceptance of the laparoscopic approach for appendectomy, which will be discussed in this chapter.[3] New imaging modalities, including computed tomography and ultrasound, have improved preoperative diagnosis and reduced the traditional 20% negative appendectomy rate associated with diagnosis on the basis of physical examination alone.[4] Increasing use of clinical scoring systems has further refined diagnostic accuracy.[5,6] Controversies persist, however, particularly regarding the utility of interval appendectomy for complex appendicitis,[7] the use of irrigation in laparoscopic appendectomy,[8] and guidelines for nonoperative versus operative management.[9]

Historically, patients and surgeons have been reluctant to approach appendicitis nonoperatively, and randomized clinical trials demonstrate very high dropout or crossover rates from nonoperative arms.[10] As a result, most studies evaluating appendicitis are small and observational, with few randomized controlled trials. Similarly, the data on appendiceal cancers, which are rare but clinically relevant, exist primarily in the form of case series.[11] This chapter will review the available evidence directing the management of appendicitis and appendiceal malignancy, with the caveat that data quality is poor. Despite the paucity of rigorous studies, the importance of appendiceal disease to general surgery practice warrants careful consideration of the available data.

Retro.

a. Laparoscopic versus Open Appendectomy

Laparoscopic versus open appendectomy: Outcomes comparison based on a large administrative database.

Guller U, Hervey S, Purves H, Muhlbaier LH, Peterson ED, Eubanks S, Pietrobon R

Ann Surg. 2004;239(1):43–52.

SYNOPSIS

Takeaway Point: Laparoscopic appendectomy is associated with decreased length of hospital stay, decreased in-hospital morbidity, and increased rate of routine discharge compared with open appendectomy.

Commentary: Despite numerous case series and small randomized clinical trials, for years after the introduction of laparoscopic appendectomy there was no clear consensus regarding the comparative effectiveness of the laparoscopic versus open approach. This is the first study comparing length of hospital stay, in-hospital mortality and morbidity, and rate of routine discharge in patients undergoing laparoscopic and open appendectomy, using a representative US nationwide database. Overall, the authors report significant benefits to the laparoscopic approach. Although this is a retrospective database study with no long-term follow-up, this study contributed to the nationwide adoption of laparoscopic appendectomy as standard of care for acute appendicitis.

ANALYSIS

Introduction: The first laparoscopic appendectomy was performed in 1981. Since its introduction into surgical practice, numerous case series and small single institution trials have compared laparoscopic appendectomy (LA) with open appendectomy (OA), but no consensus regarding the effectiveness of each procedure has been reached.

Objectives: To compare the short-term impact of LA and OA based on a large administrative database.

Methods

Trial Design: Retrospective review of a large nationwide administrative database.

Participants

Inclusion Criteria: Patients in Nationwide Inpatient Sample (NIS) database with procedure codes for laparoscopic or open appendectomy.

Exclusion Criteria: Appendicolithiasis, appendicopathia oxyurica, and incidental appendectomies or primary diagnosis other than appendicitis.

Intervention: Laparoscopic versus open appendectomy.

Endpoints

Primary Endpoint: Length of hospital stay, in-hospital complications, in-hospital mortality, rate of routine discharge.

Secondary Endpoints: Above endpoints stratified by presence of abscess or perforation.

Sample Size: 43,757 patients selected from the Nationwide Inpatient Sample (NIS) of 1000 community hospitals in 22 US states in 1997; 7618 underwent laparoscopic appendectomy and 36,139 underwent open appendectomy.

Statistical Analysis: Student's t-tests, χ^2 test, analysis of variance, multiple linear regression models, exponentiating estimated log-transformed length of stay, multiple logistic regression analyses.

Results

Baseline Data: Patients in the laparoscopic group were more likely Caucasian (63.5% vs. 56.7%, p 0.003) and female (49.8% vs. 39.6%, $p < 0.0001$) with higher median income (p 0.02). Patients who underwent open appendectomy were overall sicker, with a higher Devo Index ($p < 0.0001$) and significantly higher rates of hypertension, congestive heart failure, and diabetes. Patients in the open group also had higher rates of appendiceal perforation (21% vs. 16.1%, $p < 0.0001$) and appendiceal abscess (14% vs. 7%, $p < 0.0001$).

Outcomes: After adjusting for other risk factors, the laparoscopic appendectomy group had a shorter median hospital stay ($p < 0.0001$), higher rate of routine discharge ($p < 0.0001$), lower overall complication rate ($p\ 0.02$), decreased rate of gastrointestinal complications ($p\ 0.02$), and lower rate of infections ($p < 0.001$). When stratified by presence of appendiceal abscess or perforation, patients undergoing laparoscopic appendectomy still had shorter length of stay ($p < 0.001$), and higher rate of routine discharge ($p < 0.0001$).

Discussion

Conclusion: Laparoscopic appendectomy has significant advantages over open appendectomy, including decreased hospital length of stay, decreased in-hospital morbidity, and increased rate of routine discharge.

Limitations: Adults only, retrospective database study, outpatient follow-up data not captured, patients with perforation and abscess more likely to undergo open than laparoscopic procedures. Patients with appendicoliths were excluded which may impact generalizability. Large administrative database, so some miscoding is possible.

Retro. Cohort

b. Interval Appendectomy ~~Saved~~ .

Routine interval appendectomy is not justified after initial nonoperative treatment of acute appendicitis.

Kaminski A, Liu IL, Applebaum H, Lee SL, Haigh PI

Arch Surg. 2005;140(9):897–901.

SYNOPSIS

Takeaway Point: Interval appendectomy following initial nonoperative treatment of acute appendicitis may not be justified.

Commentary: Classically, interval appendectomy is performed 6–10 weeks after initial nonoperative management of acute appendicitis. Small case series have demonstrated recurrence rates of anywhere between 5[12] and 35%.[13] This is a retrospective cohort study examining the natural history of patients treated nonoperatively for an initial episode of acute appendicitis. The authors utilize an insurance database and determine that overall recurrence rate after nonoperative management for acute appendicitis is 5%, with a mean follow-up time of 4 years. Given the low recurrence rate, the authors argue that routine interval appendectomy is not justified. This is a database study, and has a number of important limitations. The number of false-positive diagnoses cannot be ascertained, as patients were identified on the basis of ICD-9 code and no imaging confirmation was required. The study includes both children and adults, and does not specify differences in antibiotic duration or treatment regimens. Additionally, patients have a wide range of follow-up, and 4 years may be insufficient, especially in a pediatric population, to judge the true risks and benefits of foregoing interval appendectomy. Despite these limitations, this remains one of the largest studies to date on the subject of interval appendectomy after nonoperative management of acute appendicitis, and provides important evidence on the natural history of this disease.

ANALYSIS

Introduction: Initial nonoperative management in patients presenting with acute appendicitis complicated by abscess or phlegmon has been shown to be safe and effective. The risk of recurrent appendicitis ranges from 5 to 37% in small studies with limited follow-up periods. In the pediatric population, interval appendectomy after initial nonoperative management is common, despite lack of strong evidence to support this practice.

Objectives: To determine whether interval appendectomy is justified following initial nonoperative treatment of acute appendicitis.

Methods
Trial Design: Retrospective cohort study.

Participants
Inclusion Criteria: ICD-9 code for acute appendicitis, initial nonoperative management.

Exclusion Criteria: None.

Intervention: Interval appendectomy or nonoperative treatment with or without percutaneous drainage of abscess.

Endpoints
Primary Endpoints: Recurrent appendicitis following nonoperative management.

Secondary Endpoint: Hospital length of stay.

Sample Size: 32,938 patients were initially identified with acute appendicitis from 12 acute care hospitals in the Southern California Kaiser Permanente Discharge Abstract Database between January 1992 and December 2004; of these, 1012 were managed nonoperatively.

Statistical Analysis: Cox proportional hazards regression modeling, Kaplan–Meier method with log-rank test, Wilcoxon rank sum test.

Results

Baseline Data/Outcomes: 1012 patients were treated initially with nonoperative management; of these 148 had an interval appendectomy. Of the 864 that did not have interval appendectomy, 39 had a recurrence (5%).

Of these, 22 underwent appendectomy, 2 underwent cecectomy, 2 underwent right hemicolectomy, and 13 were treated nonoperatively for a second time. Median length of stay for the second hospitalization in the recurrent appendicitis group was 4 days compared with 6 days in the interval appendectomy group (p 0.006); however, the median cumulative length of stay (including the first and second hospital stays) in the patients who recurred was the same as those who underwent interval appendectomy. Patients were followed for a median of 4 years, with follow-up ranging from 6 months to 12 years. 26 patients were lost to follow-up.

Discussion

Conclusion: For patients with acute appendicitis initially treated nonoperatively, the recurrence rate is low and routine interval appendectomy is not justified.

Limitations: Retrospective study, does not separate children and adults, does not specify differences in antibiotic duration/treatment regimens between treatment groups, does not account for patients with follow-up at outside hospitals. Significant variations in follow-up time and no breakdown of recurrence rate by year. Diagnosis of acute appendicitis was based on ICD-9 codes and the rate of false positive diagnoses cannot be determined.

---

c. Malignancies of the Appendix

Malignancies of the appendix: Beyond case series reports.

McGory ML, Maggard MA, Kang H, O'Connell JB, Ko CY

Dis Colon Rectum. 2005;48(12):2264–2271.

SYNOPSIS

Takeaway Point: A substantial number of patients with appendiceal carcinoma, both carcinoid and noncarcinoid, may not receive adequate surgical resection.

Commentary: While prior discussions of appendiceal cancer have focused on carcinoid tumors, this study shows that noncarcinoid tumors are far more common. The literature to date shows no clear consensus on optimal treatment for noncarcinoid appendiceal cancer. As these are rare tumors, it is difficult to perform a study with a large sample size, which is why reviewing the SEER database is advantageous in this population. There are, however, limitations encountered when using this database, including the fact that tumor location, patient comorbidities, reason for appendectomy, and information regarding adjuvant chemotherapy/radiation are not included in the database. Additionally, SEER collected data on operations between 1973 and 2001; during and since that time, recommendations for appendiceal cancer have changed. This paper highlights the difficulty in obtaining high quality evidence for a rare disease, and the need for further studies and better clinical guidelines.

ANALYSIS

Introduction: Appendiceal carcinomas are extremely rare, with an incidence of less than 1 per 1,000,000 people per year. The majority of these tumors are diagnosed incidentally during routine appendectomy. Most current guidelines recommend appendectomy for carcinoid tumors ≤1 cm, and right hemicolectomy for all noncarcinoid invasive subtypes as well as for carcinoids ≥2 cm or located at the base of the appendix or invading the mesoappendix. The recommendations for management of carcinoid tumors are much more homogeneous than those for noncarcinoid tumors, as these are rare cancers and difficult to study.

Objectives: To evaluate the epidemiology and survival outcomes of five histologic types of appendiceal carcinoma, accounting for tumor size.

Methods

Trial Design: Retrospective review of Surveillance, Epidemiology, and End Results (SEER) database.

Participants

Inclusion Criteria: All appendiceal cancer patients in SEER database.

Exclusion Criteria: None.

Intervention: None (retrospective database review).

Endpoints

Primary Endpoint: Tumor incidence, stage, 5-year survival determined for each histological type.

Secondary Endpoints: Appropriateness of operative procedure by tumor type and size.

Sample Size: 2514 cases of appendiceal cancer obtained from SEER database between the years 1973 and 2001: mucinous (38%), adenocarcinoma (26%), carcinoid (17%), goblet (15%), and signet (4%). SEER is a national population-based tumor registry reflecting 11 regional registries, comprising 14% of the population designed to reflect the overall characteristics of the United States.

Statistical Analysis: Kaplan–Meier estimator for observed 5-year survival, survival data compared between groups using log-rank χ^2 test of equality; χ^2 and two-sided Fisher exact test.

Results

Baseline Data: Carcinoid had the youngest age at presentation in comparison to other subtypes ($p < 0.001$), and the highest proportion of females (71%, $p < 0.001$). Average tumor size at presentation was 5.2 cm for mucinous, 2.5 cm for carcinoid, and 2.4 cm for goblet. Carcinoid and goblet tumors had the highest proportion of localized disease at presentation, and mucinous and signet had the lowest proportion of localized disease, but also highest proportion of distant disease at presentation. Distribution of tumor histology was different with regard to tumor size: most common tumor type presenting at >2 cm was mucinous, whereas the most common tumor type presenting at <1 cm was goblet.

Outcomes: Non-stage-specific survival rates were highest for carcinoid (83%) and lowest for signet (18%). In terms of appropriateness of procedure, 28% of carcinoids >2 cm underwent appendectomy alone. Only 40% of T4 tumors were removed via en bloc resection, where 35% underwent colectomy without en bloc resection, and 25% underwent appendectomy alone.

Discussion

Conclusion: A substantial number of patients with appendiceal carcinoma, both carcinoid and noncarcinoid, may not receive adequate surgical resection. The authors propose treating all appendiceal masses with right hemicolectomy, as only a small percent are carcinoids <2 cm, and therefore only this small percentage would be over treated.

Limitations: SEER collects data on the most definitive surgery for a cancer diagnosis. If, for example, a patient had an initial appendectomy, followed by a colectomy, the last surgery would be considered "definitive." This may result in underestimating the number of appendectomies performed. The database includes operations between 1973 and 2001, during which time recommendations for appendiceal cancer have changed. This is not accounted for in the analysis. Tumor location (base vs. tip of appendix), adjuvant chemotherapy/radiation, reason for appendectomy, and patient comorbidities are not included in the SEER database.

---

d. Interval Appendectomy for Perforated Appendicitis

Early vs interval appendectomy for children with perforated appendicitis. ℞𝒞𝒯.

Blakely ML, Williams R, Dassinger MS, Eubanks JW 3rd, Fischer P, Huang EY, Paton E, Culbreath B, Hester A, Streck C, Hixson SD, Langham MR Jr

Arch Surg. 2011;146(6):660–665.

SYNOPSIS

Takeaway Point: Early appendectomy for children with perforated appendicitis significantly reduces time away from normal activities and is associated with significantly fewer adverse events when compared with interval appendectomy.

Commentary: This is the first adequately powered randomized trial to compare early versus interval appendectomy for perforated appendicitis. Perforated appendicitis has been treated with either urgent operation, or nonoperative management with antibiotics and interval appendectomy in 6–8 weeks. The authors demonstrate that early appendectomy for these children is associated with faster recovery and fewer adverse events. The results of this pediatric trial are not necessarily generalizable to an adult population, or to patients with a well-formed abscess at time of presentation. Despite these limitations, this large randomized trial represents a significant addition to the literature on appendicitis management.

ANALYSIS

Introduction: The standard of care for treatment of acute nonperforated appendicitis is early appendectomy. The optimal treatment for acute perforated appendicitis, however, is controversial.

Retrospective studies have shown improved outcomes and shorter hospital length of stay with interval appendectomy; however, no adequately powered randomized trial has compared this to immediate operation.

Objectives: To compare the effectiveness and adverse event rates of early versus interval appendectomy in children with perforated appendicitis.

Methods

Trial Design: Nonblinded randomized controlled trial.

Participants

Inclusion Criteria: Age <18 with clinical diagnosis of perforated appendicitis defined by history, physical exam, laboratory values, and imaging.

Exclusion Criteria: Initial treatment at another institution, delayed presentation with a well-formed abscess or mass on examination, family transient to the area, inability to complete follow-up.

Intervention: Early (within 24 hours of admission) versus interval (6–8 weeks after diagnosis) appendectomy.

Endpoints

Primary Endpoint: Time away from normal activities.

Secondary Endpoints: Intraabdominal abscess, surgical site infection, total length of hospital stay, need for central line, need for interventional radiology (IR) procedure, complication rates from IR procedures, other adverse events.

Sample Size: 131 patients at a single tertiary referral urban children's hospital from October 2006 to August 2009, 64 randomized to early appendectomy and 67 randomized to interval appendectomy.

Statistical Analysis: Sample size calculation, intention-to-treat analysis, χ^2 test, Fisher exact test, and t-tests.

Results

Baseline Data: Baseline characteristics were well balanced between the groups. Mean age was 10.5 years for early appendectomy group and 9.9 for interval appendectomy group.

Outcomes: Early appendectomy reduced time away from normal activities when compared with interval appendectomy ($p < 0.001$). Total length of stay for early appendectomy was 9.0 days compared to 11.2 days for interval appendectomy (p 0.03). There was no difference in the total duration of intravenous antibiotics between the groups. The overall adverse event rate was 55% for interval appendectomy compared to only 30% with early appendectomy (p 0.003). Intraabdominal abscess subsequent to admission, small bowel obstruction, recurrent appendicitis, and unplanned readmission were more likely in the interval appendectomy group. Seven patients (11%) in the early appendectomy group had a diagnosis other than perforated appendicitis at time of operation, compared with one patient in the interval group.

Discussion

Conclusion: Early appendectomy for children with perforated appendicitis without preoperative well-formed abscess significantly reduces time away from normal activities and is associated with significantly lower adverse event rates when compared with interval appendectomy.

Limitations: Pediatric population. Does not address appendicitis with abscess formation or phlegmon. A moderate number of patients (11%) in the early appendectomy group had diagnoses other than perforated appendicitis at time of operation.

---

e. Irrigation in Laparoscopic Appendectomy

Irrigation versus suction alone during laparoscopic appendectomy for perforated appendicitis: A prospective randomized trial.

St Peter SD, Adibe OO, Iqbal CW, Fike FB, Sharp SW, Juang D, Lanning D, Murphy JP, Andrews WS, Sharp RJ, Snyder CL, Holcomb GW, Ostlie DJ

Ann Surg. 2012;256(4):581–585.

SYNOPSIS

Takeaway Point: There is no benefit to irrigation versus suction alone during laparoscopic appendectomy for children with perforated appendicitis.

Commentary: The efficacy of irrigating the peritoneal cavity during appendectomy for perforated appendicitis is controversial. Most studies on the topic are not randomized, and focus on open surgery, which now constitutes a minority of cases. This study represents the first prospective randomized trial comparing irrigation to suction alone in laparoscopic appendectomy for perforated appendicitis. Although limited to the pediatric population, this single-institution randomized clinical trial provides good evidence against routine irrigation during appendectomy for perforated appendicitis.

ANALYSIS

Introduction: Historically, peritoneal irrigation with or without antibiotic solution has been recommended for peritoneal contamination. Several studies have attempted to examine the utility of irrigation for perforated appendicitis, but these have been small, retrospective trials focused on open appendectomies, and yielded conflicting results.

Objectives: To determine whether there is a difference in postoperative abscess rates in children undergoing laparoscopic appendectomy for perforated appendicitis using irrigation versus suction alone.

Methods

Trial Design: Prospective randomized controlled trial.

Participants

Inclusion Criteria: Age <18 with perforated appendicitis (defined as a fecalith in the abdomen or a rent seen in the appendix).

Exclusion Criteria: Uncomplicated appendicitis.

Intervention: Minimum 500 mL irrigation with sterile saline versus suction alone during laparoscopic appendectomy for perforated appendicitis. Antibiotic prophylaxis and wound closure was standard for both groups.

Endpoints

Primary Endpoint: Postoperative abscess.

Secondary Endpoints: Time to starting clear liquids or regular diet, time to discharge from hospital, hospital charges, mean postoperative maximum daily temperatures, return admission for small bowel obstruction.

Sample Size: 220 patients between December 2008 and July 2011 at one center with 7 surgeons, 110 randomized to irrigation and 110 to suction alone.

Statistical Analysis: Sample size calculation, two-tailed Student t-test, two-tailed Fisher exact, and χ^2 with Yates correction.

Results

Baseline Data: The two groups were well matched for baseline characteristics, including age (mean age 9.7 for suction only group, 10.4 for irrigation group), sex, days of symptoms, and white blood count at admission.

Outcomes: There was no significant difference in abscess rate with irrigation versus suction alone (18.3% vs. 19.1%, p 1.0). Hospital costs, time to advancing diet, time to discharge, and mean maximum daily temperatures were statistically equivalent. There was no significant difference between the two groups in readmission for small bowel obstruction. Irrigation was associated with a trend towards longer operative time (42.8 vs. 38.7 minutes, p 0.056).

Discussion

Conclusion: Irrigation during laparoscopic appendectomy for perforated appendicitis is an additional step in the operation that holds no benefit, and the practice is not recommended.

Limitations: Pediatric population only, only immediate appendectomy. No long-term follow-up.

---

f. Duration of Postoperative Antibiotic Treatment

Duration of antibiotic treatment after appendectomy for acute complicated appendicitis.

van Rossem CC, Schreinemacher MH, Treskes K, van Hogezand RM, van Geloven AA

Br J Surg. 2014;101(6):715–719.

SYNOPSIS

Takeaway Point: There is no difference in infectious complications between 3 and 5 days of postoperative antibiotic treatment following appendectomy for complicated appendicitis.

Commentary: To prevent wound infection or intraabdominal abscess, patients with complicated appendicitis are generally prescribed a variable course of postoperative antibiotics. The authors present an observational cohort study comparing two hospitals with different antibiotic protocols; one hospital prescribes 3 days of postoperative antibiotics, and the other prescribes 5 days. They report no difference in infectious complications between the sites. It is worth noting that during the enrollment period, laparoscopic technique was introduced and in the final years became the prevailing technique. Additionally, all patients were given postoperative intravenous antibiotic regimen, requiring either a prolonged length of stay or discharge with a peripherally inserted central catheter. While the study has significant limitations, in the absence of a prospective trial, most surgeons now prescribe only three days of postoperative antibiotics following appendectomy for complex appendicitis.

ANALYSIS

Introduction: Wound infection and intraabdominal abscess are more common after complicated appendicitis than in cases without perforation or abscess. While complicated appendicitis is frequently treated with appendectomy and postoperative antibiotics, there is no consensus on appropriate antibiotic duration.

Objectives: To compare rates of postoperative infection in adults treated with 3 versus 5 days of antibiotics following appendectomy for acute complicated appendicitis.

Methods

Trial Design: Observational cohort study.

Participants

Inclusion Criteria: Adult patients with complex appendicitis (perforation or purulence) who underwent laparoscopic or open appendectomy for suspected acute appendicitis.

Exclusion Criteria: Patients with uncomplicated appendicitis.

Intervention: Three versus 5 days of intravenous cefuroxime and metronidazole, depending on hospital site.

Endpoints

Primary Endpoint: Development of postoperative infection (superficial wound infection or deep intraabdominal infection) for which readmission, reintervention, or additional antibiotic treatment was necessary.

Secondary Endpoints: Infectious complications.

Sample Size: 267 patients at two hospital locations in the Netherlands between January 2004 and December 2010 with complicated appendicitis. By hospital protocol, location A prescribed 3 days of postoperative antibiotics (126 patients treated at location A), and location B (141 patients) prescribed 5 days of antibiotics. Because some patients were given more or less antibiotic than hospital protocol, the analysis was performed based on antibiotic received, rather than location. 135 patients received 3 days of postoperative antibiotics, and 123 received 5 days.

Statistical Analysis: Student's t-test for normally distributed variables; Mann–Whitney U test; χ^2 test; univariate and multivariable logistic regression model.

Results

Baseline Data: The groups had a similar age and gender distribution. Patients at location B (assigned to 5 days of antibiotics) were significantly more likely to undergo an open procedure (89.4% vs. 42.9%, $p < 0.001$) and had significantly shorter operating time for either open (42 vs. 74 minutes) or laparoscopic (53 vs. 82 minutes, $p < 0.001$) cases.

Outcomes: There was no difference in postoperative wound infection or intraabdominal abscesses in the 3-day antibiotic treatment group versus the 5-day antibiotic treatment group. Laparoscopic approach was found to have higher rate of developing postoperative intraabdominal abscesses in univariable analysis, but not in multivariable analysis. The open approach had a higher rate of postoperative superficial wound infections.

Discussion
Conclusion: Three days of antibiotic treatment following appendectomy for complicated appendicitis is as effective as 5 days in reducing postoperative infections.

Limitations: Retrospective study, at two separate locations, each with its own practices and protocols. Patients were analyzed by number of antibiotic days received, not intention-to-treat analysis based on location protocol, but reason for protocol violations are not explained.

---

g. NOTA Study

The NOTA Study (Non Operative Treatment for Acute Appendicitis): Prospective study on the efficacy and safety of antibiotics (amoxicillin and clavulanic acid) for treating patients with right lower quadrant abdominal pain and long-term follow-up of conservatively treated suspected appendicitis.

Di Saverio S, Sibilio A, Giorgini E, Biscardi A, Villani S, Coccolini F, Smerieri N, Pisano M, Ansaloni L, Sartelli M, Catena F, Tugnoli G

Ann Surg. 2014;260(1):109–117.

SYNOPSIS

Takeaway Point: Nonoperative management of acute appendicitis is safe and effective, with a recurrence rate of 13.8% at 2 years.

Commentary: The majority of surgical textbooks in the United States recommend appendectomy for acute appendicitis, as it is a curative operation with low associated morbidity. There are potential complications to any surgery, however, and a recent prospective study in Sweden showed that the rate of postoperative complications after appendectomy was equal to the rate of relapse in antibiotic-treated patients at one year.[14] While nonoperative management is becoming more popular, the safety and long-term risks are not well established. The current study evaluates the outcomes of patients treated nonoperatively, and also utilizes a clinical scoring system to identify patients best suited for nonoperative management. The majority of patients with nonperforated appendicitis were successfully managed conservatively, with an 11.9% immediate failure rate and a 13.8% recurrence rate at 2 years. The study does have significant limitations, including utilizing a clinical scoring system (Alvarado score) that overpredicts appendicitis in women, in a predominantly female population group. Additionally, the study was observational only, and not all patients had confirmatory imaging. While this does not resolve the debate regarding nonoperative versus surgical management of appendicitis, it does provide compelling evidence for conservative treatment in appropriately selected patients.

ANALYSIS

Introduction: Appendectomy carries risks of bleeding, infection, incisional hernia, and anesthesia complications, as well as considerable hospital costs. Previous small studies comparing outcomes after nonoperative management (NOM) of appendicitis with appendectomy have had contradictory results, and there is no algorithm to determine which patients are most likely to benefit from nonoperative management.

Objectives: To evaluate the outcome of patients treated nonoperatively with antibiotics and to assess the reliability of the initial clinical evaluation in predicting which nonoperatively treated patients should have been treated surgically.

Methods

Trial Design: Prospective, observational cohort study.

Participants: Patients who presented to the emergency department with clinically suspected nonruptured acute appendicitis.

Inclusion Criteria: Age >14, lower abdominal pain or right iliac fossa pain, clinical diagnosis of attending general surgeon, confirmed by either Alvarado and/or Appendicitis Inflammatory Response (AIR) scores.

Exclusion Criteria: Diffuse peritonitis, penicillin allergy, ongoing antibiotic therapy, history of appendectomy, pregnancy, inflammatory bowel disease (IBD) history, or suspicion of IBD.

Intervention: All patients had CBC, CRP, and abdominal US and/or abdominal CT scan at the discretion of the surgeon. Standardized NOM included a 5–7-day course of amoxicillin and clavulanate. Reassessment as an outpatient was performed at 5 days. Telephone follow-up was done at 7 and 15 days, 6 months, and 1 and 2 years.

Endpoints

Primary Endpoints: Readmission due to lack of clinical improvement and/or increasing abdominal pain, incidence of appendicitis recurrences within two years, safety of antibiotic treatment.

Secondary Endpoints: Minor complications, abdominal pain after discharge, length of hospital stay, number of follow-up clinic appointments, number of sick leave days.

Sample Size: 159 patients from one center in Bologna, Italy between January 1, 2010, and December 31, 2010.

Statistical Analysis: Descriptive statistics, χ^2 test, Student's paired t-test, Mann–Whitney U-test.

Results

Baseline Data: 159 patients were enrolled to undergo NOM, 41 men and 118 women. 73% had an abdominal ultrasound, and 76% of these were positive for acute appendicitis. 17% of patients underwent CT scan; 78% of scans were positive for nonperforated appendicitis.

Outcomes: Failure of NOM was 11.9% in the first 7 days, and all of these patients ($n = 19$) received operation. Of these, one patient had an intraabdominal abscess, and six had surgical site infection. At 6 months, 17 recurrent episodes (10.7%) were reported. Another three patients recurred at one year. Overall, 22 recurrent episodes occurred in 2 years of follow-up, and 14 of these were successfully treated with antibiotics alone; the remaining 8 required surgery. No major side effects were reported with antibiotic treatment. Mean hospital length of stay was 0.4 days, and mean sick leave was 5.8 days. Mean number of outpatient follow-up visits was 1.3. No postoperative complication was recorded among patients who failed NOM.

Discussion

Conclusion: Antibiotic therapy for suspected acute nonperforated appendicitis reduces the need for operation and results in shorter sick leave time. On 2-year follow-up, 13.8% of patients had developed recurrence and most were safely treated with another course of antibiotics.

Limitations: The Alvarado score can significantly overpredict appendicitis in females, and the majority of the patients in the study were female. A significant number of patients had imaging that did not support the diagnosis of appendicitis, which may have confounded the outcomes. Study applies only to nonperforated appendicitis. No formal cost-benefit analysis. Observational, single-institution study.

h. Surgery versus Conservative Treatment for Appendiceal Abscess

Laparoscopic surgery or conservative treatment for appendiceal abscess in adults? A randomized controlled trial.

Mentula P, Sammalkorpi H, Leppäniemi A

Ann Surg. 2015;262(2):237–242.

SYNOPSIS

Takeaway Point: Laparoscopic surgery is a safe and feasible first-line option for treatment of appendiceal abscess, and is associated with fewer readmissions and additional interventions than conservative treatment.

Commentary: This is the first randomized prospective trial comparing acute surgery to nonoperative management in the adult population for appendiceal abscess. The management of initial treatment for adults presenting with appendiceal abscess is controversial, and initial medical management (antibiotics with percutaneous drainage with or without interval appendectomy) has been favored in previous literature. The authors demonstrate that laparoscopic surgery is a safe and feasible first-line option for treatment of appendiceal abscess, and is associated with fewer readmissions and additional interventions than conservative treatment. The results of this trial do not inform us of complications occurring past 60 days. Despite this, this prospective randomized trial represents a significant addition to the literature on appendicitis management.

ANALYSIS

Introduction: Approximately 7% of adult patients with acute appendicitis present with an appendiceal abscess, and management is controversial. Two prior meta-analyses demonstrated a lower complication and morbidity rate with a conservative approach, but the scant available prospective data present a mixed picture.

Objectives: To compare recovery time after immediate laparoscopic surgery versus conservative management for appendiceal abscess.

Methods
Trial Design: Single-center randomized controlled trial with two parallel groups designed to identify superiority.

Participants

Inclusion Criteria: Adult patients presenting with appendiceal abscess of at least 2 cm on CT, US, or both.

Exclusion Criteria: Antimicrobial therapy for >24 hours prior to randomization, attempted drainage prior to randomization, age >80 or <18, pregnancy, allergy to cefuroxime or metronidazole, severe chronic disease that would substantially increase operative mortality, previous major intraabdominal surgery that could have caused intraabdominal adhesions, carrier of a resistant bacterial strain, history of institutionalization or hospitalization for ≥2 weeks before randomization, suspicion of malignant disease, and patients with clinically diffuse peritonitis.

Intervention: Both groups received intravenous cefuroxime 1.5 g three times per day and metronidazole 500 mg three times per day until the patient was afebrile for 24 hours and CRP was declining and below 150 mg/L. After discharge patients were given oral cephalexin 500 mg three times per day and metronidazole 500 mg three times per day for 7 days.

Conservative Group: If largest diameter of abscess was ≥3 cm, ultrasound-guided percutaneous drainage of the abscess was attempted as soon as possible. If this was not feasible, needle aspiration of the abscess was attempted.

Laparoscopy Group: Laparoscopic appendectomy within 8 hours of randomization, abscess was entered and drained with a suction device, and the appendix was removed through an endocatch bag. If no appendix was found, laparoscopic drainage of the abscess was considered an adequate treatment.

Endpoints

Primary Endpoint: Hospital stay, both primary as well as readmission, within 60 days.

Secondary Endpoints: Need for additional interventions, residual abscess on day 7 after randomization, complications, number of recurrent abscesses within 60 days of randomization, and rate of failure of attempted procedure (drainage or appendectomy).

Sample Size: 60 patients at a single tertiary referral center from February 2011 to August 2014, 30 randomized to laparoscopic group and 30 randomized to conservative group.

Statistical Analysis: Two sample t-tests, Mann–Whitney U, Fisher exact test, intention-to-treat analysis.

Results
Baseline Data: Baseline characteristics were well balanced between the groups. Median age was 45 for the laparoscopy group and 46 for the conservative group.

Outcomes: Median total hospital stay during 60 days from randomization was 4 days, and this did not differ significantly between the laparoscopic and conservative groups. The rate of readmission was higher in the conservative group (p 0.026), with more patients in the conservative group needing additional interventions (p 0.042). Residual or recurrent abscess rate was statistically similar between the groups. The overall rate of uneventful recovery within 60 days was 90% in the laparoscopy group and 50% in the conservative group (p 0.002).

Discussion
Conclusion: Laparoscopic surgery is a safe and feasible first-line option for treatment of appendiceal abscess, and is associated with fewer readmissions and additional interventions than conservative treatment.

Limitations: Does not account for longer-term complication, or recurrent appendicitis of stump past 60 days. Did not take location or accessibility of abscess into account (ie, presence of intervening bowel precluding percutaneous drainage). Results may not be generalizable as this study was single-site and mostly single-surgeon.

REFERENCES
1. Williams GR. Presidential Address: A history of appendicitis with anecdotes illustrating its importance. *Ann Surg.* 1983;197(5):495–506.
2. Lowry SF, Davidov T, Shiroff AM. Appendicitis and appendiceal abscess. In: Fischer J, ed. *Fischer's Mastery of Surgery*, 6th ed. Philadelphia: Lippincott Williams & Wilkins; 2012:149.
3. Guller U, Hervey S, Purves H, Muhlbaier LH, Peterson ED, Eubanks S, et al. Laparoscopic versus open appendectomy: Outcomes comparison based on a large administrative database. *Ann Surg.* 2004;239(1):43–52.

4. Drake FT, Flum DR. Improvement in the diagnosis of appendicitis. *Adv Surg.* 2013;47:299–328.

5. Alvarado A. A practical score for the early diagnosis of acute appendicitis. *Ann Emerg Med.* 1986;15:557–564.

6. Andersson M, Andersson RE: The appendicitis inflammatory response score: A tool for the diagnosis of acute appendicitis that outperforms the Alvarado score. *World J Surg.* 2008;32:1843–1849.

7. BlakComely ML, Williams R, Dassinger MS, Eubanks JW 3rd, Fischer P, Huang EY, et al. Early vs interval appendectomy for children with perforated appendicitis. *Arch Surg.* 2011;146(6):660–655.

8. St Peter SD, Adibe OO, Iqbal CW, Fike FB, Sharp SW, Juang D, et al. Irrigation versus suction alone during laparoscopic appendectomy for perforated appendicitis: A prospective randomized trial. *Ann Surg.* 2012;256(4):581–585.

9. Di Saverio S, Sibilio A, Giorgini E, Biscardi A, Villani S, Coccolini F, et al. The NOTA Study (Non Operative Treatment for Acute Appendicitis): Prospective study on the efficacy and safety of antibiotics (amoxicillin and clavulanic acid) for treating patients with right lower quadrant abdominal pain and long-term follow-up of conservatively treated suspected appendicitis. *Ann Surg.* 2014;260(1):109–117.

10. Liang MK et al. The appendix. In: Brunicardi FC et al. *Schwartz's Principles of Surgery*, 10th ed. New York: McGraw-Hill; 2014 (no page given; available via AccessSurgery at http://accesssurgery.mhmedical.com.proxy1.lib.tju.edu/content.aspx?bookid=980&Sectionid=59610872; accessed 6/23/15).

11. McGory ML, Maggard MA, Kang H, O'Connell JB, Ko CY. Malignancies of the appendix: Beyond the case series reports. *Dis Colon Rectum.* 2005;48(12):2264–2271.

12. Kaminski A, Liu IL, Applebaum H, Lee SL, Haigh PI. Routine interval appendectomy is not justified after initial nonoperative treatment of acute appendicitis. *Arch Surg.* 2005;140(9):897–901.

13. Eriksson S, Granstrom L. Randomized controlled trial of appendicotomy versus antibiotic therapy for acute appendicitis. *Br J Surg.* 1995;82(2):166–169.

14. Hansson J, Korner U, Khorram-Manesh A, et al. Randomized clinical trial of antibiotic therapy versus appendectomy. *Br J Surg.* 2000;96:473–481.

13

Bariatric Surgery

Yulia Zak • Denise Gee

Over 15 million adult Americans (6.6% of the population) had a BMI > 40 kg/m^2 in 2013, and the rate of obesity continues to rise.[1] Obesity is associated with increased morbidity and mortality.[2] Approximately 179,000 weight loss procedures were performed in the United States in 2013, and strong data now demonstrate that bariatric surgery decreases morbidity and mortality in obese patients.[3]

The first published bariatric case series was performed in the early 1960s by Payne and colleagues.[4] The authors described the jejunocolic bypass, an operation aimed purely at malabsorption, that consisted of dividing the proximal jejunum 35–50 cm from the ligament of Treitz and anastomosing it to the proximal transverse colon.[4] Although this resulted in successful weight loss, virtually all the patients suffered from diarrhea, dehydration, and severe electrolyte imbalances.[5] In an attempt to avoid these complications, jejunoileal bypass replaced the jejunocolic, with an anastomosis performed 10 cm proximal to the ileocecal valve, and with the bypassed small intestine anastomosed to the transverse or sigmoid colon. This operation, however, was also fraught with complications, including diarrhea, dehydration, vitamin and mineral deficiencies, protein depletion, polyarthralgia, hepatic insufficiency, and ultimately, weight regain.[6,7]

The high morbidity rate of these procedures led to the exploration of weight loss operations that combined malabsorption with restriction. Biliopancreatic diversion with partial distal gastrectomy and Roux-en-Y reconstruction became popular in the 1970s. Subsequently, the biliopancreatic diversion with duodenal switch, where a sleeve gastrectomy maintained the integrity of the pylorus and proximal duodenum, became popular in the late 1990s. These procedures led not only to significant excess weight loss, but also to very high rates of remission of diabetes mellitus, hypertension, and hyperlipidemia.[8–10] The Roux-en-Y gastric bypass configuration (RYGB) also appeared in the 1970s, proving to be superior to jejuno-ileal bypass with regard to its complication rates.[11,12] Unfortunately these operations still carried significant malabsorptive side effects, leading some surgeons to favor purely restrictive procedures, such as nonadjustable vertical banded gastroplasty (VBG), and later, adjustable gastric banding (AGB). These are less successful than the RYGB in weight loss and reduction of obesity-related comorbidities such as diabetes mellitus. They also have their own procedure-related complications, including staple line dehiscence or stoma stenosis after VBG, and band slippage or erosion with the AGB.[6,13,14]

The final bariatric procedure that was initially conceived as a solely restrictive solution, but which has since been shown to induce concurrent metabolic changes, is the standalone sleeve gastrectomy, in which the fundus and the lateral 80% of the body of the stomach is resected. It was initially used in superobese patients with BMI > 50 as a first stage before proceeding with duodenal switch or gastric bypass. However, over the last 10 years the laparoscopic version of this operation [laparoscopic sleeve gastrectomy (LSG)] has become the most prevalent surgical approach to morbid obesity, surpassing the laparoscopic RYGB and AGB. Although unequivocal long-term data about the outcomes of LSG has yet to be published, middle-term data discussed in this chapter demonstrate that it is a safe procedure with weight loss outcomes better than those after gastric banding, although slightly worse than those after RYGB.[15,16]

The improved safety profile of the most frequently performed weight loss procedures today, LRYGB and LSG, is due in part to a major focus on quality improvement measures such as American College of Surgeons Bariatric Surgery Center Network (ACS-BSCN) and the Metabolic and Bariatric Surgery Accreditation and Quality Improvement Program (MBSAQIP), and in part due to the evolution of laparoscopy and advanced surgical techniques and technology. The studies below detail the outcomes of the most prevalent weight loss surgical techniques today, as well as their impact on what has become one of the most important public health issues.

---

a. Weight Loss and Ghrelin

Plasma ghrelin levels after diet-induced weight loss or gastric bypass surgery.

Cummings DE, Weigle DS, Frayo RS, Breen PA, Ma MK, Dellinger EP, Purnell JQ

NEJM. 2002;346(21):1623–1630.

SYNOPSIS

Takeaway Point: Bariatric surgery suppresses ghrelin levels, which may contribute to weight loss.

Commentary: Meal volume restriction induces early satiety after gastric bypass, facilitating weight loss. The other mechanisms for weight loss after bariatric surgery, however, have not been clearly explained. The authors presented a matched control trial that examined the effect of weight loss associated with Roux-en-Y gastric bypass versus diet alone on the 24-hour ghrelin profile. They discovered that bariatric surgery patients have markedly decreased levels of ghrelin, which, unlike those in matched weight controls, do not oscillate in relation to meals. This provides major insight into one mechanism by which bariatric surgery leads to long-term appetite suppression and weight loss. Additionally, it sheds light on why diet-induced weight loss is extremely difficult to maintain, by demonstrating that plasma ghrelin levels *rise* after such weight loss.

ANALYSIS

Introduction: Ghrelin is a peptide hormone secreted in the stomach and duodenum that circulates under fasting conditions and acts on the hypothalamus to stimulate appetite. It also participates in long-term regulation of body weight. Given that gastric bypass excludes most of the stomach and the duodenum, the authors postulated that RYGB may reduce circulating ghrelin levels. This, in turn, may contribute to the durability of weight loss after bariatric surgery, as compared with diet-induced weight loss.

Objectives: To compare 24-hour plasma ghrelin levels in subjects before and after gastric bypass, before and after diet-induced weight loss, and normal-weight subjects.

Methods

Trial Design: Matched control study.

Participants

Inclusion Criteria: Age ≥ 18, stable body weight for at least 3 months.

Exclusion Criteria: Chronic medical or psychiatric illness, pregnancy, tobacco use, substance abuse, consumption of more than two alcoholic drinks per day, aerobic exercise >30 minutes 3 times per week, and previous gastrointestinal surgery.

Intervention: Subjects were admitted for an overnight fast, and plasma ghrelin levels were measured every 30 minutes between 8 AM and 9 PM (with three meals during the day), then hourly until 8 AM. The ghrelin profiles were compared between the subjects who had undergone a Roux-en-Y gastric bypass 9–31 months previously, BMI-matched obese subjects who had recently lost weight through a supervised dieting program, and a control group of normal-weight subjects.

Endpoints

Primary Endpoint: 24-hour plasma ghrelin profiles.

Secondary Endpoints: Weight loss, leptin levels, insulin levels, blood pressure, insulin sensitivity, lipid profiles.

Sample Size: 13 obese subjects who had undergone a 6-month dietary program for weight loss, 5 subjects after gastric bypass, and 10 normal-weight controls at a single university.

Statistical Analysis: Two-tailed, paired Student's t-tests, univariate linear regression.

Results

Baseline Data: Aside from the difference in BMI between the normal-weight group and the two obese subjects groups, there were no baseline differences.

Outcomes: Plasma ghrelin levels in obese patients rose just before and fell shortly after each meal. These fluctuations were not present in the gastric bypass group. The subjects who lost an average of 17% of body weight through dieting experienced a 24% increase in the area under the curve of the ghrelin 24-hour profile (p 0.006). In contrast, this area was 77% lower in the subjects who had undergone gastric bypass than in normal-weight controls ($p < 0.0001$), and 72% lower than in obese controls (p 0.01). The gastric bypass patients retained normal postprandial elevations of insulin and diurnal variations in leptin levels. In the diet group, weight loss was associated with significant decreases in adipocyte volume, leptin levels, fasting insulin levels, and blood pressure, in addition to improvement in insulin sensitivity and lipid levels.

Discussion

Conclusion: Circulating ghrelin levels increase with diet-induced weight loss and drastically decrease after gastric bypass. This likely contributes to the weight-reducing effect of the operation.

Limitations: The patients in the surgical group underwent gastric bypass a mean of 1.4 ± 0.4 years previously. Therefore, no conclusions regarding the long-term trend of ghrelin levels after bariatric surgery are appropriate at this time. Since only gastric bypass patients were included in the study, it is also unclear whether the findings can be extrapolated to other bariatric procedures. Furthermore, exclusion of patients with chronic illnesses may limit the generalizability to the obese population, which has high rates of chronic conditions such as diabetes mellitus, hypertension, and hyperlipidemia. The sample size was small.

b. SOS 10-Year Risk Factors after Bariatric Surgery

Lifestyle, diabetes, and cardiovascular risk factors 10 years after bariatric surgery.

Sjöström L, Lindroos AK, Peltonen M, Torgerson J, Bouchard C, Carlsson B, Dahlgren S, Larsson B, Narbro K, Sjöström CD, Sullivan M, Wedel H, Swedish Obese Subjects Study Scientific Group

NEJM. 2004;351(26):2683–2693.

SYNOPSIS

Takeaway Point: Bariatric surgery results in long-term weight loss and improvement in associated comorbidities.

Commentary: The Swedish Obese Subjects (SOS) trial is the largest prospective study of bariatric surgery outcomes to date. The authors' 10-year data show the dramatic effect of surgical weight loss on patients' morbidity and mortality. Specifically, this study addressed the effect of bariatric surgery on obesity-related comorbidities, and demonstrated long-term sustainability of this impact. It is interesting to note that not all risk factors seem to improve permanently (eg, hyperlipidemia), and the mechanisms for these changes have not been entirely elucidated. Overall, however, these findings have been essential in validating bariatric surgery interventions as favorable and lasting options for the treatment of morbid obesity.

ANALYSIS

Introduction: It is known that obesity is linked to increased morbidity and mortality. The former is postulated to result largely from associated comorbidities, including diabetes, hypertension, and hyperlipidemia. Surgically induced weight loss, however, had not been previously shown to have a long-lasting effect on these conditions.

Objectives: To assess changes in cardiovascular risk factors over 2-and 10-year follow-up periods in bariatric patients and medically treated matched controls.

Methods

Trial Design: Prospective, matched control surgical intervention trial.

Participants

Inclusion Criteria: BMI ≥34 for men or ≥38 for women, age 37–60. The subjects were matched according to an algorithm composed of 18 demographic and clinical variables.

Exclusion Criteria: Previous surgery for gastric or duodenal ulcer, previous bariatric surgery, gastric ulcer during the past 6 months, ongoing malignancy, active malignancy during the past 5 years, myocardial infarction during the past 6 months, bulimic eating pattern, drug or alcohol abuse, psychiatric or cooperation problems contra-indicating bariatric surgery, and other contraindicating conditions such as continuous glucocorticoid or anti-inflammatory treatment.

Intervention: The surgical patients and their matched controls had physical exams and laboratory workup performed at each scheduled visit. Surgically treated patients underwent gastric banding, vertical banded gastroplasty, or gastric bypass. Matched controls received nonstandardized medical treatment for their obesity and existing comorbidities.

Endpoints

Primary Endpoint: Overall mortality (addressed in the main SOS study; see **c**, below).

Secondary Endpoints: Changes in body weight, risk factors, energy intake, and physical activity; incidence of risk factors at time of follow-up in subjects who did not have these conditions at baseline; rates of improvement in comorbidities over the 2- and 10-year follow-up periods in those patients who had them at baseline.

Sample Size: 4047 subjects who had been enrolled into the SOS study from 25 surgical departments in Sweden and followed for at least 2 years, and 1703 subjects who had been enrolled for at least 10 years before January 2004. Follow-up was 86.6% at 2 years and 74.5% at 10 years.

Statistical Analysis: Analysis of covariance, logistic regression.

Results

Baseline Data: At the time of the matching examination, the patients in the surgery group were heavier (119.2 vs. 116.1 kg,

$p < 0.001$), younger (46.1 vs. 47.4 years, $p = 0.005$), and had a higher plasma insulin level (22.8 vs. 20.9 mU/L, $p = 0.009$).

Outcomes: Bariatric surgery patients lost significantly more weight, and this difference was maintained at 2 and 10 years of follow-up (+0.1% in controls vs. −23.4% in surgery group, and +1.6% in controls vs. −16.1% in surgery group, respectively; $p < 0.001$). Surgical patients also had a lower energy intake and higher proportion of physically active subjects than did the control group over the 10-year period. There were significant decreases in serum glucose, insulin, uric acid, triglycerides, total cholesterol, and systolic/diastolic blood pressure, with a favorable increase in high-density lipoprotein (HDL) cholesterol at 2 years ($p < 0.05$). These differences remained significant for glucose, insulin, uric acid, triglycerides, HDL, and diastolic blood pressure at 10 years ($p < 0.05$), reflecting recovery from diabetes, hyperuricemia, hypertriglyceridemia, and hypertension. The new incidence rates of diabetes, hypertriglyceridemia, and hyperuricemia were also lower in the surgically treated group than in the control group at 2 and 10 years.

Discussion

Conclusion: Obese patients experience greater long-term weight loss, more physical activity, lower energy intake, and recovery from risk factors such as diabetes, hyperuricemia, hypertriglyceridemia, low HDL, and hypertension after bariatric surgery when compared to standard lifestyle management.

Limitations: Incomplete follow-up at 10 years could have contributed to bias, as could lack of randomization and the presence of some heterogeneity between the groups. Medical management was not standardized and ranged from "sophisticated lifestyle intervention and behavior modification to, in some practices, no treatment whatsoever" (p. 2685).

---

c. Swedish Obese Subjects Study

Effects of bariatric surgery on mortality in Swedish obese subjects.

Sjöström L, Narbro K, Sjöström CD, Karason K, Larsson B, Wedel H, Lystig T, Sullivan M, Bouchard C, Carlsson B, Bengtsson C, Dahlgren S, Gummesson A, Jacobson P, Karlsson J, Lindroos AK, Lönroth H, Näslund I, Olbers T, Stenlöf K, Torgerson J, Agren G, Carlsson LM, Swedish Obese Subjects Study

NEJM. 2007;357(8):741–752.

SYNOPSIS

Takeaway Point: Bariatric surgery is associated with long-term weight loss and decreased mortality.

Commentary: The authors present a large, multi-institution, prospective, controlled trial comparing overall mortality of obese subjects undergoing bariatric surgery with those who received conventional medical treatment. Although the trial was not powered to prove that weight loss itself was linked to improved survival, it clearly showed that bariatric surgery was associated with sustained weight loss and lower mortality in long-term follow-up. Further investigations should examine the mechanisms of this effect; however, this study widely established bariatric surgery as a valid life-prolonging intervention. It is possible that the positive effect on significant medical comorbidities such as diabetes mellitus, hypertension, and hyperlipidemia that has been demonstrated by some of the trials discussed in this chapter (see **h**, below and **b**, above) may contribute to the reduction in mortality.

ANALYSIS

Introduction: Although a number of large long-term investigations have demonstrated an association between obesity and increased mortality, definitive data regarding the effect of weight loss on survival was not available prior to the publication of this study. Several retrospective cohort studies had suggested that intentional weight loss may be associated with lower rates of mortality, but prospective data from large sample sizes were lacking.

Objectives: To examine the effects of intentional weight loss on mortality by evaluating whether bariatric surgery is associated with lower mortality than conventional nonoperative treatment of obesity.

Methods
Trial Design: Prospective matched control trial.

Participants
Inclusion Criteria: Age 37–60, BMI $\geq$ 34 for men and $\geq$ 38 for women.

Exclusion Criteria: Previous surgery for gastric or duodenal ulcer, previous bariatric surgery, gastric ulcer during the past 6 months, ongoing malignancy, active malignancy during the past 5 years, myocardial infarction during the past 6 months, bulimic eating pattern, drug or alcohol abuse, psychiatric or cooperation problems contraindicating bariatric surgery, and other contraindicating conditions such as continuous glucocorticoid or anti-inflammatory treatment.

Intervention: Of the 2010 patients in the surgical cohort, 376 received a gastric band, 1369 underwent vertical banded gastroplasty, and 265 underwent a Roux-en-Y gastric bypass. 2037 matched controls were treated with a conventional medical approach beginning the day of the surgical cohort's operation.

Endpoints

Primary Endpoint: Death rate.

Secondary Endpoints: Causes of death, weight change.

Sample Size: 4047 obese subjects at 25 surgical departments in Sweden were recruited between 1987 and 2001.

Statistical Analysis: Wald test, Cox proportional-hazards models, Kaplan–Meier method, multivariate Cox proportional-hazards models, χ^2 test.

Results

Baseline Data: At the time of the matching examination, the two groups were similar in all characteristics except weight (the surgery group were on average 2.3 kg heavier, $p < 0.001$), age (surgery group 1.3 years younger, $p < 0.001$), and smoking prevalence (higher in the surgery group, $p < 0.001$). At the time of the baseline examination 4 weeks prior to surgery, the intervention group had gained more weight, while the control group had lost weight. This resulted in further divergence of variables, including serum glucose, triglycerides, total cholesterol, transaminases, and blood pressure, all favoring the control group.

Outcomes: 1471 patients who underwent bariatric surgery and 1444 who received conventional medical treatment were followed for a mean of 10.9 ± 3.5 years (ranging from 4 years 9 months to 18 years 2 months). During that time, the surgery group had a significantly lower overall mortality rate (HR 0.76, 95% CI 0.59–0.99, p 0.04), with 6.3% of the control group and 5.0% of the intervention group dying during the follow-up period. The mean weight change in the control group was $\pm 2\%$. The mean weight loss was $25 \pm 11\%$ after gastric bypass, $16 \pm 11\%$ after vertical banded gastroplasty, and $14 \pm 14\%$ after gastric banding at 10 years. There was no relationship between the degree of weight loss and rate of mortality, or the type of operative intervention and rate of death. Univariate analyses showed that serum triglyceride and glucose levels were the strongest predictors of mortality. In multivariate analyses, age and smoking were the strongest predictors. Cardiovascular causes were the most common, with cancer as the second most common etiology.

Discussion

Conclusion: Bariatric surgery in obese subjects was associated with a reduction in overall mortality, as compared with conventional treatment in contemporaneously matched, obese controls.

Limitations: The study was not randomized, with some heterogeneity between the matched groups. The trial was also not powered to determine whether a specific surgical approach or degree of weight loss was responsible for improved survival. It also could not draw definitive conclusions about the benefits provided to different age groups.

---

d. Laparoscopic Gastric Bypass versus Gastric Band

A prospective randomized trial of laparoscopic gastric bypass versus laparoscopic adjustable gastric banding for the treatment of morbid obesity: Outcomes, quality of life, and costs.

Nguyen NT, Slone JA, Nguyen XM, Hartman JS, Hoyt DB

Ann Surg. 2009;250(4):631–641.

SYNOPSIS

Takeaway Point: Laparoscopic gastric banding is a safe procedure with fewer complications than Roux-en-Y gastric bypass; however, it is significantly less effective in achieving long-term weight loss.

Commentary: Prior to the development of the laparoscopic adjustable gastric band, Roux-en-Y gastric bypass (RYGB) was the gold standard for weight loss–directed surgical intervention. However, gastric bypass is a procedure that is difficult to reverse and has a low but significant rate of long-term complications (internal hernias, marginal ulcers, anastomotic strictures, vitamin/mineral deficiency, etc). Therefore, the gastric band became a promising approach with the advantages of reversibility and no requirement for intestinal reconstruction. It had been previously shown to result in significant weight loss when compared to medical treatment.[17,18] The authors present one of the largest prospective randomized trials comparing the two modalities, and were able to show that while gastric banding is safer than the bypass, it falls short in providing desired weight loss. These results have been confirmed by published systematic reviews.[19] Although this study did not examine the effect of the procedure on obese patients' comorbidities, its results have since been replicated[20] and have contributed to the drastic decline in use of the laparoscopic gastric band in recent years.

ANALYSIS

Introduction: The laparoscopic adjustable gastric band was approved for use by the FDA in 2001, and by the time this article was published, it was the second most commonly performed bariatric procedure after gastric bypass. It was developed as the least invasive and first reversible surgical procedure for weight loss. There were no definitive data, however, regarding its long-term risks and outcomes.

Objectives: To evaluate the outcomes, convalescence, quality of life, and costs of laparoscopic Roux-en-Y gastric bypass versus laparoscopic adjustable gastric banding.

Methods
Trial Design: Prospective randomized trial.

Participants

Inclusion Criteria: BMI 40–60 kg/m² or 35 kg/m² with comorbidities, acceptable surgical risk, age 18–60.

Exclusion Criteria: Large ventral hernia, hiatal hernia, previous gastric or bariatric surgery.

Intervention: Patients were randomized to undergo laparoscopic gastric bypass or gastric banding. All patients had a Gastrografin swallow study performed on postoperative day 1. Gastric banding patients had band adjustments in clinic every 3–4 months. Nutritionist and social worker meetings, as well as regular support group meetings, were held for all patients.

Endpoints

Primary Endpoint: Percent of excess weight loss.

Secondary Endpoints: Operative time, estimated blood loss, length of hospital stay, number of patients requiring ICU stay, time to return to normal activities, morbidity, mortality, early and late surgical complications, quality of life, cost.

Sample Size: 111 patients were randomized to and underwent gastric bypass, and 86 patients underwent gastric banding between November 2002 and September 2007 at a single bariatric center.

Statistical Analysis: Two-sample t-test, Fisher exact test, χ^2 test, ANOVA, unpaired t-tests, univariate analysis.

Results

Baseline Data: Mean BMI was 47 ± 5.5 in the gastric bypass group versus $45.5 \pm 5.4 \, kg/m^2$ in the gastric banding group (p 0.01), while the mean age was 41.4 ± 11.0 versus 45.8 ± 9.8 ($p < 0.01$), respectively. Other baseline characteristics were similar between the two groups.

Outcomes: Mean follow-up was 4.2 years for gastric bypass and 3.6 years for the laparoscopic gastric band group. Operative time was significantly less for the gastric band versus gastric bypass (68.2 ± 24.7 vs. 136.9 ± 31.9 minutes, $p < 0.01$), as were blood loss (21.9 ± 14.1 vs. 80.9 ± 49.1 mL, $p < 0.01$), length of hospital stay (1.5 ± 1.1 vs. 3.1 ± 1.5 days, $p < 0.01$), and time to return to work (14.0 ± 10.1 vs. 21.0 ± 13.6 days, $p < 0.01$). Early (15.3% vs. 4.7%, $p = 0.02$) and late (13.5% vs. 0%, $p < 0.01$) minor complications, as well as late major complications (26.1% vs. 11.6%, $p = 0.01$), were significantly higher after gastric bypass than after the band. There were more 30-day readmissions after gastric bypass (5.4% vs. 0%, $p = 0.04$), but no significant differences in early or late reoperations or mortality (0.9% for bypass and 0% for band at 1 year). Mean excess weight loss was significantly higher in the gastric bypass patients when compared to the band patients both at 2 years ($68.9 \pm 16.1\%$ vs. $41.8 \pm 20\%$, $p < 0.05$) and at 4 years ($68.4 \pm 19.5\%$ vs. $45.4 \pm 27.6\%$, $p < 0.05$). Failure to lose weight occurred in 16.7% of patients in the gastric band group versus 0% in the bypass group. Operative direct costs were similar between the two groups, although total costs were higher after gastric bypass ($p < 0.01$). There were no differences in quality of life at one year between the groups.

Discussion

Conclusion: Compared with gastric bypass, gastric banding is associated with shorter operative time and length of hospital stay, fewer perioperative complications, and lower immediate cost. However, it results in significantly less weight loss and has a higher treatment failure rate.

Limitations: There were several baseline differences between the study populations. Also, more patients dropped out of the gastric band group (39) than from the gastric bypass cohort (14), due to patient refusal to proceed with the randomized selection or lack of insurance coverage, which could have led to selection bias.

e. Laparoscopic Gastric Bypass versus Duodenal Switch

Randomized clinical trial of laparoscopic gastric bypass versus laparoscopic duodenal switch for superobesity.

Søvik TT, Taha O, Aasheim ET, Engström M, Kristinsson J, Björkman S, Schou CF, Lönroth H, Mala T, Olbers T

Br J Surg. 2010;97(2):160–166.

SYNOPSIS

Takeaway Point: In superobese patients, laparoscopic duodenal switch results in greater weight loss than Roux-en-Y gastric bypass in the first year.

Commentary: The authors carried out a randomized multi-institution trial comparing the outcomes of laparoscopic Roux-en-Y gastric bypass (LRYGB) and laparoscopic duodenal switch (LDS) in patients with BMI 50–60. The study demonstrated that LDS results in significantly more excess weight loss at one year postoperatively, with comparable perioperative and long-term complication rates. Unfortunately, the trial was limited by its relatively small sample size and lack of long-term follow-up. However, it has established LDS as an acceptable alternative to LRYGB in the surgical management of superobese patients.

ANALYSIS

Introduction: Although both laparoscopic Roux-en-Y gastric bypass (LRYGB) and duodenal switch (LDS) have been shown to be effective interventions for weight loss, gastric bypass has been traditionally preferred because of the higher risk of nutritional deficiencies with the duodenal switch. However, previously published data showed that long-term weight loss failure and/or regain rates are as high as 35–43% in superobese (BMI > 50) gastric bypass patients,[21,22] while some non-randomized middle-term data suggested that duodenal switch may result in superior weight loss.

Objectives: To compare outcomes of LRYGB with those of LDS in superobese patients.

Methods

Trial Design: Prospective randomized trial.

Participants

Inclusion Criteria: BMI 50–60 kg/m^2 at referral, age 20–50 years.

Exclusion Criteria: Previous bariatric or major abdominal surgery, disabling cardiopulmonary disease, malignancy, oral steroid treatment, conditions associated with poor compliance (drug abuse or severe psychiatric illness).

Intervention: Subjects were randomized to undergo LRYGB or LDS. In LRYGB, the biliopancreatic limb was standardized at 50 cm distal to the ligament of Treitz, and the alimentary limb was measured to 150 cm. In LDS, the gastric sleeve was created using a nasogastric tube of 30–32 French, the common limb was measured to 100 cm from the cecum, and the alimentary limb was 200 cm long. Perioperative care and diet advancement was the same for both groups.

Endpoints

Primary Endpoint: Weight loss after surgery.

Secondary Endpoints: Perioperative and long-term complications, changes in body composition and comorbidities, nutritional status, quality of life.

Sample Size: 31 patients underwent LRYGB and 29 patients underwent LDS at two participating institutions in Norway and Sweden between March 2006 and August 2007.

Statistical Analysis: χ^2 test, Fisher's exact test, Student's t-test, Mann–Whitney U-test.

Results

Baseline Data: There were more patients with depression in the LDS group (p 0.045). Otherwise, patients' baseline characteristics were similar between groups.

Outcomes: There were no deaths, and rates of perioperative and long-term complications and readmissions were similar in the two groups. Patients who underwent LDS lost significantly more excess weight at 6 weeks (28.1% vs. 22.3%), 6 months (56.9% vs. 44.0%), and 1 year (74.8% vs. 54.4%; all $p \leq 0.001$). Two LDS patients (vs. zero LRYGB patients) experienced a significant metabolic disturbance during the follow-up period.

Discussion

Conclusion: In superobese patients with BMI > 50, both LRYGB and LDS can be performed with acceptable safety, but LDS results in greater weight loss in the first year.

Limitations: Relatively small sample sizes and lack of long-term follow-up limits the authors' ability to make definitive conclusions that would radically change current practice. The same limitation may have also resulted in inability to determine a true difference in perioperative and long-term complications, which should factor into the surgeon's choice of a procedure for superobese patients.

f. ACS-BSCN Outcomes

First report from the American College of Surgeons Bariatric Surgery Center Network: Laparoscopic sleeve gastrectomy has morbidity and effectiveness positioned between the band and the bypass.

Hutter MM, Schirmer BD, Jones DB, Ko CY, Cohen ME, Merkow RP, Nguyen NT

Ann Surg. 2011;254(3):410–420.

SYNOPSIS

Takeaway Point: Laparoscopic sleeve gastrectomy (LSG) is more effective than laparoscopic adjustable gastric band (LAGB) but less effective than laparoscopic or open Roux-en-Y gastric bypass (LRYGB, ORYGB) with regard to weight loss and reduction in comorbidities. The same relationship exists for procedure-related morbidity and complication rates for up to one year.

Commentary: The authors present the first report from the American College of Surgeons Bariatric Surgery Center Network Accreditation Program (ACS-BSCN), which was launched in 2005 with the goal to improve the quality and safety of bariatric care. ACS-BSCN has since merged with the American Society for Metabolic and Bariatric Surgery (ASMBS) accreditation structure to create a single unified accreditation program for bariatric centers, termed the Metabolic and Bariatric Surgery Accreditation and Quality Improvement Program (MBSAQIP). The program encompasses almost 600 hospitals across the United States and provides access to "big data," which, many hope, has the potential to influence not only the standards of practice and outcomes but also public policy and insurance coverage decisions. Since the inception of the program, significant improvements in bariatric procedure-related mortality and patient safety have already been documented.[23–25]

ANALYSIS

Introduction: At the time of this publication, no large-scale data were available regarding the clinical effectiveness and morbidity of laparoscopic sleeve gastrectomy as a standalone procedure, compared to the other established bariatric operations. Smaller scale observational studies suggested that LSG has outcomes and complication rates positioned between the band and the bypass.

Objectives: To analyze one-year data from ACS-BSCN pertaining to outcomes of LSG, LAGB, and laparoscopic and open Roux-en-Y gastric bypass.

Methods

Trial Design: Prospective, multi-institution, observational study.

Participants

Inclusion Criteria: All the cases of LSG, LAGB, LRYGB, or ORYGB entered into the ACS-BSCN database by accredited facilities.

Exclusion Criteria: Revisional procedures, biliopancreatic diversions with duodenal switch, "mini-loop" gastric bypass, other bariatric procedures, cases with missing operative dates or nonsensical data.

Intervention: Prospectively maintained database with data entered at baseline and at 30 days, 6 months, 1 year, and yearly after the patient undergoes LSG, LAGB, LRYGB, or ORYGB.

Endpoints

Primary Endpoint: Procedure-specific morbidity and mortality.

Secondary Endpoints: Procedure-specific weight loss and reduction in weight-specific comorbidities.

Sample Size: 28,616 patients from 109 hospitals, whose data were submitted between July 2007 and September 2010. There were 944 LSG, 12,193 LAGB, 14,491 LRYGB, and 988 ORYGB cases.

Statistical Analysis: χ^2 tests, ANOVA, t-tests, multivariate logistic regression models.

Results

Baseline Data: There was a higher percentage of super obese (BMI > 50) patients in the LSG group (30.2%) versus the LAGB group (16.42%) and LRYGB group (25.95%). LSG patients also had a higher proportion of comorbidities when compared to LAGB, but lower comorbidities than LRYGB. LSG group also had significantly more patients with prior operations when compared to the other groups.

Outcomes: LSG had significantly higher conversion, 30-day morbidity (including anastomotic/staple line leaks, strictures, bleeding, infection, etc), readmission, and reoperation rates than

LAGB, and lower conversion and reoperation rates compared to LRYGB. LSG had higher rates of organ space infection, renal insufficiency, and sepsis than LRYGB. It had lower rates of strictures, intestinal obstruction, and anastomotic ulcers than LRYGB; and a comparable rate of all other postoperative bariatric specific complications. After risk adjustment, there were no significant differences in mortality among the four procedures. Reduction in BMI at 6 months and 1 year was lowest for LAGB (5.02 and 7.05 kg/m^2, respectively), highest for LRYGB/ORYGB (10.82 and 15.34 kg/m^2), with LSG positioned in-between (8.75 and 11.87 kg/m^2, $p < 0.05$). At one year, diabetes resolved or improved in 44% of LAGB patients, 55% of LSG patients, and 83% of LRYGB patients. Similar patterns were seen for resolution of hypertension (44%, 68%, and 79%, respectively), hyperlipidemia (33%, 35%, and 66%), and obstructive sleep apnea (38%, 62%, and 66%). A slightly lower rate of resolution of GERD was seen in the LSG, at 50% compared with 64% resolution after LAGB and 70% after LRYGB.

Discussion

Conclusion: LSG is a safe operation with complication rates intermediate between those of LAGB and LRYGB. Its effectiveness in inducing weight loss and treatment of comorbidities is better than that of LAGB but less than that of LRYGB.

Limitations: The study period was relatively short and represents a narrow snapshot of the practices in bariatric surgery during that time. Therefore, some of the findings, including the proportion of the individual surgical procedures performed, are not accurate today. The data are skewed toward high-volume academic medical centers that have ACS-BSCN accreditation. Small numbers of patients with data regarding specific comorbidities limit interpretation of outcomes. This is also an observational study, so selection bias may have affected outcomes.

g. SM-BOSS

Early results of the Swiss Multicentre Bypass or Sleeve Study (SM-BOSS): A prospective randomized trial comparing laparoscopic sleeve gastrectomy and Roux-en-Y gastric bypass.

Peterli R, Borbèly Y, Kern B, Gass M, Peters T, Thurnheer M, Schultes B, Laederach K, Bueter M, Schiesser M

Ann Surg. 2013;258(5):690–694.

SYNOPSIS

Takeaway Point: Laparoscopic sleeve gastrectomy leads to similar excess weight loss at one year when compared to Roux-en-Y gastric bypass, and has a trend toward fewer complications.

Commentary: As the use of the laparoscopic adjustable gastric band has declined, sleeve gastrectomy has taken over and is now the most common bariatric procedure in the United States, outnumbering even the gastric bypass. Sleeve gastrectomy does not require creation of intestinal anastomoses, which avoids some of the most feared complications of gastric bypass. It is also a less complex surgical procedure that requires less time to perform. On the other hand, some authors argue that although LSG has a lower overall complication rate, the nature of its complications (staple line leaks and strictures) can be deleterious and very difficult to treat. Other considerations that may make one procedure better or worse for a given patient are still being established. For example, the potential exacerbating impact of LSG on gastroesophageal reflux disease (GERD; briefly touched on by the authors) is still controversial. The definitive comparison of long-term weight loss with LSG versus LRYGB has also not been established. The authors present a randomized trial comparing LSG with LRYGB that is intended to obtain such data. The trial is ongoing, and these are results of 100% complete follow-up at one year, with additional partial data up to 3 years postoperatively. The final long-term results of SM-BOSS are eagerly awaited and will provide important contributions to the bariatric surgical community.

ANALYSIS

Introduction: Laparoscopic sleeve gastrectomy (LSG) was initially developed as the first stage in the two-stage duodenal switch operation for weight loss. When it was noted that patients lost weight after sleeve gastrectomy alone, it gained popularity as a technique that was significantly simpler than gastric bypass and had lower associated morbidity.

Objectives: To compare the efficacy and safety of laparoscopic sleeve gastrectomy versus Roux-en-Y gastric bypass.

Methods

Trial Design: Multicenter randomized trial.

Participants

Inclusion Criteria: BMI > 40 or > 35 kg/m^2 with at least one comorbidity, age 18–65, and failure of nonsurgical treatment over 2 years.

Exclusion Criteria: Contraindications to major abdominal surgery, severe symptomatic GERD despite medication, large hiatal hernia, expected dense adhesions, need for endoscopic surveillance of the duodenum, and inflammatory bowel disease.

Intervention: Patients were randomized to either LSG or LRYGB. The procedures were performed using standardized techniques (35 Fr bougie for calibration of the gastric sleeve, 150 cm antecolic Roux limb with a linear or circular 25 mm stapled gastrojejunostomy, and 50 cm biliopancreatic limb for the gastric bypass). Pre- and postoperative care was standardized and the same for both groups.

Endpoints

Primary Endpoint: Weight loss over a 5-year period.

Secondary Endpoints: Perioperative morbidity and mortality, comorbidity remission, quality of life (using the Gastrointestinal Quality of Life Index).[26]

Sample Size: 217 patients from four bariatric centers in Switzerland enrolled between January 2007 and November 2011, with 107 patients in the sleeve gastrectomy and 110 patients in the gastric bypass arms.

Statistical Analysis: Student's t and Fisher exact two-sided tests.

Results

Baseline Data: Baseline characteristics were similar between the groups.

Outcomes: Median follow-up was 2 years. The mean operative time was less for LSG than for LRYGB (87.2 ± 52.3 vs. 108 ± 42.3 min, p 0.003). There was a nonsignificant trend toward more perioperative complications in the LRYGB group (17.2% vs. 8.4%, p 0.02). There was no significant difference in weight loss between LSG and LRYGB at 1 or 2 years. Both procedures resulted in similar rates of improvement in comorbid conditions including hypertension, hyperlipidemia, type 2 diabetes, obstructive sleep apnea, back pain, and depression. The LRYGB group had a higher rate of GERD remission (75% vs. 50%, p 0.008), while LSG patients had a trend toward a higher rate of new-onset GERD (12.5% vs. 4%, p 0.12). Quality of life was equal between the groups.

Discussion

Conclusion: LSG is associated with fewer short-term complications than LRYGB, and is equally effective with regard to weight loss and reduction in comorbidities at 1 year, except for incidence of GERD.

Limitations: Relatively short-term follow-up prohibits definitive conclusions about long-term outcomes. The trial was initially powered to detect a difference in 5-year follow-up.

---

h. Bariatric Surgery and Diabetes

Bariatric surgery versus intensive medical therapy for diabetes—3-year outcomes.

Schauer PR, Bhatt DL, Kirwan JP, Wolski K, Brethauer SA, Navaneethan SD, Aminian A, Pothier CE, Kim ES, Nissen SE, Kashyap SR, STAMPEDE Investigators

NEJM. 2014;370(21):2002–2013.

SYNOPSIS

Takeaway Point: Bariatric surgery leads to significantly greater improvements in glycemic control in obese patients with type 2 diabetes compared with medical therapy alone.

Commentary: The authors present data from a randomized controlled trial comparing traditional medical therapy for type 2 diabetes mellitus with Roux-en-Y gastric bypass and sleeve gastrectomy. While the number of subjects in each group is relatively small, the results are impressive not only in the magnitude of impact of the surgical approaches as compared to medical intervention but also in the durability of this effect. Because this trial included patients with BMI as low as 27 and showed that the glycemic changes were of similar magnitude in subjects with relatively low BMI, this study raised the question of whether bariatric surgery is underutilized. Should it be used for patients outside of the current NIH Consensus Criteria of BMI > 40 or ≥ 35 with comorbid conditions?[27] It also raised inquiries about the possible utility of bariatric surgery as a primary treatment for uncontrolled diabetes mellitus. Last, this study showed that gastric bypass may be a better surgical option for uncontrolled diabetic patients than sleeve gastrectomy, which has influenced mainstream bariatric surgical practice.

ANALYSIS

Introduction: The STAMPEDE (Surgical Treatment and Medications Potentially Eradicate Diabetes Efficiently) randomized controlled trial had previously shown that bariatric surgical interventions were superior to medical therapy alone in improving glycemic control and reducing the need for antiglycemic medications in obese diabetics after 1-year follow-up.[28] The current study presents follow-up at 3 years.

Objectives: To examine the long term durability of bariatric surgery as compared with intensive medical therapy for treating diabetes mellitus.

Methods
Trial Design: Randomized controlled trial.

Participants
Inclusion Criteria: Age 20–60, HbA1c > 7.0%, BMI 27–43.

Exclusion Criteria: Previous bariatric surgery or other complex abdominal surgery; or poorly controlled medical or psychiatric disorders.

Intervention: Patients were randomized to one of three groups: intensive medical therapy alone, medical therapy plus Roux-en-Y gastric bypass, and medical therapy plus sleeve gastrectomy. Medical therapy was adjusted for all groups at scheduled regular intervals with the goal of achieving HbA1c ≤ 6%.

Endpoints
Primary Endpoint: HbA1c ≤ 6%.

Secondary Endpoints: Weight, use of glucose-lowering medications, blood pressure, lipid levels, renal function, carotid intima-media thickness, adverse events/complications, quality of life.

Sample Size: 150 patients between March 2007 and November 2011 at a single academic center. Of these, 40 received maximal medical therapy, 48 underwent gastric bypass, and 49 had sleeve gastrectomy.

Statistical Analysis: χ^2 test, ANOVA, mixed model for repeated measures, multivariable logistic model.

Results
Baseline Data: There were no significant baseline differences between the groups.

Outcomes: Of the initial 150 patients, 137 were evaluated at the 3-year point (91.3%). HbA1c ≤ 6% was achieved in 5% of patients in the medical treatment group, 38% of the gastric bypass group ($p < 0.001$), and 24% of the sleeve gastrectomy group (p 0.01). Median fasting glucose levels were lower in each of the surgical groups when compared to the medical intervention group ($p < 0.01$). There was more glycemic relapse (HbA1c ≤ 6% at 1 year but not at 3 years) in the medical therapy group (80%) than in the gastric bypass group

(24%, p = 0.03). Reductions in the use of glucose-lowering medications were also greater in the surgical groups, with gastric bypass more effective than sleeve gastrectomy (p < 0.05) and each operation more effective than medical therapy alone (p < 0.001). Similar trends were found for reduction in body weight (24.5 ± 9.1% after gastric bypass, 21.1 ± 8.9% after sleeve gastrectomy, 4.2 ± 8.3% after medical therapy, p < 0.001), BMI, waist circumference, waist-to-hip ratio, triglyceride levels, and albuminuria. Although surgical patients had a significant decrease in medication use for hyperlipidemia and hypertension, there were no significant differences in blood pressure or LDL levels among the groups at 3 years, or carotid intima-media thickness at 2 years. Finally, there were significant improvements in quality-of-life (QOL) assessments for the two surgical groups versus the medical therapy group. There were no major surgical complications.

Discussion

Conclusion: Bariatric surgery, as compared with intensive medical therapy alone, results in superior and sustained glycemic control and weight reduction 3 years after intervention.

Limitations: Relatively small sample size and length of follow-up could mask additional differences between the two surgical groups that may be evident on longer follow-up.

REFERENCES

1. Sturm R, Hattori A. Morbid obesity rates continue to rise rapidly in the United States. *Int J Obesity* (London). 2013;37(6):889–891.

2. Sjöström LV. Mortality of severely obese subjects. *Am J Clin Nutr*. 1992;55(2 Suppl):516S–523S.

3. Sjöström L et al. Effects of bariatric surgery on mortality in Swedish obese subjects. *NEJM*. 2007;357(8):741–752.

4. Payne JH, DeWind LT, Commons RR. Metabolic observations in patients with jejunocolic shunts. *Am J Surg*. 1963;106:273–289.

5. Moshiri M, Osman S, Robinson TJ, Khandelwal S, Bhargava P, Rohrmann CA. Evolution of bariatric surgery: A historical perspective. *Am J Roentgenol*. 2013;201(1):W40–W48.

6. Baker MT. The history and evolution of bariatric surgical procedures. *Surg Clin N Am*. 2011;91(6):1181–1201.

7. Brown R, O'Leary J, Woodward E. Hepatic effects of jejunoileal bypass for morbid obesity. *Am J Surg*. 1974;127:53–58.

8. Scopinaro N, Adami GF, Marinari GM, Gianetta E, Traverso E, Friedman D, et al. Biliopancreatic diversion. *World J Surg*. 1998;22(9):936–946.

9. Hess DS, Hess DW. Biliopancreatic diversion with a duodenal switch. *Obesity Surg.* 1998;8(3):267–282.

10. Marceau P, Biron S, Marceau S, Hould FS, Lebel S, Lescelleur O, et al. Long-term metabolic outcomes 5 to 20 years after biliopancreatic diversion. *Obesity Surg.* 2015;25(9):1584–1593.

11. Griffen WO Jr, Young VL, Stevenson CC. A prospective comparison of gastric and jejunoileal bypass procedures for morbid obesity. *Ann Surg.* 1977;186(4):500–509.

12. Deitel M. A synopsis of the development of bariatric operations. *Obesity Surg.* 2007;17(6):707–710.

13. Capella JF1, Capella RF. The weight reduction operation of choice: Vertical banded gastroplasty or gastric bypass? *Am J Surg.* 1996;171(1):74–79.

14. Nguyen NT, Slone JA, Nguyen XM, Hartman JS, Hoyt DB. A prospective randomized trial of laparoscopic gastric bypass versus laparoscopic adjustable gastric banding for the treatment of morbid obesity: Outcomes, quality of life, and costs. *Ann Surg.* 2009;250 (4):631–641.

15. Hutter MM, Schirmer BD, Jones DB, Ko CY, Cohen ME, Merkow RP, et al. First report from the American College of Surgeons Bariatric Surgery Center Network: laparoscopic sleeve gastrectomy has morbidity and effectiveness positioned between the band and the bypass. *Ann Surg.* 2011;254(3):410–420.

16. Peterli R, Borbèly Y, Kern B, Gass M, Peters T, Thurnheer M, et al. Early results of the Swiss Multicentre Bypass or Sleeve Study (SM-BOSS): A prospective randomized trial comparing laparoscopic sleeve gastrectomy and Roux-en-Y gastric bypass. *Ann Surg.* 2013;258(5):690–694.

17. O'Brien PE, Dixon JB, Laurie C, Skinner S, Proietto J, McNeil J, et al. Treatment of mild to moderate obesity with laparoscopic adjustable gastric banding or an intensive medical program: A randomized trial. *Ann Intern Med.* 2006;144(9):625–633.

18. Dixon JB, O'Brien PE, Playfair J, Chapman L, Schachter LM, Skinner S, et al. Adjustable gastric banding and conventional therapy for type 2 diabetes: A randomized controlled trial. *JAMA.* 2008;299(3):316–323.

19. Colquitt JL, Pickett K, Loveman E, Frampton GK. Surgery for weight loss in adults. *Cochrane Database Syst Rev.* Aug. 8, 2014;8: CD003641.

20. Angrisani L, Cutolo PP, Formisano G, Nosso G, Vitolo G. Laparoscopic adjustable gastric banding versus Roux-en-Y gastric bypass: 10-year results of a prospective, randomized trial. *Surg Obesity Relat Disease.* 2013;9(3):405–413.

21. Christou NV, Look D, Maclean LD. Weight gain after short- and long-limb gastric bypass in patients followed for longer than 10 years. *Ann Surg.* 2006;244(5):734–740.

22. MacLean LD, Rhode BM, Nohr CW. Late outcome of isolated gastric bypass. *Ann Surg.* 2000;231(4):524–528.

23. Nguyen NT, Nguyen B, Nguyen VQ, Ziogas A, Hohmann S, Stamos MJ. Outcomes of bariatric surgery performed at accredited vs nonaccredited centers. *J Am Coll Surg.* 2012;215(4):467–474.

24. Kwon S, Wang B, Wong E, Alfonso-Cristancho R, Sullivan SD, Flum DR. The impact of accreditation on safety and cost of bariatric surgery. *Surg Obesity Relat Disease.* 2013;9(5):617–622.

25. Morton JM, Garg T, Nguyen NT. Does hospital accreditation matter for bariatric surgery? *Ann Surg.* 2014;260(3):504–509.

26. Eypasch E, Williams JI, Wood-Dauphinee S, et al. Gastrointestinal Quality of Life Index: Development, validation and application of a new instrument. *Br J Surg.* 1995;82:216–222.

27. Cummings DE, Cohen RV. Beyond BMI: The need for new guidelines governing the use of bariatric and metabolic surgery. *Lancet Diabetes Endocrinol.* 2014;2(2):175–181.

28. Schauer PR, Kashyap SR, Wolski K, Brethauer SA, Kirwan JP, Pothier CE, et al. Bariatric surgery versus intensive medical therapy in obese patients with diabetes. *NEJM.* 2012;366(17):1567–1576.

14

Vascular Surgery

Laura Peterson • Matthew Corriere

Vascular surgery is a constantly evolving specialty, and evidence-based care is a rapidly moving target. Treatment of vascular disease has changed dramatically over the 24 years since the North American Symptomatic Carotid Endarterectomy Trial (NASCET),[1] the earliest clinical trial referenced in this chapter, was published. Although new medications, procedures, and strategies have greatly expanded the number of treatment options available to vascular surgeons and their patients, they also create challenges in generalizing prospective trial results and applying them to individual patients.

Several studies covered in this chapter compare medical versus procedure-based management strategies for vascular disease. When interpreting study results, it is important to remember that within clinical practice these treatments are typically utilized in an additive fashion; that is, procedure-based treatments are often performed in addition to (rather than instead of) aggressive medical therapy. It can be challenging, however, to determine how advances in medical therapy should impact procedural intervention criteria when trial-based head-to-head comparisons include outdated approaches. The NASCET[1] and Asymptomatic Carotid Artery Stenosis (ACAS)[2] trials exemplify this phenomenon. Although both of these studies were well designed and contributed important evidence to guide management of symptomatic and asymptomatic carotid stenosis, respectively, advances in medical therapy since their publication (including more standardized approaches to cardiovascular risk reduction, routine use of statin therapy, and availability of more aggressive antiplatelet regimens) have likely narrowed the gap in outcomes between medical and procedure-based treatment. Although many practitioners using contemporary medical therapy for carotid stenosis have transitioned to more conservative utilization of procedural intervention (particularly for asymptomatic disease) based on improved medical treatment outcomes, updated evidence is not available to precisely define objective management criteria. New randomized trials comparing contemporary medical therapy alone with and without procedural intervention for carotid stenosis are currently underway, and it is foreseeable that additional trials may be warranted in the future as medical and procedural treatments continue to advance. Similar challenges exist for healthcare providers trying to use results from randomized trials comparing medical versus procedural management to guide treatment of venous thromboembolism[3,4] and symptomatic renal artery stenosis,[5] particularly when medical options are unacceptable or have failed.

Prospective trials comparing different approaches to procedural intervention (often open surgical vs. endovascular) are another valuable source of clinical evidence. Randomized comparisons between open and endovascular treatment of carotid stenosis, abdominal aortic aneurysm (AAA), and peripheral arterial disease (PAD) are abundant in the vascular surgery literature, and we include examples of each in this chapter.[6–8] None of the included studies was the first randomized comparison published between the treatments under consideration, but rather the most recent contribution to a larger group of randomized studies, many of which may have different inclusion criteria, endpoints, and conclusions. Those seeking to gain a more comprehensive understanding of the issues, controversies, and limitations related to these trials should refer to the previous randomized trials referenced in the discussion of each included study. Because device innovation and redesign proceed at a pace that exceeds high-quality evidence from randomized clinical trials, providers often have access to next-generation devices without direct evidence to guide how (or if) the new technology should affect treatment selection. The trials in this chapter exemplify the importance of using randomized studies to critically evaluate outcomes associated with new treatments, many of which demonstrate similar long-term outcomes between treatments that differ significantly in cost, invasiveness, and perioperative adverse events.

The articles and references included in this chapter should be considered as a means of accessing key evidence, controversies, and unanswered questions for readers in vascular surgery. Readers seeking a broader overview of evidence-based care should also refer to published consensus guidelines, which rely heavily on comparative effectiveness, observational, and case-control study designs in addition to randomized trials.[9-13]

a. NASCET

Beneficial effect of carotid endarterectomy in symptomatic patients with high-grade carotid stenosis.

North American Symptomatic Carotid Endarterectomy Trial Collaborators

NEJM. 1991;325(7):445–453.

SYNOPSIS

Takeaway Point: Carotid endarterectomy (CEA), in conjunction with medical therapy, reduces the risk of significant ipsilateral fatal and nonfatal stroke in patients with symptomatic high-grade stenosis of 70–99%.

Commentary: Carotid endarterectomy has been used in the treatment of carotid artery stenosis since the 1950s. Prior to NASCET and its European counterpart, the European Carotid Surgery Trial (ECST),[14] evaluation of CEA in comparison with best medical management had not been undertaken in patients with symptomatic carotid artery stenosis. NASCET demonstrated the clear benefit of CEA compared to medical management for patients with symptomatic carotid artery stenosis of 70–99%. The absolute 2-year reduction in ipsilateral fatal and nonfatal stroke was 17%. The exclusion criteria in NASCET were relatively robust and excluded all patients over the age of 80 as well as those with any cardiac rhythm disorder. It is also important to recall that the best medical management of the NASCET era included aspirin at doses of 1300 mg. Studies are presently underway to evaluate the effectiveness of CEA against more modern medical management.

ANALYSIS

Introduction: The role of carotid endarterectomy (CEA) in the treatment of patients with symptomatic carotid artery stenosis has long been questioned, due to initial negative trials and high complication rates. Improved medical therapy, in particular antiplatelet drugs, raised further questions regarding the appropriate role of CEA.

Objectives: To determine whether carotid endarterectomy reduces the risk of stroke among patients with a recent adverse cerebrovascular event and ipsilateral stenosis.

Methods

Trial Design: Multicenter randomized controlled trial.

Participants

Inclusion Criteria: Patients <80 years old with a previous transient ischemic attack, monocular blindness, or nondisabling stroke within the preceding 120 days and an associated stenosis of 70–99% of the ipsilateral internal carotid artery by arteriography. Participating medical centers had to have a rate of <6% for stroke and death occurring within 30 days of operation for at least 50 consecutive CEAs performed in the preceding 24 months.

Exclusion Criteria: No angiographic information; intracranial lesions more severe than extracranial lesion; kidney, liver, or lung failure; cancer likely to cause death in the next 5 years; disabling cerebral infarction on either side; symptoms attributed to nonatherosclerotic disease; cardiac valvular or rhythm disorders that could produce cardiogenic symptoms; prior ipsilateral CEA.

Intervention: Patients were given antiplatelet treatment with 1300 mg aspirin and appropriate medical management of their comorbidities. Patients randomized to the surgery arm received CEA in addition to medical management. Patients were assessed at 30 days, every 3 months for the first year, and every 4 months until death or stroke.

Endpoints

Primary Endpoint: Fatal or nonfatal stroke ipsilateral to the carotid lesion.

Secondary Endpoints: Any stroke, any stroke or death, major or fatal ipsilateral stroke, any major or fatal stroke, any major stroke or death.

Sample Size: 662 patients were enrolled between January 1, 1988 and February 21, 1991 at 50 medical centers in the United States and Canada. 331 were randomized to the medical arm and 328 to the surgical arm.

Statistical Analysis: Mantel–Haenszel χ^2 test and Kaplan–Meier survival curves. All p values were reported as two-tailed.

Results

Baseline Data: Three patients in the analysis group were excluded because they did not meet entry criteria. There were no significant differences between the medical and surgical arm.

Outcomes: Twenty-one medical patients (6.3%) underwent CEA and one surgical patient refused CEA. In the 30 days after randomization, there was a 5.8% rate of perioperative total stroke and death in the surgical group and a 2.1% rate of severe stroke and/or death. In the medical group, the overall stroke rate was 0.9% at 32 days from randomization. The 24-month risk of any fatal or nonfatal ipsilateral stroke in the surgical group was 9% versus 26% in the medical group, resulting in an absolute risk reduction of 17% ($p < 0.001$) and a relative risk reduction of 65%. The overall number needed to treat to prevent an ipsilateral stroke was six. Among patients who did not die or have a major stroke in the first 30 days, the risk of any major or fatal stroke within 24 months was 12.2% in the medical group and 1.2% in the surgical group for an absolute risk reduction of 10.6% ($p < 0.001$).

Discussion

Conclusion: CEA in addition to medical therapy reduces the risk of ipsilateral fatal and nonfatal stroke in patients with symptomatic high-grade stenosis of 70–99%.

Limitations: Excluded significant number of patients based on comorbidities. This study allowed enrollment only from centers with both high volume and low stroke rates, potentially decreasing reproducibility of these results at centers with less volume or expertise.

---

b. ACAS

Endarterectomy for asymptomatic carotid artery stenosis.

Executive Committee for the Asymptomatic Carotid Atherosclerosis Study

JAMA. 1995;273(18):1421–1428.

SYNOPSIS

Takeaway Point: Carotid endarterectomy (CEA) reduces the 5-year risk of stroke compared to medical management alone in patients with asymptomatic carotid artery stenosis of >60%.

Commentary: The ACAS trial addresses the need for surgical intervention in asymptomatic carotid artery disease. The study was designed to evaluate the 5-year stroke risk reduction of surgical intervention compared to medical management alone. Medical management in this study was the addition of aspirin as well as best treatment guidelines for all medical conditions. Advances in best medical management have occurred in the decade since ACAS was published. Presently, research is being undertaken to better understand how current medical therapy regimens compare to CEA in asymptomatic patients. The study was halted after a median of 2.7 years of follow-up as the surgical arm reached a relative risk reduction of 53% (p 0.004) as compared to the medical arm. The authors noted that women had a higher perioperative complication rate of stroke and death as compared to men and their 5-year relative risk reduction was only 17%. At present, initial screening is recommended by the Society of Vascular Surgery in patients who are older than 55 and who have cardiovascular risk factors. The consensus is that asymptomatic patients should have a yearly ultrasound to follow the progression of disease.

ANALYSIS

Introduction: Progression from asymptomatic to symptomatic carotid artery disease is variable, with the concern that patients may present with a devastating neurologic event. Prior studies have not addressed surgical treatment of asymptomatic disease.

Objectives: To determine whether the addition of carotid endarterectomy to aggressive medical management can reduce the incidence of cerebral infarction in patients with asymptomatic carotid artery stenosis.

Methods

Trial Design: Prospective randomized multicenter trial.

Participants

Inclusion Criteria: Age 40–79 years with hemodynamically significant carotid stenosis documented by one of three criteria: (1) arteriography within the previous 60 days indicating stenosis with at least 60% reduction in diameter, (2) ultrasound evaluation with a frequency or velocity greater than the instrument specific cutoff point with 95% positive predictive value (PPV), or (3) ultrasound examination showing a frequency or velocity greater than the instrument specific 90% PPV cutoff point confirmed by ocular pneumoplethysmography.

Exclusion Criteria: Previous cerebrovascular events in the distribution of the relevant carotid artery, contraindications to aspirin therapy, "a disorder that could seriously complicate surgery," a condition that could lead to disability or death within 5 years.

Intervention: The patients in the medical therapy study arm were given 325 mg aspirin daily. The surgical arm included aspirin, a preoperative arteriogram, and a carotid endarterectomy (CEA).

Endpoints

Primary Endpoints: Stroke or transient ischemic attack (TIA) occurring in the distribution of the study artery at any time point. All strokes or deaths occurring within 30 days after randomization in the surgical group and 42 days after randomization in the medical group.

Secondary Endpoints: Ipsilateral TIA, or perioperative TIA, stroke, or death.

Sample Size: 1662 patients at 39 centers between 1987 and 1993. Three patients were lost to follow up and excluded from analysis. 825 patients were in the surgical and 834 in the medical therapy arms. 101 patients in the surgical arm received medical therapy alone and 45 in the medical arm underwent CEA. In the surgical arm 414 patients underwent arteriography prior to CEA.

Statistical Analysis: Intention-to-treat analysis. Two-sided test of the null hypothesis, χ^2 test, Kaplan–Meier estimates.

Results

Baseline Data: Baseline characteristics were similar between medical and surgical treatment groups, although a history of prior stroke or TIA was more prevalent in the medical treatment group.

Outcomes: During the perioperative period 19 patients (2.3%) in the surgical group and 3 patients (0.4%) in the medical group had a stroke or died. Only 414 patients in the surgical arm underwent arteriography prior to CEA. In this group there was a complication rate of 1.2%. The authors estimated that if all CEA patients in the study had undergone arteriography, there would be a combined perioperative stroke or death rate of 2.7%. The estimated 5-year risk of ipsilateral stroke and any perioperative stroke was 11% in the medical group and 5.1% in the surgical group (p 0.004). The relative risk reduction was 53%.

Discussion

Conclusion: Carotid endarterectomy (CEA) confers a 53% 5-year relative stroke risk reduction as compared to full-strength aspirin therapy alone in treatment of asymptomatic carotid artery stenosis greater than 60%.

Limitations: Although arteriography was mandated by study protocol for all CEA patients, only 414 patients underwent this. In patients who received arteriography, 33 were excluded as the degree of stenosis was found to be <60%. Women were underrepresented in this study. They also had a higher perioperative stroke or death rate. The relative 5-year risk reduction for women was only 17%. There was also a high crossover rate of 9% with the majority in the CEA group.

---

c. PREPIC

A clinical trial of vena caval filters in the prevention of pulmonary embolism in patients with proximal deep vein thrombosis.

Decousus H, Leizorovicz A, Parent F, Page Y, Tardy B, Girard P, Laporte S, Faivre R, Charbonnier B, Barral FG, Huet Y, Simonneau G

NEJM. 1998;338(7):409–415.

Takeaway Point: Placement of inferior vena cava filters reduces short-term rates of symptomatic and asymptomatic pulmonary embolism but has no effect on long-term prevention of pulmonary embolism, and is associated with an increased risk of recurrent deep-vein thrombosis.

Commentary: Patients who develop proximal deep-vein thrombosis (DVT) are at risk of subsequent pulmonary embolism (PE) due to proximal clot migration. With the development of easily used percutaneous caval filters, over 30,000 filters were being placed annually in the United States in the early 1990s.[15] Prior to this study there was little evidence to support or refute this practice. This study examined the effectiveness of inferior vena cava (IVC) filters in patients who were receiving therapeutic anticoagulation. At the time of the PREPIC study, the third edition of the American College of Chest Physicians consensus statement regarding the treatment of venous thromboembolic disease recommended caval filters for patients who had DVTs or PEs who had contraindications to therapeutic anticoagulation or failure of anticoagulation therapy.[16] The 2 × 2 factorial design in this study allowed the authors to examine both the benefit and risk of prophylactic IVC filter placement, as well as the effect of low-molecular-weight heparin versus unfractionated heparin on the study's primary and secondary outcomes.

ANALYSIS

Introduction: Patients who develop proximal deep-vein thrombosis are at risk for subsequent pulmonary embolism. The use of caval filters as a risk reduction strategy in this population had previously not been well examined.

Objectives: To evaluate the benefits and risks of prophylactic filter placement in addition to anticoagulant therapy in patients with proximal deep-vein thrombosis (DVT) who were considered at high risk for pulmonary embolism (PE).

Methods
Trial Design: A 2 × 2 factorial designed multicenter randomized trial.

Participants

Inclusion Criteria: Patients >18 years of age with acute proximal DVT confirmed by venography, with or without synchronous symptomatic PE, or at high risk for a PE (high risk was defined by the treating provider).

Exclusion Criteria: Previous filter placement, contraindication/ failure of anticoagulation, therapeutic anticoagulant for >48 hours, indications for thrombolysis, short life expectancy, iodine allergy, hereditary thrombophilia, severe renal or hepatic disease, or pregnancy.

Intervention: Patients were randomized to either IVC filter or no filter, and to low- molecular-weight heparin or unfractionated heparin. All patients underwent ventilation–perfusion scanning within 48 hours of enrollment to determine presence of existing PE. If ventilation–perfusion scanning was abnormal, they underwent pulmonary arteriography to confirm PE. All patients underwent either pulmonary angiography or ventilation–perfusion scan between 8 and 12 days after randomization to detect asymptomatic PE.

Endpoints

Primary Endpoint: Occurrence of PE within the first 12 days after randomization.

Secondary Endpoints: Recurrent DVT, death, major filter complications, and major bleeding.

Sample Size: 400 patients were recruited between September 1991 and February 1995 at 44 French medical centers. 200 patients were randomly assigned filters and 200 were in the no-filter group. 195 patients were assigned to receive low-molecular-weight heparin and 205 to receive unfractionated heparin.

Statistical Analysis: Intention-to-treat analysis. χ^2 test, Fisher's exact test, and Student's t-test. Kaplan–Meier analysis was performed to examine the cumulative rate of events. Statistical significance was assessed with the Mantel–Haenszel method.

Results

Baseline Data: Baseline characteristics across treatment groups were equivalent. 28 patients did not have screening tests performed for asymptomatic PE.

Outcomes: Within the first 12 days from randomization there were more PEs in the no-filter group compared to the filter group (4.8% vs. 1.1%, p 0.03) but there was no difference in symptomatic PEs at the end of 2 years. Patients assigned to filter had more recurrent DVTs than those in the no-filter group (20.8% vs. 11.6% OR 1.87; 95% CI 1.1–3.2; p 0.02). There was no difference in thromboembolism, mortality, or major bleeding between the low-molecular-weight heparin compared with unfractionated heparin.

Discussion

Conclusion: In addition to heparin therapy, the use of a permanent caval filter reduces the short-term occurrence of symptomatic or asymptomatic PEs without an observed effect on immediate or long-term mortality. Filters were also associated with an increase in recurrent DVTs.

Limitations: The anticoagulation protocol did not extend beyond 3 months, potentially introducing bias related to long-term DVT rates. Ventilation–perfusion scanning was used to diagnose PE; the sensitivity and specificity of this test are affected by a variety of factors that may have resulted in incorrect classification (including missed events for patients with small PE). CTA is presently considered the gold standard for PE diagnosis in clinical practice.

---

d. VA Small Aneurysm Trial

Immediate repair compared with surveillance of small abdominal aortic aneurysms.

Lederle FA, Wilson SE, Johnson GR, Reinke DB, Littooy FN, Acher CW, Ballard DJ, Messina LM, Gordon IL, Chute EP, Krupski WC, Busuttil SJ, Barone GW, Sparks S, Graham LM, Rapp JH, Makaroun MS, Moneta GL, Cambria RA, Makhoul RG, Eton D, Ansel HJ, Freischlag JA, Bandyk D, Aneurysm Detection and Management Veterans Affairs Cooperative Study Group

NEJM. 2002;346(19):1437–1444.

SYNOPSIS

Takeaway Point: Early intervention in abdominal aortic aneurysms (AAAs) of 4.0–5.4 cm conveys no survival advantage compared to surveillance alone.

Commentary: Prior to this trial the elective surgical repair of abdominal aortic aneurysms remained controversial. Elective repair had been recommended for patients who had aneurysms of ≥4.0 cm in diameter who did not have medical contraindications.[17] The authors randomized patients at all national Veterans Affairs Medical Centers who were between 50 and 79 years of age who had AAA of 4.0–5.4cm in size to either immediate repair or surveillance. They found no survival advantage to immediate repair of AAAs. The patient population was predominately male (>98%), and this study has been criticized about the extrapolation of its results to women.

ANALYSIS

Introduction: The size for surgical intervention in the treatment of abdominal aortic aneurysms (AAAs) has been controversial. Prior studies had not evaluated the survival effect of early intervention.

Objectives: To determine whether early surgical intervention or observation results in higher rates of survival for patients with small abdominal aortic aneurysms (AAAs).

Methods
Trial Design: Prospective randomized multicenter clinical trial.

Participants

Inclusion Criteria: Age 50–79 years with an abdominal aortic aneurysm measuring 4.0–5.4 cm in diameter by CT within 12 weeks of randomization.

Exclusion Criteria: Prior aortic surgery; evidence of rupture of the aneurysm; expansion of the aneurysm of ≥1.0 cm in the last year or ≥0.7 cm in the last 6 months; suprarenal or juxtarenal aortic aneurysm; thoracic aortic aneurysm; severe heart, lung, or liver disease; a serum creatinine ≥2.5; a history of major surgical procedure or angioplasty in the past 3 months; expected survival of <5 years; severe debilitation.

Intervention: In the immediate repair group patients underwent standard open surgical repair with interposition of a synthetic graft within 6 weeks of randomization. In the surveillance group patients were followed without repair until the aneurysm reached at least 5.5 cm in diameter or enlarged by ≥1.0 cm in a year or ≥0.7 cm in 6 months. They underwent ultrasound evaluation or CT every 6 months.

Endpoints

Primary Endpoint: Rate of death from any cause.

Secondary Endpoints: Rate of death related to abdominal aortic aneurysm defined as death caused directly or indirectly by rupture or repair.

Sample Size: Between 1992 and 2000, 5038 patients with aneurysm were considered for randomization. Of these 1136 met criteria and were included in this study. 569 patients were assigned to the immediate repair group and 567 to surveillance.

Statistical Analysis: Intention to treat analysis. Cumulative survival curves were generated by the product limit method with log-rank test. Cox proportional-hazards model, χ^2 tests, Student's t-tests.

Results

Baseline Data: The two groups did not differ significantly at baseline with the exception of a slightly higher creatinine in the immediate repair group (1.2 ± 0.3 vs. 1.0 ± 0.3, p 0.02). Greater than 98% of the population was male.

Outcomes: Mean duration of follow-up was 4.9 years. In the immediate repair group 92.6% underwent aneurysm repair, and 72.1% of these repairs were performed within the proscribed 6 weeks after randomization. In the surveillance group 61.6% underwent surgical repair by the end of the study; 9% of patients in the surveillance group who underwent repair did not meet study criteria for repair. There was no significant difference between the two groups in the primary outcome of the rate of death from any cause (relative risk 1.21 for repair vs. surveillance; 95% CI 0.95–1.54). The rate of death due to AAA was not reduced by immediate repair. Operative mortality associated with repair was 2% at 30 days.

Discussion

Conclusion: Immediate repair of AAA of 4.0–5.4 cm in male patients provides no survival advantage over surveillance.

Limitations: This study did not have equal gender distribution and is limited as to what can be concluded for female patients. Over half of the patients in the surveillance group underwent operative intervention prior to the conclusion of the study with 9% not meeting criteria for open intervention as defined by the study.

---

e. AAA Expansion

Abdominal aortic aneurysm expansion: Risk factors and time intervals for surveillance.

Brady AR, Thompson SG, Fowkes FG, Greenhalgh RM, Powell JT, UK Small Aneurysm Trial Participants

Circulation. 2004;110(1):16–21.

SYNOPSIS

Takeaway Point: Imaging surveillance of abdominal aortic aneurysm (AAA) can be performed safely at 24-month intervals for aneurysms ≤4.0 cm in diameter, and at 12-month intervals for those between 4.1 and 4.5 cm, with less than 1% risk of expansion to 5.5 cm or greater.

Commentary: This trial provides an examination of the expansion rate of abdominal aortic aneurysms (AAAs) in a large national cohort. Previous studies had been limited by small sample sizes. Chance overestimation of an aneurysm measurement can end surveillance by prompting elective surgery, making the last measurement of a series biased toward higher values. Linear regression models are affected by this bias. In contrast, this study utilized random effects linear and quadratic growth models to improve estimations. The trial demonstrated that longer surveillance intervals were safe for patients with small AAAs, and that interventions to reduce cardiovascular risk factors are unlikely to substantially change aneurysm growth rates. The VA small aneurysm study (see **d,** above) had previously established that early intervention on small AAAs provided no mortality benefit. This information in conjunction with the results of this study further limit the need for aggressive surveillance.

ANALYSIS

Introduction: Aneursym growth in patients with abdominal aortic aneurysm (AAA) is variable. Surveillance intervals are inconsistent between centers, and the risk factors for expansion are incompletely understood. Prior studies have demonstrated that elective surgery for AAAs of less than 5.5 cm provides no mortality advantage, and that AAAs of this size have a low rate of rupture (~1% per year).

Objectives: To characterize average and interpatient variability in AAA expansion to inform surveillance protocols, and to investigate a predefined set of cardiovascular characteristics and risk factors for association with aneurysm growth.

Methods
Trial Design: Prospective cohort trial.

Participants

Inclusion Criteria: Patients with AAA referred to vascular surgeons for AAA surveillance.

Exclusion Criteria: Patients with only one AAA measurement.

Intervention: AAA surveillance by ultrasound. All patients were followed every 3 months if ≥5.0 cm or every 6 months if <5.0 cm. This was continued until surgery, death, or end of study follow-up.

Endpoints

Primary Endpoint: Aneurysm growth rate.

Secondary Endpoints: Cardiovascular characteristics associated with increased aneurysm growth rate.

Sample Size: 2366 patients at 93 UK hospitals between 1991 and 1998. 623 patients were excluded because of a single AAA measurement. A total of 9125 AAA measurements were obtained on the remaining 1743 patients.

Statistical Analysis: Random effects linear and quadratic growth models.

Results

Baseline Data: Mean age of 69.4 years (range 58–77), with 1356 (78%) male. The mean AAA diameter at baseline was 4.3 cm (±0.7 cm). 614 patients were active tobacco users, 971 were former users, and 105 were never users.

Outcomes: The average linear expansion rate across all patients was 2.6 mm/year (95% CI 2.5–2.6). There was wide variation between individual patients (95% reference range from −1.0 to 6.1 mm/year). Surveillance imaging intervals of 36, 24, 12, and 3 months for patients with AAA diameters of 3.5, 4.0, 4.5, and 5.0 cm, respectively, yielded less than a 1% chance of expansion to >5.5 cm. Patients who self-reported current tobacco use had significantly faster AAA expansion, by 0.4 mm/year ($p < 0.001$). Other cardiovascular risk factors were not associated with a significantly faster growth rate.

Discussion

Conclusion: AAA ≤4.0 cm can be evaluated every 24 months, and AAA 4.1–4.5 cm at every 12 months, with less than 1% risk of expansion to ≥5.5 cm. While current smokers do have a faster expansion rate, it is not significant enough to warrant different surveillance intervals.

Limitations: Follow-up for study participants ranged from 1.4 to 2.5 years. 1090 patients' surveillance period was terminated because of dissipation of the study protocol rather than the specified endpoints of repair or death.

---

f. PREVENT III

Technical factors affecting autogenous vein graft failure: Observations from a large multicenter trial.

Schanzer A, Hevelone N, Owens CD, Belkin M, Bandyk DF, Clowes AW, Moneta GL, Conte MS

J Vasc Surg. 2007;46(6):1180–1190.

SYNOPSIS

Takeaway Point: Small vein diameter, conduit choice, and graft origin are significant technical predictors of early primary patency (PP) and secondary patency (SP) loss of vascular bypass grafts.

Commentary: The PREVENT III study was initially designed to test the effect of a molecule that inhibits cell cycle gene expression on the development of neointimal hyperplasia. The initial results of that trial demonstrated no efficacy of the study drug on PP or SP for vascular bypass grafts.[18] The authors were left with a robust multicenter dataset with technical information on 1400 infrainguinal bypasses. Previous prospective studies had all been single institutions with less robust datasets. This study provided a broad representation of the current practice of autogenous vein infrainguinal bypass for limb salvage and identified key surgical variables. The authors examined technical variables affecting 30-day and 1-year PP, primary assisted patency (PAP), and SP. The variables with the most detrimental effects on both 30-day and 1-year PP and SAP were vein diameter <3 mm and conduit type.

ANALYSIS

Introduction: The influence of operator dependent variables on the outcomes of lower-extremity bypass surgery had previously been limited to single-institution retrospective studies.

Objectives: To utilize the PREVENT III database to assess the influence of specific technical factors on early (30 days) and midterm (1 year) outcomes of autogenous vein in infrainguinal bypass (IB).

Methods
Trial Design: Phase III multicenter randomized double-blinded placebo-controlled trial.

Participants

Inclusion Criteria: Patients >18 years old who underwent IB with autogenous vein for chronic limb ischemia (CLI). CLI was defined as gangrene, a nonhealing ischemic ulcer, or ischemic rest pain.

Exclusion Criteria: In situ reconstruction or claudication as an indication for IB surgery.

Intervention: Patients were randomized to receive topical bypass vein treatment with edifoligide, an experimental DNA molecule that inhibits cell cycle gene expression, or a placebo. Technical variables related to the surgery were recorded, including conduit diameter (as measured by the narrowest point), graft type, vein length, bypass configuration, and conduit orientation. Patients were followed for one year from the time of surgery with postoperative graft ultrasound at 1, 3, 6, and 12 months. The study protocol also identified "high risk" grafts as any vein with a diameter of <3 mm or any non-single-segment conduit.

Endpoints

Primary Endpoint: *Primary patency* (PP) defined as uninterrupted patency, *primary assisted patency* (PAP) defined as a graft requiring intervention prior to occlusion, and *secondary patency* (SP) defined as a graft requiring intervention after occlusion.

Secondary Endpoints: Limb salvage (LS) and death.

Sample Size: From November 2001 through October 2003, 1404 patients from 83 different medical centers in Canada and the United States were enrolled in this study. 702 patients were enrolled in the edifoligide and 702 in the placebo group.

Statistical Analysis: Univariate comparisons using Fisher exact test and Kaplan–Meier curves with log-rank test. All variables that were found to be significant on univariate analysis were introduced into a multivariate Cox proportional-hazards model. Wilcoxon rank sum test was used for nonparametric data.

Results

Baseline Data: Baseline data between drug and placebo groups were described previously.[15] High-risk grafts were used in 339 (24%) of the bypasses.

Outcomes: For the study cohort there was a 9.0% loss of PP and a 3.9% loss of SP at 30 days. Significant technical predictors of early loss of PP were conduit diameter of <3 mm (p 0.007), composite vein (p 0.001) and graft origin at the superficial femoral artery (p 0.028). At one year the strongest predictor for the loss of PP,

PAP, and SP was graft diameter <3 mm (hazard ratio (HR) 2.35, 2.68, and 2.90, respectively). The use of any non-single segment great saphenous vein (GSV) bypass conduit was associated with a 1.5 HR loss of PP, PAP, and SP. Vein length of 50–60 cm had a HR of 1.5 and >60 cm a HR of 1.33 when compared to grafts <40 cm in PP only. Graft origin had a similar association with PP only. Common and superficial femoral artery-origin grafts demonstrated inferior 1 year PP when compared with popliteal artery origin grafts.

Discussion

Conclusion: Small vein diameter, conduit choice, and graft origin are significant technical predictors of early PP and SP loss. At one year, vein diameter <3 mm and conduit type are associated with loss of PP, SP, and SAP while graft length and origin affect PP alone.

Limitations: This study was not specifically designed to assess the impact of technical variables on outcomes. The methods for recording these variables were not standardized. In situ grafts were completely excluded given the original intent of the study. There were too few adverse events at 30 days to perform multivariate analysis.

---

g. BASIL

Bypass versus Angioplasty in Severe Ischaemia of the Leg (BASIL) trial: An intention-to-treat analysis of amputation-free and overall survival in patients randomized to a bypass surgery-first or a balloon angioplasty-first revascularization strategy.

Bradbury AW, Adam DJ, Bell J, Forbes JF, Fowkes FG, Gillespie I, Ruckley CV, Raab GM, BASIL Trial Participants

J Vasc Surg. 2010;51(5 Suppl):5S–17S.

SYNOPSIS

Takeaway Point: In all patients with severe leg ischemia, there is no overall difference in amputation-free survival or overall survival when treated with bypass surgery or balloon angioplasty first, although bypass surgery conveys an overall survival advantage for patients who survive past 2 years after intervention.

Commentary: The BASIL study was the first multicenter randomized controlled trial to evaluate bypass surgery (BSX)- and balloon angioplasty (BAP)-first revascularization strategies in patients who present with severe limb ischemia due to infrainguinal disease. In 2005, an intention-to-treat analysis was performed demonstrating that short-term amputation-free survival (AFS) and overall survival (OS) were similar between the two treatment strategies. In post hoc analysis, performed on the survival curves, there was a suggestion that after 2 years, AFS and OS were higher after BSX.[19] The follow-up was extended to a minimum of 3 years in this patient cohort. The end analysis demonstrated that there was no difference in survival between the two groups when the entire time period was evaluated. However, patients who underwent BSX as a first revascularization attempt had improved OS after the 2-year time period. Because of significant controversy over the interpretation of this trial, and a high rate of crossover between groups, a second "treatment received" analysis was published. This analysis showed that BAP had a higher immediate failure rate (20% vs. 2.6%, p 0.01). In this analysis, AFS (p 0.006), but not OS (p 0.06), was worse in patients who underwent BSX after failed BAP.[20]

ANALYSIS

Introduction: Patients with infrainguinal severe limb ischemia present a clinical treatment dilemma. It is unclear which patients should undergo traditional open surgery versus endovascular intervention.

Objectives: To evaluate the long-term amputation-free survival and overall survival in patients randomized to bypass surgery or balloon angioplasty for severe limb ischemia.

Methods
Trial Design: Multicenter randomized controlled trial.

Participants

Inclusion Criteria: Patients with severe leg ischemia (SLI) due to infrainguinal disease. SLI was defined as ischemic rest pain and/or night pain requiring opiate analgesia and/or tissue loss of presumed arterial origin for >2 weeks. Patients could be randomized only if there was "genuine doubt" by the surgeon about whether BSX- or BAP-first revascularization would benefit the patient most.

Exclusion Criteria: Patient was unfit for urgent or immediate revascularization by either means.

Intervention: Patients were randomized to either BSX- or BAP-first revascularization.

Endpoints

Primary Endpoint: *Amputation-free survival* (AFS), defined as patient alive without amputation of trial leg at the trans-tibial level or above, and overall survival (OS).

Secondary Endpoints: Post-procedural morbidity, reintervention, health-related quality of life (HRQOL), use of hospital resources.

Sample Size: 452 patients with SLI were randomized at 27 UK hospitals between August 1999 and June 2004; 228 patients were randomized to BSX and 224 to BAP.

Statistical Analysis: Intention-to-treat analysis and one-sided *t*-test; Cox proportional-hazards model to examine AFS and OS with time-dependent hazards ratio (HR) to compare treatments before and after 2 years from randomization.

Results

Baseline Data: Baseline characteristics were similar between the two groups. Only one-third of patients were on a statin, and only one-third received antiplatelet therapy where indicated. A minimum of 3 years' follow-up was captured for all except four patients.

Outcomes: For the follow-up period as a whole, AFS did not differ between groups with 3.84 years for BSX and 3.62 years for BAP (difference 0.22y; 95% CI −0.34–0.78). OS was also similar at 4.48 years for BSX and 4.25 years for BAP (difference 0.23y; 95% CI −0.33–0.79). However, using time-dependent Cox proportional-hazards analysis for patients who survived to 2 years after randomization, BSX was associated with a significant increase in subsequent mean OS of 7.3 months (*p* 0.02) and a nonsignificant increase in restricted mean AFS of 5.9 months (*p* 0.06).

Discussion

Conclusion: Overall, there is no significant difference in AFS and OS between BSX and BAP. In patients who survive past 2 years, BSX provides a statistically significant increase in OS.

Limitations: Appropriate medical therapy was not adequately used in this patient population. There was no standard follow-up protocol. In the BAP group only nine patients received stents. This study has been criticized for omission of stenting from the endovascular treatment approach, which may have affected outcomes associated with endovascular treatment. There was significant controversy over interpretation of this trial, and a "treatment received" analysis was published simultaneously with the intention-to-treat analysis.

h. CREST

Stenting versus endarterectomy for treatment of carotid-artery stenosis.

Brott TG, Hobson RW II, Howard G, Roubin GS, Clark WM, Brooks W, Mackey A, Hill MD, Leimgruber PP, Sheffet AJ, Howard VJ, Moore WS, Voeks JH, Hopkins LN,K Cutlip DE, Cohen DJ, Popma JJ, Ferguson RD, Cohen SN, Blackshear JL, Silver FL, Mohr JP, Lal BK, Meschia JF

NEJM. 2010;363(1):11–23.

SYNOPSIS

Takeaway Point: Carotid artery stenting (CAS) and carotid endarterectomy (CEA) have equivalent rates of periprocedural death and 4-year ipsilateral stroke rates. In the periprocedural period, however, CAS is associated with a higher rate of stroke, and CEA with a higher rate of myocardial infarction (MI).

Commentary: This randomized trial compared CEA and CAS in patients with carotid artery atherosclerosis. While CAS and CEA were comparable in terms of the primary outcomes (composite measure of periprocedural morbidity/mortality, and 4-year ipsilateral stroke rate), they differed in the rates of periprocedural stroke and myocardial infarction. In particular, the assessment of periprocedural myocardial infarction has generated some discussion. Cardiac enzyme levels were routinely measured and a MI was defined as twice the laboratory upper limit of normal regardless of symptoms. Some have argued that these criteria for MI diagnosis were overly inclusive, as they may capture asymptomatic patients without the echocardiogram or ECG changes used in clinical practice to confirm MI. Ultimately, this study helped delineate which patients benefit for consideration of either CAS or CEA in treatment of their carotid atherosclerosis. The periprocedural rates of stroke and death in this study were the best reported to date, potentially reflecting a skilled and experienced group of providers and/or improved medical management. The CREST trial did not include a control group randomized to medical therapy without procedural intervention and this additional comparison is presently being evaluated in the CREST 2 trial. Residents wishing to examine historic trials for a more complete review of the topic should be directed to the SPACE, CASES-PMS, and CAVATAS trials.[21–23] The CAVATAS was an early study examining the effect of balloon angioplasty without stent placement as compared to CEA. It demonstrated no significant differences between the two groups but was criticized for the high periprocedural stroke rate. SPACE evaluated CAS versus CEA. It failed to prove noninferiority of CAS, and the authors recommended against the use of CAS in treatment of carotid artery stenosis. SPACE was criticized because of the experience of the interventionists allowed to participate. CREST's stricter requirements for participating surgeons and interventionalists were likely based on these concerns.

ANALYSIS

Introduction: Carotid endarterectomy (CEA) has been established as an effective treatment for extracranial carotid atherosclerosis. Carotid artery stenting (CAS) is an alternative treatment choice for this disease process.

Objectives: To compare the outcomes of CAS with those of CEA among patients with symptomatic or asymptomatic extracranial carotid stenosis.

Methods

Trial Design: Multicenter randomized controlled trial.

Participants

Inclusion Criteria: Symptomatic was defined as presence of amaurosis fugax, a minor nondisabling stroke, or transient ischemic attack within 180 days of randomization. Anatomic inclusion criteria for symptomatic patients included stenosis of ≥50% by arteriography or ≥70% by US, computed tomography angiography (CTA), or magnetic resonance angiography (MRA). Anatomic inclusion criteria for asymptomatic patients were stenosis ≥60% by angiography, ≥70% by US, or ≥80% by CTA or MRA if US was in the 50–69% range. Additionally, all participates had to be suitable anatomic candidates for both revascularization techniques.

Exclusion Criteria: Previous stroke severe enough to preclude assessment of clinical endpoints, chronic atrial fibrillation, paroxysmal atrial fibrillation within the preceding 6 months or that necessitated anticoagulation therapy, unstable angina, or MI within the previous 30 days.

Intervention: CEA versus CAS.

Endpoints

Primary Endpoint: Composite of any periprocedural stroke, MI, or death, or ipsilateral stroke within 4 years after randomization.

Secondary Endpoints: Death, stroke (any, major/minor, ipsilateral/nonipsilateral), myocardial infarction.

Sample Size: 2522 patients were randomized at 108 centers between 2000 and 2008. Asymptomatic patients were recruited from 2005 onward. 1271 were randomized to receive carotid stenting and 1251 to CEA.

Statistical Analysis: Intention-to-treat survival analysis and longitudinal random-effect growth curve models.

Results

Baseline Data: Of the 1271 patients randomized to CAS, 36 (2.8%) withdrew consent, 73 (5.7%) underwent CEA, and 33 (2.6%) were lost to follow-up. In the 1251 patients randomized to CEA, 64 (5.1%) withdrew consent, 13 (1.0%) underwent CAS, and 47 (3.8%) were lost to follow-up.

Outcomes: Composite primary endpoints were similar between the two groups during the periprocedural period (7.2% CAS and 6.8% CEA, p 0.51). However, individual endpoints differed between intervention groups. All-cause mortality was equivalent (0.7% CAS vs. 0.3% CEA, p 0.18), but there was a higher rate of stroke in the CAS group (4.1% CAS vs. 2.3% CEA, p 0.01) and myocardial infarction in the CEA group (1.2% CAS vs. 2.3% CEA, p 0.03). The 4-year incidence of ipsilateral stroke was similar between groups (2.0% CAS vs. 2.4% CEA).

Discussion

Conclusion: CAS and CEA have similar outcomes for periprocedural death and 4-year ipsilateral stroke. In the periprocedural period, CAS has a higher rate of stroke and CEA a higher rate of myocardial infarction.

Limitations: Rigorous criteria ensured highly skilled and experienced surgeons and interventionalists performed all procedures; the results, therefore, may not be reproducible in settings with greater heterogeneity among providers. The addition of asymptomatic patients and antiplatelet therapy potentially lowered statistical power of results. This study did not evaluate the use of medical therapy alone.

---

i. Long-Term Results of OVER

Long-term comparison of endovascular and open repair of abdominal aortic aneurysm.

Lederle FA, Feischlag JA, Kyriakides TC, Matsumura JS, Padberg FT Jr, Kohler TR, Kougias P, Jean-Claude JM, Cikrit DF, Swanson KM, OVER Veterans Affairs Cooperative Study Group

NEJM. 2010 Nov;367(21):1988–1997.

SYNOPSIS

Takeaway Point: Endovascular and open repair of abdominal aortic aneurysm (AAA) have similar long-term survival.

Commentary: The authors report here on the long-term results of the OVER trial. This is a Veteran's Affairs study that randomized patients to either endovascular or open repair of AAA. Previous studies had shown a survival advantage to endovascular repair, both during the perioperative period and at 2 years. This study demonstrated that the short-term survival advantage became nonsignificant after 3 years. Subgroup analyses suggested specific benefits associated with endovascular repair for younger participants and with open repair for older participants. These results generated discussion regarding the implications of method of AAA repair on cost, imaging, and mortality. Many surgeons anticipated that the OVER results might significantly change treatment selection approaches and/or criteria for AAA repair.[24] Residents wishing to have a more complete review of the literature should examine The UK EVAR trial.[25]

ANALYSIS

Introduction: Previous studies have looked at the survival advantage of endovascular repair versus open abdominal aortic aneurysm (AAA) repair in the perioperative and short-term intervals, but long-term outcomes are unknown.

Objectives: To evaluate the long-term morbidity and mortality of endovascular AAA as compared to traditional open repair.

Methods
Trial Design: Randomized multicenter trial.

Participants

Inclusion Criteria: Patients ≥49 years of age with one of the following: an aneurysm of ≥5.0 cm, an associated iliac artery aneurysm ≥3.0 cm, maximum diameter of ≥4.5 cm with rapid enlargement (0.7 cm in 6 months or 1.0 cm in 12 months), or a saccular appearance.

Exclusion Criteria: Prior abdominal aortic surgery, need for urgent repair, unwilling to consent or follow-up, or not a candidate for either procedure.

Intervention: Open AAA repair (OR) or endovascular AAA repair (EVAR).

Endpoints

Primary Endpoint: Long-term mortality from any cause.

Secondary Endpoints: Secondary therapeutic procedures that resulted directly or indirectly from the initial procedure, postrepair hospitalizations, uncorrected aortoiliac abnormalities noted on imaging at the conclusion of the study, and health-related quality-of-life factors.

Sample Size: A total of 881 patients were enrolled at 42 Veterans Affairs centers between 2002 and 2008. 449 patients underwent OR and 437 underwent EVAR.

Statistical Analysis: Intention-to-treat analysis, Kaplan–Meier survival curves, Cox proportional-hazards model, χ^2 and t-tests, longitudinal mixed-effects models.

Results

Baseline Data: Baseline data were similar for both groups. Mean diameter of AAA was 5.7 cm.

Outcomes: 96% of patients underwent their assigned repair. In 2% of patients the assigned repair was attempted but could not be completed. At 2- and 3-year analysis, patients undergoing EVAR had fewer deaths than the OR group (p 0.04 and p 0.05). There were six aneurysm ruptures in the EVAR group at follow-up compared to zero in the OR group (p 0.03). There was no difference in the number of secondary procedures in either group. At the end of follow-up, 146 deaths occurred in each group (hazard ratio with EVAR vs OR 0.97, 95% CI 0.77 to 1.22; p 0.81). Subgroup analysis with patients ≤70 years demonstrated an overall survival advantage with EVAR (hazard ratio, 0.65; 95% CI 0.43–0.98; p 0.04). In patients >70 years of age, survival was better with OR (hazard ratio, 1.31; CI 0.99–1.73; p 0.06). There were no differences in health-related quality of life.

Discussion

Conclusion: While there is an initial survival advantage of EVAR over OR, this dissipates after 3 years. EVAR conveys a survival advantage in patients ≤70 years while OR yields better long-term survival in those age >70.

Limitations: This study had a >99% male population. The results cannot be wholly extrapolated to women. The study was not powered for the subgroup analyses.

j. CaVenT

Long-term outcome after additional catheter-directed thrombolysis versus standard treatment for acute ilio-femoral deep vein thrombosis (the CaVenT study): A randomized controlled trial.

Enden T, Haig Y, Kløw NE, Slagsvold CE, Sandvik L, Ghanima W, Hafsahl G, Holme PA, Holmen LO, Njaastad AM, Sandbæk G, Sandset PM, CaVenT Study Group

Lancet. 2012 Jan;379(9810):31–38.

SYNOPSIS

Takeaway Point: Catheter-directed thrombolysis (CDT) with alteplase in addition to medical therapy reduces the long-term risk of postthrombotic syndrome (PTS) in patients with deep venous thrombosis (DVT) of the iliofemoral system.

Commentary: This is the first study to evaluate in a randomized fashion the effect of catheter-directed thrombolysis (CDT) on long-term development of PTS. The authors performed a random-ized group trial comparing standard medical management with CDT with alteplase. They focused their results on the 24-month presence of PTS and demonstrated an absolute risk reduction of 14.4% with CDT as compared to medical management alone.

ANALYSIS

Introduction: Acute DVT proximal to the popliteal vein confers a high risk of postthrombotic syndrome (PTS). The impact of CDT in addition to medical thrombolysis on development of PTS is unknown.

Objectives: To examine whether additional treatment with CDT using alteplase reduced development of PTS.

Methods

Trial Design: Multicenter randomized controlled trial.

Participants

Inclusion Criteria: Age 18–75 years, onset of symptoms within 21 days, and a DVT localized in the upper half of the thigh, the common iliac, or iliofemoral segment.

Exclusion Criteria: Anticoagulation for >7 days, contraindica-tions to thrombolytic therapy, Hg <8.0 g/dL, platelets <100, severe renal failure, severe hypertension, pregnancy, less than 14 days posttrauma or surgery, history of subarachnoid or intracereberal bleeding, life expectancy less than 24 months, drug abuse, psychiatric disorders, previous ipsilateral DVT, malignant disease requiring chemotherapy, any thrombolytic therapy in the previous 7 days.

Intervention: Patients were randomized to either medical therapy (low-molecular-weight heparin plus warfarin followed by warfarin alone), or CDT with alteplase plus medical therapy.

Endpoints

Primary Endpoint: Iliofemoral patency after 6 months. Frequency of PTS after 24 months.

Secondary Endpoints: Clinically relevant bleeding related to CDT, recurrent venous thromboembolism (VTE), PTS at 6 months.

Sample Size: Between 2006 and 2009, 209 patients were enrolled at 20 centers in Norway. 108 patients were placed in the medical arm and 101 in the CDT arm.

Statistical Analysis: Intention-to-treat analysis. Two-sided uncorrected χ^2 test, two-sided t-test or Mann–Whitney test.

Results

Baseline Data: The baseline demographics of the groups were similar. The mean age was 51.5 years ± 15.8 and 37% of the population was female.

Outcomes: The absolute risk reduction of PTS at 24 months with CDT compared to medical therapy was 14.4% (95% CI 0.2 –27.9; p 0.047) and the number needed to treat was 7. Iliofemoral patency rates were improved in the CDT arm (65.9%) over the medical therapy arm (47.4%; p 0.012).

Discussion

Conclusion: CDT in addition to medical therapy improves iliofemoral patency and reduces the risk of PTS in patients who have had an upper thigh, iliac, or iliofemoral DVT.

Limitations: Although 20 centers were used for recruitment of patients, only 4 had CDT capabilities. Four patients were included in the CDT arm who either failed to meet inclusion criteria or had exclusion criteria. The endpoint evaluator scoring presence of PTS was not blinded to the leg ipsilateral to the previous DVT.

k. CORAL

Stenting and medical therapy for atherosclerotic renal-artery stenosis.

Cooper CJ, Murphy TP, Cutlip DE, Jamerson K, Henrich W, Reid DM, Cohen DJ, Matsumoto AH, Steffes M, Jaff MR, Prince MR, Lewis EF, Tuttle KR, Shapiro JI, Rundback JH, Massaro JM, D'Agostino RB Sr, Dworkin LD, CORAL Investigators

NEJM. 2014;370(1):13–22.

SYNOPSIS

Takeaway Point: Renal artery stent placement does not improve cardiovascular and renal outcomes as compared to medical management alone for hypertension associated with renal artery stenosis.

Commentary: The annual number of renal artery stents placed increased 364% between 1996 and 2000 in the Medicare patient population.[26] The ASTRAL trial, which preceded CORAL, randomized patients with atherosclerotic renal artery stenosis to receive either medical therapy or revascularization with angioplasty or stenting.[27] ASTRAL demonstrated that there was no difference in either renal function or blood pressure between the two treatment groups. ASTRAL did not examine clinical outcomes. The authors in this study evaluated the effect of renal artery stenting plus medical management as compared to medical management alone on a composite primary endpoint of adverse renal and cardiovascular clinical outcomes. No differences were seen in either the composite primary outcome or separated secondary outcomes. From the results of this study it was shown that the best medical therapy without stenting should be the preferred treatment for the majority of patients with atherosclerotic renal artery disease. Design of this study benefitted from standardized medical therapy that included a run-in phase prior to randomization, overcoming a major limitation of previous investigations. Only a minority of participants had severe chronic kidney disease (~50% had stage ≥3 CKD), which may have impacted renal outcomes (as participants with normal preoperative renal function may have had potential to worsen but no potential to improve).

ANALYSIS

Introduction: Renal artery stenosis is present in 1–5% of patients with hypertension. Previous studies regarding renal artery stent placement in this population have not demonstrated improvement in blood pressure or renal function, but no trial has specifically assessed clinical outcomes.

Objectives: To determine the effects of renal artery stenting on the incidence of cardiovascular and renal adverse events.

Methods

Trial Design: Multicenter randomized controlled trial.

Participants

Inclusion Criteria: Severe renal artery stenosis and hypertension on two antihypertensive medications, or chronic renal disease with an estimated glomerular filtration rate (GFR) of <60 mL/minute. Severe renal artery stenosis was defined angiographically as either stenosis of at least 80% but less than 100% of an artery, or greater than 60% but less than 80% with a systolic pressure gradient of at least 20 mmHg.

Exclusion Criteria: Fibromuscular dysplasia, chronic renal disease from a nonischemic nephropathy, creatinine >4.0 mg/dL, kidney length ≤7 cm.

Intervention: The medical management group received antiplatelet therapy, amlodipine–atorvastatin, and unless contraindicated, the angiotensin II type 1 receptor–blocker candesartan, with or without hydrochlorothiazide. The stenting group had placement of a renal artery stent in addition to medical management.

Endpoints

Primary Endpoint: The occurrence of a major cardiovascular or renal event. This was defined as a composite of the following: death from cardiovascular or renal causes, stroke, myocardial infarction, hospitalization for congestive heart failure, progressive renal insufficiency, or the need for permanent renal replacement.

Secondary Endpoints: Each component of the primary endpoint was separated and evaluated as a single endpoint.

Sample Size: 947 patients were enrolled from 2005 to 2010 at 10 sites; 467 patients were randomized to stent plus medical therapy, and 480 were randomized to medical therapy only.

Statistical Analysis: Intention-to-treat analysis, χ^2 and Fisher's exact test, Student's t-test, Kaplan–Meier curves, Cox proportional-hazards model.

Results

Baseline Data: Baseline characteristics were generally similar, with the exception of a higher prevalence of myocardial infarction, history of heart failure, and tobacco use in the medical therapy group.

Outcomes: 94.6% of patients in the stent group received stents, which resulted in a mean reduction of renal stenosis from 68 ± 11% to 16 ± 8% ($p < 0.001$). 19 patients assigned to medical therapy alone crossed over to the stent group. There was no significant difference in the composite primary endpoint between the stent and medical therapy groups (35.1% vs. 35.8%; HR 0.94; 95% CI 0.76–1.17, p 0.58). There were no significant between-group differences when the components of the primary endpoint were separated and reviewed individually. There was a modest reduction in the stent group in systolic blood pressure on longitudinal analysis of –2.3 mmHg (95% from CI –4.4 to –0.2 mmHg; p 0.03).

Discussion

Conclusion: Renal artery stenting plus medical management does not improve clinical outcomes over medical management alone.

Limitations: Mean renal artery stenosis was 67%, suggesting that many patients did not have severe disease (60% was the minimum for trial eligibility). Debate continues regarding the appropriate severity of stenosis for intervention, and how a more severe minimum cutoff point potentially would have influenced the findings. It is important to note that a subgroup analysis of patients with greater than 80% stenosis revealed no benefit associated with stenting, although sample size estimates used for trial design were not based on this test.

I. IRONIC

Improved quality of life after 1 year with an invasive versus noninvasive treatment strategy in claudicants: One-year results of the Invasive Revascularization Or Not in Intermittent Claudication (IRONIC) trial.

Nordanstig J, Taft C, Hensäter M, Perlander A, Osterberg K, Jivegård L

Circulation. 2014;130(12):939–947.

SYNOPSIS

Takeaway Point: Invasive treatment in patients with intermediate claudication improves patient quality-of-life metrics and intermittent claudication distance but not maximum walking difference as compared to noninvasive management.

Commentary: Appropriate use of procedural intervention for peripheral arterial disease, especially intermittent claudication, is a controversial topic. Increasing scrutiny related to unnecessary procedures has been accompanied by calls for more conservative approaches to revascularization in patients with claudication, particularly those who continue to smoke or have not attempted (and failed) both pharmacotherapy and exercise therapy. Unfortunately, not all providers consistently behave as responsible stewards of patients' interests, clinical evidence, or value-based care. In many care environments, these concepts may be contrary to provider incentives of which patients are seldom aware.

Within this environment, the results of the IRONIC trial provide a timely and highly relevant counterpoint, demonstrating associations between an invasive treatment strategy and improved one-year outcomes (including both quality of life and claudication distance). Using a relatively novel approach to treatment randomization, the investigators designed their study on the basis of strategies (invasive vs. noninvasive) rather than specific procedures. Noninvasive treatment included educational materials, structured exercise training advice, and pharmacotherapy (consisting of an antiplatelet medication plus cilostazol); this approach closely resembles the initial therapy recommended by clinical practice guidelines endorsed by many medical societies, which use a single algorithm for all patients that reserves revascularization for those patients failing all other options. The IRONIC results, however, suggest that existing clinical guidelines may not maximize symptomatic treatment responses, at least among patients with moderate symptoms (those with either very mild or severe symptoms were excluded from the study). Overtreatment is a significant problem that is receiving justified scrutiny, but a "one size fits all" approach to treatment selection has potential negative consequences if the pendulum swings too far toward conservative management. Although rigid adherence to existing clinical practice guidelines would certainly have the potential to reduce unnecessary procedures, the IRONIC results suggest that this approach would also achieve inferior quality-of-life and lower extremity function for many patients.

ANALYSIS

Introduction: The quality of evidence for invasive revascularization in intermittent claudication is low. Prior studies have focused on patency outcomes without taking into consideration patient quality-of-life.

Objectives: To evaluate whether an invasive treatment strategy for intermittent claudication versus medical therapy improves health-related quality-of-life metrics after one year.

Methods

Trial Design: Single-center prospective parallel randomized trial.

Participants

Inclusion Criteria: Stable (≥6 months) intermittent claudication symptoms in patients ≤80 years of age.

Exclusion Criteria: Activity limiting medical condition, very mild claudication symptoms or disease requiring invasive treatment, weight >120 kg, inability to speak Swedish.

Intervention: All patients received aspirin or clopidogrel, statin therapy, and cilostazol. Cilostazol was discontinued at 3 months if no clinical effect was noted. Hypertension and diabetes were managed according to national guidelines. All patients were given structured exercise advice but were not supervised. The recommendations of the Trans-Atlantic inter-Society Consensus document on management of peripheral arterial disease (TASC II) were applied when choosing optimal strategy for revascularization in the invasive treatment (IT) group. A combination of endovascular, hybrid, and open surgical techniques were therefore used depending on the patient's disease burden.

Endpoints

Primary Endpoint: Health-related quality-of-life (HRQOL) score on SF-36, a generic HRQOL questionnaire, and VascQoL, a vascular-specific questionnaire.

Secondary Endpoints: Maximum walking distance (MWD) and intermittent claudication distance (ICD).

Sample Size: 158 patients were randomized, 79 to invasive therapy (IT) with 70 receiving intervention, and 79 to noninvasive therapy (NIT) with 73 receiving this intervention.

Statistical Analysis: Intention-to-treat analysis. Student's t-test for intergroup comparisons of normally distributed values. Mann–Whitney U-test for skewed distributions. Wilcoxon signed-rank test for skewed data and χ^2 test for discrete variables. The Cohen criteria for interpreting effect size calculations.

Results

Baseline Data: Demographic and risk factor profiles at baseline showed no significant differences between groups.

Outcomes: Loss to follow-up was 10% ($n = 8$) in the IT and 4% ($n = 3$) in the NIT group at one year. In the NIT group six patients required invasive intervention due to progression of disease ($n = 5$) or presentation with acute ischemia ($n = 1$). There was a larger improvement on the SF-36 in the IT versus the NIT ($p < 0.001$). With regard to intragroup changes, both the IT and NIT improved on the VascQoL ($p < 0.001$ vs. < 0.01). The change in ICD on treadmill was larger in the IT versus NIT (p 0.003) group, while there was no difference in the MWD between treatment groups.

Discussion
Conclusion: Patients with intermittent claudication who undergo invasive treatment have an improved health quality-of-life (QOL) score on both a generic and a disease-specific quality-of-life evaluation at one year.

Limitations: This study did not evaluate the direct effect of specific invasive treatments on patient quality-of-life. It was not powered to evaluate subtle differences in invasive treatment choices. These results cannot be applied to patients with mild or severe intermittent claudication. Further, the effects on quality of life metrics at one year may not be consistent beyond that time interval.

REFERENCES

1. North American Symptomatic Carotid Endarterectomy Trial Collaborators. Beneficial effect of carotid endarterectomy in symptomatic patients with high-grade carotid stenosis. *NEJM.* 1991;325 (7):445–453.

2. Executive Committee for the Asymptomatic Carotid Atherosclerosis Study. Endarterectomy for asymptomatic carotid artery stenosis. *JAMA.* 1995;273(18):1421–1428.

3. Decousus H, Leizorovicz A, Parent F, et al. A clinical trial of vena caval filters in the prevention of pulmonary embolism in patients with proximal deep-vein thrombosis. Prevention du Risque d'Embolie Pulmonaire par Interruption Cave Study Group. *NEJM.* 1998;338 (7):409–415.

4. Enden T, Haig Y, Klow NE et al. Long-term outcome after additional catheter-directed thrombolysis versus standard treatment for acute iliofemoral deep vein thrombosis (the CaVenT study): A randomised controlled trial. *Lancet.* 2012;379(9810):31–38.

5. Cooper CJ, Murphy TP, Cutlip DE, et al. Stenting and medical therapy for atherosclerotic renal-artery stenosis. *NEJM.* 2014;370 (1):13–22.

6. Brott TG, Hobson RW 2nd, Howard G, et al. Stenting versus endarterectomy for treatment of carotid-artery stenosis. *NEJM*. 2010;363 (1):11–23.

7. Lederle FA, Freischlag JA, Kyriakides TC, et al. Outcomes following endovascular vs open repair of abdominal aortic aneurysm: A randomized trial. *JAMA*. 2009;302(14):1535–1542.

8. Bradbury AW, Adam DJ, Bell J, et al. Bypass versus Angioplasty in Severe Ischaemia of the Leg (BASIL) trial: An intention-to-treat analysis of amputation-free and overall survival in patients randomized to a bypass surgery-first or a balloon angioplasty-first revascularization strategy. *J Vasc Surg*. 2010;51(5 Suppl):5S–17S.

9. Hirsch AT, Haskal ZJ, Hertzer NR, et al. ACC/AHA 2005 Practice Guidelines for the management of patients with peripheral arterial disease (lower extremity, renal, mesenteric, and abdominal aortic): A collaborative report from the American Association for Vascular Surgery/Society for Vascular Surgery, Society for Cardiovascular Angiography and Interventions, Society for Vascular Medicine and Biology, Society of Interventional Radiology, and the ACC/AHA Task Force on Practice Guidelines (Writing Committee to Develop Guidelines for the Management of Patients with Peripheral Arterial Disease): endorsed by the American Association of Cardiovascular and Pulmonary Rehabilitation; National Heart, Lung, and Blood Institute; Society for Vascular Nursing; TransAtlantic Inter-Society Consensus; and Vascular Disease Foundation. *Circulation*. 2006;113 (11):e463–e654.

10. Norgren L, Hiatt WR, Dormandy JA, Nehler MR, Harris KA, Fowkes FG. Inter-Society Consensus for the Management of Peripheral Arterial Disease (TASC II). *J Vasc Surg*. 2007;45(Suppl S):S5–S67.

11. Chaikof EL, Brewster DC, Dalman RL, et al. The care of patients with an abdominal aortic aneurysm: The Society for Vascular Surgery practice guidelines. *J Vasc Surg*. 2009;50(4 Suppl):S2–S49.

12. Kearon C, Kahn SR, Agnelli G, Goldhaber S, Raskob GE, Comerota AJ. Antithrombotic therapy for venous thromboembolic disease. *Chest*. 2008;133(6):454s–545s.

13. Conte MS, Pomposelli FB, Clair DG, et al. Society for Vascular Surgery practice guidelines for atherosclerotic occlusive disease of the lower extremities: Management of asymptomatic disease and claudication. *J Vasc Surg*. 2015;61(3 Suppl):2S–41S.

14. European Carotid Surery Trialists' Collaborative Group. Randomised trial of endarterectomy for recently symptomatic carotid stenosis: Final results of the MRC European Carotid Surgery Trial (ECST). *Lancet*. 1998;352(9113):1379–1387.

15. Magnant JG, Walsh DB, Juravsky LI, Cronenwett JL. Current use of inferior vena cava filters. *J Vasc Surg*. 1992;16:701–706.

16. Hyers TM, Hull RD, Weg JG. Antithrombotic therapy for venous thromboembolic disease. *Chest.* 1995;108(4 Suppl):335S–351S.

17. Hollier LH, Taylor LM, Ochsner J. Recommended indications for operative treatment of abdominal aortic aneurysms: Report of a subcommittee of the Joint Council of the Society for Vascular Surgery and the North American Chapter of the International Society for Cardiovascular Surgery. *J Vasc Surg.* 1992;15:1046–1056.

18. Conte MS, Bandyk DF, Clowes AW, Moneta GL, Seely L, Lorenz TJ, et al. Results of PREVENT III: A multicenter, randomized tiral of edifoligide for the prevention of vein graft failure in lower extremity bypoass surgery. *J Vasc Surg.* 2006;43:742–751.

19. Adam DJ, Beard JD, Cleveland T, Bell J, Bradbury AW, Forbes JF, et al. Bypass versus angioplasty in severe ischaemia of the leg (BASIL): Multicenter, randomized controlled trial. *Lancet.* 2005;366:1925–1934.

20. Bradbury AW, Adam DJ, Bell J, Forbes JF, Fowkes FG, Gillespie I, et al.; BASIL trial Participants. Bypass versus Angioplasty in Severe Ischaemia of the Leg (BASIL) trial: Analysis of amputation free and overall survival by treatment received. *J Vasc Surg.* 2010;51 (5 Suppl):18S–31S.

21. Beckman JA. Is the dream of EVAR over? *NEJM.* 2012;367(21): 2041–2043.

22. Katzen BT, Criado FJ, Ramee SR, et al. Carotid artery stenting with emboli protection surveillance study: Thirty-day results of the CASES-PMS study. *Catheter Cardiovasc Intervent.* 2007;70:316–323.

23. CAVATAS Investigators. Endovascular versus surgical treatment in patients with carotid stenosis in the Carotid and Vertebral Artery Transluminal Angioplasty Study (CAVATAS): A randomised trial. *Lancet.* 2001;357:1729–1737.

24. Ringleb PA, Allenberg J, Bruckmann H, et al. 30 day results from the SPACE trial of stent-protected angioplasty versus carotid endarterectomy in symptomatic patients: A randomised non-inferiority trial. *Lancet.* 2006;368:1239–1247.

25. The United Kingdom EVAR Trial Investigators. Endovascular versus open repair of abdominal aortic aneurysm. *NEJM.* 2010;362:1863–1871.

26. Murphy TP, Soares G, Kim M. Increase in utilization of percutaneous renal artery interventions by Medicare beneficiaries, 1996-2000. *Am J Roentgenol.* 2004;183:561–568.

27. The ASTRAL Investigators. Revascularization versus medical therapy for renal-artery stenosis. *NEJM.* 2009;361:1953–1962.

15

Soft Tissue and Skin

Laura Mazer • Laura Rosenberg • Alex Haynes

Malignancies of the skin and soft tissue are among the most common cancers diagnosed in the United States.[1] While the majority of these neoplasms are basal and squamous cell cancers with very low mortality, the incidence of malignant melanoma is increasing, and this potentially fatal malignancy was the fifth and seventh most common cancer in men and women, respectively, in 2015.[2] Across the country, nearly 10,000 deaths will occur annually from this disease.

Treatment of melanoma has changed dramatically over the last several decades. Emphasis on early detection and diagnosis has led to more prompt identification of melanoma, with approximately half of new diagnoses being in situ disease.[2] A series of studies initiated in the 1970s have documented the safety of smaller resection margins (1–2 cm vs. the historical 5 cm), sparing patients the accompanying morbidity and healthcare costs.[3–6] A series of seminal articles have extended our understanding of nodal management, including the role of sentinel node biopsy, for early identification of nodal metastases without the morbidity of anatomic nodal dissection.[7,8]

Accompanying the changes in surgical management have been innovations in the systemic treatment of melanoma. Adjuvant interferon has been shown to reduce recurrences and improve survival, albeit modestly.[9] The biggest changes in systemic treatment for metastatic melanoma have come with the introduction of targeted therapy (BRAF and MEK inhibition) and immunotherapy targeted at the CTLA-4 and PD-1 pathways. New research seeks to better understand how to incorporate these therapies with surgery, either as adjuvant therapy for high-risk stage II and III patients, or in combination with metastectomy in stage IV disease.

Soft tissue sarcoma represents a more rare, but important set of malignancies that the general surgeon will encounter. Almost 12,000 cases of sarcoma are identified in the United States every year with approximately 4870 deaths.[2] Because of the relative rarity and heterogeneity of these malignancies, rigorous clinical trials have been more difficult to produce. However, beginning with the work at the National Cancer Institute in the 1970s and 1980s, the previous practice of amputation for soft tissue sarcoma of the extremities has been replaced with a limb-sparing approach, often in conjunction with radiotherapy. Knowledge gained from the management of extremity soft tissue sarcoma has been extrapolated to tumors arising in the retroperitoneum, which constitute about 12% of all sarcomas. Management of these tumors remains controversial, including the roles of aggressive resection of adjacent organs and the application of neoadjuvant radiation. Trials attempting to answer the latter have failed to accrue in the past, but a study is currently in progress under the guidance of the European Organization for Research and Treatment of Cancer that will hopefully add to our knowledge on this topic.

---

a. Limb-Sparing Surgery for Soft-Tissue Sarcoma

The treatment of soft-tissue sarcomas of the extremities: Prospective randomized evaluations of (1) limb-sparing surgery plus radiation therapy compared with amputation and (2) the role of adjuvant chemotherapy.

Rosenberg SA, Tepper J, Glatstein E, Costa J, Baker A, Brennan M, DeMoss EV, Seipp C, Sindelar WF, Sugarbaker P, Wesley R

Ann Surg. 1982;196(3):305–315.

SYNOPSIS

Takeaway Point: A limb-sparing approach (excision plus radiation) for soft tissue sarcoma of the extremity has equivalent survival to amputation.

Commentary: This study was the first rigorous comparison of limb-sparing surgery with radiation versus amputation for soft tissue sarcoma of the extremity. Forty-three patients were randomized between the two approaches. There were no significant differences in 5-year recurrence free (71% vs. 78%) or overall (83% and 88%) survival in the limb-sparing and amputation groups, respectively.

The findings from this study dramatically changed the management of patients with extremity sarcomas, allowing limb preservation and better functional outcomes. This paradigm of organ preservation through more conservative surgery with adjuvant (or neoadjuvant) radiation has also been applied to other anatomic locations of sarcoma (eg, retroperitoneum, head, and neck) as well as to other malignancies (eg, breast, larynx).

ANALYSIS

Introduction: Soft tissue sarcomas represent a diverse group of pathologic tumors but share a tendency to local invasion along anatomic structures, resulting in high rates of local recurrence after surgical excision. Historically, this prompted radical excision with limb amputations to achieve local control. The combination of surgical excision with postoperative radiation has been suggested as a limb-sparing alternative. This is the first study to compare the two alternatives directly.

Objectives: To compare limb-sparing surgery with radiation to radical excision and amputation for soft tissue sarcomas of the extremity.

Methods

Trial Design: Prospective randomized controlled trial.

Participants

Inclusion Criteria: Patients with diagnosis of round cell or pleomorphic liposarcoma, pleomorphic rhabdomyosarcoma, synovial cell sarcoma, fibrosarcoma, neurofibrosarcoma, leiomyosarcoma, malignant fibrous histiocytoma, or undifferentiated sarcoma distal to the shoulder or hip joints.

Exclusion Criteria: Metastatic disease, history of prior chemotherapy or radiation, other malignancy (other than basal cell), severe infection, concomitant severe disease, age <30 years with embryonal or alveolar rhabdomyosarcoma. Extensive tumor where local excision was not possible.

Intervention: Either amputation or limb-sparing resection (removal of all gross disease) followed by radiation therapy, randomization stratified by histology, grade, time from initial diagnosis, and proximal or distal lesion.

Endpoints

Primary Endpoint: Disease-free and overall survival.

Secondary Endpoint: Quality of life.

Sample Size: 43 patients enrolled between 1975 and 1981, with 16 in the amputation arm and 27 in the limb-sparing plus radiation arm.

Statistical Analysis: Mantel–Haenszel test, Kaplan–Meier curves, Fisher exact test.

Results

Baseline Data: There were no significant differences in gender, race, site, histology, or grade between the groups. Patients randomized to amputation tended to be younger.

Outcomes: Four of the 27 limb-sparing patients had positive resection margins, versus zero in the amputation group. Median follow-up was 4 years and 8 months. In that time, three amputation patients and six limb-sparing patients experienced recurrence. There was no significant difference in time to recurrence between the groups. Five-year disease-free survival (75% amputation, 71% limb-sparing) and overall survival (88% vs. 83%) were similar between the groups. There was a trend toward higher local recurrence in the limb-sparing group (p 0.06). There was no significant difference in quality-of-life parameters between the two groups.

Discussion

Conclusion: There is no difference in disease-free or overall survival between amputation and limb-sparing surgery plus radiation for soft tissue sarcoma of the extremity.

Limitations: The same cohort was also enrolled in a study of adjuvant chemotherapy. This may account for the overall improvement in outcomes compared with prior studies of extremity soft tissue sarcomas.

---

b. Narrow Margins for Thin Melanoma

Thin stage I primary cutaneous malignant melanoma. Comparison of excision with margins of 1 or 3 cm.

Veronesi U, Cascinelli N, Adamus J, Balch C, Bandiera D, Barchuk A, Bufalino R, Craig P, Marsillac JD, Durand JC, van Geel AN, Holmstrom H, Hunter JA, Horgensen OG, Kiss B, Kroon B, Lacour J, Lejeune F, MacKie R, Mechl Z, Mitrov G, Morabito A, Nosek H, Panizzon R, Prade M, Santi Pierluigi, Slooten EV, Tomin R, Trapeznikov N, Tsanov T, Urist M, Wozniak KD

NEJM. 1988;318(18):1159–1162.

SYNOPSIS

Takeaway Point: For melanomas less than 2 mm thick, 1-cm margins are as effective as 3-cm margins in obtaining local control and are associated with equivalent survival.

Commentary: This article presents the results of a large, multi-center randomized trial organized by the World Health Organization Melanoma Group of excision margins in early-stage melanoma. 610 patients with melanomas less than 2 mm Breslow thickness were randomly assigned to 1- or 3-cm margins of excision around the biopsy site. After a mean follow-up of 55 months, there was no significant difference in 5-year survival between the groups. The locoregional recurrence rates were extremely low in both groups. The results from this study helped usher in an era of more conservative resection of primary melanoma. Prior to this study, margins of 3–5 cm or even wider were advocated, leading to a great deal of local morbidity, including necessity for skin grafts and complex flap reconstructions. After these findings were published, 1-cm margins became the standard for thin melanoma.

ANALYSIS

Introduction: Prior to this study, the standard of care for excision of primary melanoma consisted of wide local excision with 3–5-cm margins. Breslow first reported favorable outcomes of narrow margins in 1977, but no randomized trial had yet compared the two approaches.

Objectives: To determine whether an excision with a 1-cm skin margin was adequate and safe in patients with cutaneous melanomas ≤2 mm thick.

Methods
Trial Design: Randomized controlled trial.

Participants

Inclusion Criteria: Patients with clinical stage I melanoma (≤2 mm thick).

Exclusion Criteria: Facial or digit melanomas, excisional biopsy > 6 weeks prior to randomization, age >65, satellite nodules, multiple primary melanomas, or history of additional cancer.

Intervention: All patients had excisional biopsy to verify thickness <2 mm, and were then randomized to excision with either 3- or 1-cm margins surrounding the scar. All participating sites had a standard protocol for management of recurrent disease during follow-up.

Endpoints

Primary Endpoint: Recurrence rate.

Secondary Endpoints: Disease-free and overall survival.

Sample Size: 612 patients enrolled between 1980 and 1985, 305 were randomized to 1-cm margins and 307 to 3-cm margins.

Statistical Analysis: χ^2 test, Kaplan–Meier curves.

Results

Baseline Data: The two groups were similar in gender, age, and location of the primary tumor. Mean thickness was 0.99 mm in the 1-cm excision group and 1.2 mm in the 3-cm excision group ($p > 0.05$).

Outcomes: At 55 months' follow-up, survival was 96.8% in the 1-cm excision group and 96% in the 3-cm excision group (p 0.58). Disease-free survival was also similar between the groups (p 0.66). There was no difference in rates of regional or distant nodal metastases.

Discussion

Conclusion: More conservative surgical excision (1 cm lateral margins) is as effective as the traditional 3 cm margins in patients with cutaneous melanoma ≤2 mm.

Limitations: No multivariate analysis was performed. Follow-up was at 55 months; this may not be long enough (especially given the very high survival rate) to demonstrate the true difference in approaches.

---

c. EST 1684

Interferon alfa-2b adjuvant therapy of high-risk resected cutaneous melanoma: The Eastern Cooperative Oncology Group Trial EST 1684.

Kirkwood JM, Strawderman MH, Ernstoff MS, Smith TJ, Borden EC, Blum RH

J Clin Oncol. 1996;14(1):7–17.

SYNOPSIS

Takeaway Point: Interferon alfa-2b (IFNα-2b) prolongs the relapse-free interval and overall survival following resection of high-risk (T4 or N1) melanoma.

Commentary: IFNα-2b had previously been found to have anti-tumor activity against metastatic melanoma. Patients with deep primary tumors or lymph node metastases have a high risk of relapse and mortality. Prior adjuvant therapies had not impacted relapse-free or overall survival. This study evaluated the use of IFNα-2b as adjuvant therapy in high-risk patients, and found that IFN prolongs both relapse-free interval and overall survival following resection. This was the first study to demonstrate the success of an adjuvant treatment for this population. IFN treatment was associated with significant toxicity, with the majority of patients requiring dose adjustments, and the risk–benefit analysis of when to use this treatment continues to be an individualized decision.

ANALYSIS

Introduction: IFNα-2b has shown antitumor activity in metastatic melanoma. In this study, it was evaluated as adjuvant therapy following resection in high-risk patients.

Objectives: To evaluate the efficacy of IFNα-2b as adjuvant therapy following resection of deep primary (T4) or regionally metastatic (N1) melanoma.

Methods
Trial Design: Phase 3, multicenter, blinded, randomized controlled trial.

Participants
Inclusion Criteria: Patients with histologically proven primary cutaneous melanoma. Patients were grouped into four categories based on extent of disease: (1) deep (>4 mm) primary melanomas (T4, N0, M0), (2) primary melanomas of any stage with occult lymph node metastasis discovered at elective lymph node dissection (Tp, N1, M0), (3) clinically detected regional lymph node involvement with synchronous primary melanoma (TcN1M0), and (4) regional lymph node recurrence after primary surgery. Groups 1–3 were required to enter the study within 56 days of first biopsy; group 4 was required to enter within 42 days of lymphadenectomy.

Exclusion Criteria: Those with staging errors; failure to perform lymphadenectomy; unknown primary site. Prior systemic therapy, distant metastatic disease, or significant comorbidities.

Intervention: Patients were randomized to either IFNα-2b at maximum tolerated doses of 20 MU/m per day IV for 5 days per week for 4 weeks, then 3 times weekly at 10 MU/m per day subcutaneously (SC) for 48 weeks, or clinical observation.

Endpoints

Primary Endpoint: Relapse-free survival; overall survival.

Secondary Endpoints: Relapse-free survival stratified by stage; association of patient characteristics (age, sex, performance status, Clark level, Breslow thickness, time to randomization, ulceration, excisional biopsy performed) with survival.

Sample Size: 280 patients enrolled between 1984 and 1990, block-randomized according to tumor stage, 143 to receive IFN, 137 to observation alone.

Statistical Analysis: Kaplan–Meier survival curves; estimated hazard plots for overall survival smoothed with a simple kernel technique; Fisher's exact test; Cox's proportional-hazards regression; stratified log-rank test; Cox model.

Results

Baseline Data: Patients largely well matched across baseline characteristics. Nonsignificant trend toward thicker primary in the observation group.

Outcomes

Primary: Median relapse-free survival time for patients who received IFN was 1.72 years, versus 0.98 years for observation alone (p 0.0023). Overall median survival time was 3.82 years for IFN patients and 2.78 years for observation (p 0.0237).

Secondary: The estimated 5-year relapse-free survival rate was 37% for IFN versus 26% for observation. The estimated 5-year survival rate was 46% for IFN and 37% for observation. There was a marked suppression of relapse and death with IFN treatment across all node-positive groups. In patients with nonpalpable but pathologically detected lymph node metastases, there was a reduction of the estimated hazard of relapse from 60% to 25% during the first year of treatment. The reduction in hazard of relapse for those with clinically palpable nodes was even more prominent. In the multivariate analysis, treatment with IFN, age, time from diagnosis or first recurrence to study entry, and tumor ulceration were all significantly associated with both relapse-free and overall survival ($p < 0.05$). Dosing delays or dose reductions were required for 50% of patients during the IV treatment phase and for 48% of patients during the SC treatment phase due to side effects. These were primarily constitutional and neuropsychiatric symptoms, as well as myelosuppression and hepatotoxicity and included two deaths from hepatic failure. Overall 74% of patients were able to continue treatment until 1 year.

Discussion

Conclusion: IFNα-2b prolongs the relapse-free interval and overall survival following resection of deep primary (T4) or regionally metastatic (N1) melanoma. Toxicity is significant, and requires dose adjustments in the majority of patients.

Limitations: Results were not analyzed according to the number of positive nodes, which other studies have recognized as a significant prognostic factor. Breslow thickness was not a prognostic factor for disease-free and overall survival, which runs contrary to other published studies. A significant percentage of patients experienced toxicity, including two patients with "lethal hepatic toxicity," but the study reported limited details regarding the full range of side effects.

---

d. Radiation for Extremity Sarcoma

Randomized prospective study of the benefit of adjuvant radiation therapy in the treatment of soft tissue sarcomas of the extremity.

Yang JC, Chang AE, Baker AR, Sindelar WF, Danforth DN, Tapalian SL, DeLaney T, Glatstein E, Steinberg SM, Merino MJ, Rosenberg SA

J Clin Oncol. 1998;16(1):197–203.

SYNOPSIS

Takeaway Point: Postoperative radiation after resection of soft tissue sarcoma of the extremity results in a significant decrease in local recurrence, but no difference in overall survival.

Commentary: This randomized trial sought to assess the effect of postoperative radiation on local recurrence and survival following limb-sparing resection of extremity soft tissue sarcoma at the Surgery Branch of the National Cancer Institute. A total of 141 patients, 91 with high-grade lesions and 50 with low-grade, underwent limb-sparing resection. Subsequently, patients with high-grade lesions were randomized to postoperative chemotherapy alone or postoperative chemotherapy plus radiation to the resection site. Patients with low-grade lesions were randomized to observation or radiation. In both cohorts, the addition of postoperative radiation reduced the risk of local recurrence, but did not significantly affect survival. There was a decrease in objective measures of limb function (joint movement, strength, edema) in patients receiving radiation, but no difference in patient-reported quality-of-life metrics. This study established the effectiveness of adjuvant radiation for local control in extremity sarcoma. Efforts to establish radiation protocols that limit toxicity have been made since this publication, as well as consideration of omission of radiotherapy for selected lesions with low risk of recurrence (eg, small low-grade lesions with negative margins).

ANALYSIS

Introduction: Although surgery remains the mainstay of treatment for soft tissue sarcomas, chemoradiation has been essential in optimizing cure rates and improving postoperative quality of life. After randomized trials demonstrating similar cure rates for limb-sparing surgery (LSS) and radiation (see **a**, above), amputation rates for extremity sarcomas have fallen dramatically. High-dose radiation therapy carries its own high costs and morbidity, and the necessity of radiation after limb-sparing surgery has not been evaluated.

Objectives: To assess the impact of postoperative external-beam radiation therapy on local recurrence (LR), overall survival (OS), and quality of life after limb-sparing resection of extremity sarcomas.

Methods

Trial Design: Prospective randomized trial.

Participants

Inclusion Criteria: Patients with extremity soft tissue tumors who underwent LSS.

Exclusion Criteria: Evidence of metastatic disease, a second malignancy, contraindications to chemotherapy or radiation therapy; patients with widely positive margins after LSS.

Intervention: Patients undergoing limb-sparing resection for high-grade lesions were randomized to chemotherapy plus adjuvant radiation therapy (XRT) or chemotherapy alone. For low-grade lesions, patients were randomized to adjuvant XRT or observation. Randomization was stratified by grade, tumor location (proximal vs. distal), and close surgical margins.

Endpoints

Primary Endpoint: Local recurrence.

Secondary Endpoints: Overall survival, quality of life.

Sample Size: 141 patients with extremity soft tissue tumors who had undergone limb-sparing surgery were randomized between 1983 and 1991; 70 to the radiation arm and 71 to no radiation. Of these, 91 had high-grade lesions (47 XRT, 44 no XRT) and 50 had low-grade lesions (26 XRT, 24 no XRT).

Statistical Analysis: Log-rank method, Kaplan–Meier curves, Fisher's exact test, and Mehta test.

Results

Baseline Data: The authors reported the results for patients with high- and low-grade tumors separately. In both the high- and low-grade cohorts, patient characteristics were similar between the two treatment groups.

Outcomes: Median follow-up was 9.6 years for the high-grade and 9.9 years for the low-grade cohort. In the high-grade cohort, rate of local recurrence was higher in the no-XRT group (0 vs. 9 events, p 0.003). The probability of metastatic disease did not differ between the treatment groups, and overall survival was similar at 10 years (75% for XRT vs. 74% for no-XRT, p 0.71). For patients with low-grade sarcomas, results were similar. Local recurrence was higher in the no-XRT group (1 vs. 8 events, p 0.016), but overall survival was not different. In the quality-of-life studies, patients receiving XRT had significantly decreased joint motion and muscle strength 12 months after surgery, but there was no overall difference in global quality-of-life assessments or performance of activities of daily living.

Discussion

Conclusion: Postoperative XRT after LSS is associated with decreased local recurrence, but does not improve overall survival.

Limitations: Study not stratified on the basis of histology. No cost–benefit analysis to compare cost of initial radiation versus cost of managing the subsequent higher rate of local recurrences (some of which required amputation).

---

e. Regional Lymph Nodes in Truncal Melanoma

Immediate or delayed dissection of regional nodes in patients with melanoma of the trunk: A randomised trial. WHO Melanoma Programme.

Cascinelli N, Morabito A, Santinami M, MacKie RM, Belli F

Lancet. 1998;351(9105):793–796.

SYNOPSIS

Takeaway Point: Elective routine regional node dissection in patients with truncal melanoma without clinical evidence of regional node metastasis does not improve 5-year survival.

Commentary: The authors present a small, international, multi-center randomized trial comparing immediate versus delayed lymph node dissection in patients with truncal melanoma with a Breslow thickness of at least 1.5 mm. There was no significant difference in overall 5-year survival between immediate and delayed dissection groups. Early detection of positive regional nodes did significantly affect survival, however. Patients with occult nodal metastases discovered on immediate dissection had a significantly higher 5-year survival rate than did patients who developed regional node metastases in follow-up and underwent delayed dissection. The study was criticized for its small sample size and wide confidence intervals, but despite these shortcomings the results furthered interest in the use of sentinel node biopsy at the time of initial surgery, since early detection and intervention might have a role in improving survival.

ANALYSIS

Introduction: The benefit of elective node dissection in patients with cutaneous melanoma without clinically detectable node metastasis is unclear. A prior trial had demonstrated a potential benefit in a subgroup of patients aged 60 or younger with primarily melanoma between 1 and 4 mm thick, but was not able to confirm a benefit for all patients. The current study attempts to further clarify the role of elective lymph node dissection in clinically node-negative melanoma.

Objectives: To evaluate the efficacy of elective dissection of regional nodes in patients with clinically localized truncal melanoma.

Methods

Trial Design: Multicenter randomized trial.

Participants

Inclusion Criteria: Patients aged 65 or younger, with primary truncal melanoma, no evidence of nodal or distant metastases, and a Breslow thickness of ≥1.5 mm.

Exclusion Criteria: Prior cancer; clinically positive nodes; primary melanoma in a previously defined area on the trunk known to drain to multiple lymphatic basins.

Intervention: After wide excision with a 3 cm margin, patients were randomized to undergo either immediate ("elective") node dissection or observation and delayed node dissection only if there was clinical evidence of regional node metastases.

Endpoints

Primary Endpoint: 5-year survival of patients according to time of node dissection.

Secondary Endpoints: 5-year survival according to status of regional nodes; subgroup analysis of survival according to sex, Breslow thickness, and age ≥ 60 years.

Sample Size: 240 patients randomized between 1982 and 1989, 122 randomized to immediate node dissection and 118 randomized to observation with delayed node dissection.

Statistical Analysis: Study designed to detect at $\alpha = 0.05$ a difference of 20% with a power of 90%, t-test, χ^2 test with Yates' correction, Kaplan–Meier method, Cox's proportional-hazards model, likelihood ratio test, Wald statistic.

Results

Baseline Data: Treatment arms were balanced for sex, tumor thickness, and age.

Outcomes

Primary: Patients undergoing delayed and immediate node dissection had 5-year survival rates of 51.3% and 61.7%, respectively. This difference was not significant (p 0.09).

Secondary: Survival of patients who underwent wide excision only (who never developed node metastases and therefore did not have delayed dissection) and survival of patients who underwent elective node dissection but were found to have no evidence of metastatic disease were similar. Survival of those found to have occult node metastases at immediate node dissection was significantly higher (48.2%) than those who underwent delayed node dissection after developing regional node metastases (26.6%) (p 0.04). Multivariate analysis demonstrated that the routine use of elective node dissection had no impact on survival. The status of regional nodes significantly affected survival (p 0.07). Those patients with regional nodes that became clinically positive during the follow-up period had the worst prognosis.

Discussion

Conclusion: Elective regional node dissection in patients with truncal melanoma with a Breslow thickness of at least 1.5 mm does not confer an overall survival benefit.

Limitations: The study's small sample size resulted in wide confidence intervals, limiting the clinical significance of the results. The small sample size did not allow for subgroup analysis; the number of patients with surgically treated positive nodes was particularly small. Direct comparison with other study results was not possible because of differences in length of follow-up, average Breslow thickness, and exclusive study of truncal melanoma.

f. Retroperitoneal Sarcoma Survival

Predictors of survival after resection of retroperitoneal sarcoma: A population-based analysis and critical appraisal of the AJCC staging system.

Nathan H, Raut CP, Thornton K, Herman JM, Ahuja N, Schulick RD, Choti MA, Pawlik TM

Ann Surg. 2009;250(6):970–976.

SYNOPSIS

Takeaway Point: The American Joint Committee on Cancer (AJCC) staging system for sarcoma does not differentiate by anatomic location, and is not a good predictor of outcomes for retroperitoneal tumors. Alternative prognostic tools are needed.

Commentary: Soft tissue sarcomas are rare tumors, and retroperitoneal lesions are found in only a minority of cases. This has made it challenging to define appropriate prognostic tools. The AJCC staging system has been developed largely from data on extremity sarcomas. Nathan et al use a large, national database—the Surveillance, Epidemiology, and End Results (SEER) program—to understand the utility of the current staging system as well as evaluate alternative predictors. The authors found only moderate predictive value from the current staging system (c 0.66). This is likely due to the fact that almost all retroperitoneal sarcomas are >5 cm and that, by definition, all are deep to the fascia. Almost none have lymph node involvement, which leaves only grade as a component of staging. Importantly, factors such as histologic subtype and relationship to adjacent organs provided important prognostic information not currently incorporated into the AJCC staging system, speaking to the heterogeneity of behavior of soft tissue sarcoma as a group of malignancies. The findings here have spurred the development of multiple prognostic models, including nomograms and other schema that help provide more patient-specific information taking into account tumor type and other individualized data.

ANALYSIS

Introduction: Complete surgical resection is the only potential cure for retroperitoneal sarcoma, but incomplete resection and recurrence are common. As such, there is interest in identifying high-risk patients who might benefit from aggressive adjuvant therapies. The AJCC 6th edition staging system for soft tissue sarcomas was developed mostly from extremity data, and its prognostic value for retroperitoneal sarcoma is unknown.

Objectives: To identify predictors of survival after resection of retroperitoneal sarcoma (RPS) and to evaluate the performance of the AJCC staging system for RPS.

Methods

Trial Design: Retrospective cohort study.

Participants

Inclusion Criteria: Patients in the 2007 SEER database diagnosed with primary RPS between 1988 and 2005.

Exclusion Criteria: Gastrointestinal stromal tumors.

Intervention: Retrospective database study, no intervention.

Endpoints

Primary Endpoint: Association of survival with various prognostic variables, including the AJCC staging system for soft tissue sarcoma.

Sample Size: 2500 patients with RPS in the SEER database; 1365 underwent curative-intent surgeries.

Statistical Analysis: Kaplan–Meier survival curves and Cox proportional-hazards models; Akaike information criteria to refine the model; sensitivity analyses; concordance index.

Results

Baseline Data: Mean age was 63, 55% female; the majority (53%) were diagnosed between 2000 and 2005. Liposarcoma was the most common subtype (50%); 26% leiomyosarcoma, 11% malignant fibrous histiocytoma. 26% were grade I, 21% grade 4, and 20% were unknown grade. 82% of tumors were greater than 5 cm; 13% were unknown size.

Outcomes: Patients who did not receive curative intent surgery had higher incidence of metastatic disease and tended to be older ($p < 0.001$) and more often male ($p < 0.001$). Overall survival in the cohort was 61% at 3 years, 47% at 5 years, and 27% at 10 years. Histological subtype ($p < 0.001$), grade ($p < 0.001$), and tumor invasion of adjacent structures ($p < 0.001$) were significant predictors of survival in the multivariate analysis. To evaluate the prognostic ability of the AJCC staging system, the authors focused on M0 patients with known tumor size: in this cohort, the T-stage (tumor size) had no prognostic value (p 0.4, c 0.50). There was no difference in survival between stage I and stage II patients, although stage III and IV patients did have significantly lower survival. The overall staging system had moderate discriminative ability (c 0.66).

Discussion

Conclusion: The AJCC staging system for soft tissue sarcoma is a poor predictor of survival in RPS; in particular, tumor size does not impact survival. Tumor aggressiveness, indicated by histological grade and local invasion, does predict survival.

Limitations: Retrospective database study; included patients over a long time period; some data on tumor grade and size were incomplete in the database.

---

g. Ipilimumab in Metastatic Melanoma

Improved survival with ipilimumab in patients with metastatic melanoma.

Hodi FS, O'Day SJ, McDermott DF, Weber RW, Sosman JA, Haanen JB, Gonzalez R, Robert C, Schadendorf D, Hassel JC, Akerley W, van den Eertwegh AJ, Lutzky J, Lorigan P, Vaubel JM, Linette GP, Hogg D, Ottensmeier CH, Lebbé C, Peschel C, Quirt I, Clark JI, Wolchok JD, Weber JS, Tian J, Yellin MJ, Nichol GM, Hoos A, Urba WJ

NEJM. 2010;363(8):711–723.

SYNOPSIS

Takeaway Point: Ipilimumab can improve overall survival in patients with previously treated metastatic melanoma, although adverse events may be severe and treatment-limiting.

Commentary: Ipilimumab is a human monoclonal antibody that blocks cytotoxic T-lymphocyte-associated antigen 4 (CTLA-4) to provoke an antitumor T-cell response, promoting antitumor immunity. This study aimed to evaluate whether ipilimumab with or without gp100 (a tumor vaccine) could improve overall survival in patients with previously treated metastatic melanoma. Ipilimumab did improve overall survival in these patients as compared to gp100 alone. While the median overall survival was only slightly improved (10 months with ipilimumab vs. 6.4 months with gp100 alone), there was a small group of patients receiving ipilimumab who experienced a sustained response, with 9 of 15 patients (60%) maintaining an objective response for 2 years. While the majority of patients may not respond to this drug, this dramatic long-term response in select patients opened a new era of therapy for metastatic melanoma. It is possible that further study may discover better targeted immunologic therapies, or more effective combination therapy regimens in the treatment of metastatic melanoma. Adverse events were sometimes severe and life-threatening, including colitis and endocrinopathies, but were generally reversible.

ANALYSIS

Introduction: Prior to this trial, no adjuvant therapy had been shown to improve overall survival for patients with metastatic melanoma. Ipilimumab is a human monoclonal antibody that blocks CTLA-4, an immune checkpoint that downregulates T-cell activation, to provoke an antitumor T-cell response. Prior studies have demonstrated activity against melanoma, both alone and in combination with glycoprotein 100 (gp100), a cancer vaccine. There has never been a phase 3 trial of this treatment, and there is no accepted standard dosing regimen.

Objectives: To evaluate the impact of ipilimumab, with or without gp100, on overall survival in patients with metastatic melanoma who had undergone prior treatment.

Methods
Trial Design: Phase 3, international, multicenter, randomized, double-blind study.

Participants
Inclusion Criteria: Adult patients with unresectable stage III or IV melanoma who had received previous therapy with dacarbazine, temozolomide, fotemustine, carboplatin, or interleukin-2; life expectancy of at least 4 months; ECOG performance status of 0 or 1; positive status for HLA-A*0201; normal hematologic, hepatic, and renal function.

Exclusion Criteria: Other cancer within 5 years; primary ocular melanoma; previous receipt of anti-CTLA-4 antibody, cancer vaccine, or immunosuppressive therapy; autoimmune disease; active, untreated metastases in the central nervous system; pregnancy or lactation; long-term use of corticosteroids.

Intervention: Patients were randomly assigned, in a 3:1:1 ratio, to (1) induction ipilimumab, at a dose of 3 mg/kg, plus a gp100 peptide vaccine; (2) ipilimumab plus placebo; or (3) gp100 plus placebo—each once every 3 weeks for four cycles.

Endpoints

Primary Endpoint: Overall survival.

Secondary Endpoints: Comparison between ipilimumab-alone and gp-100 alone groups and between the two ipilimumab groups; overall response rate; duration of response; and progression-free survival.

Sample Size: 676 patients enrolled from 125 centers in 13 countries between 2004 and 2008: 403 randomized to receive ipilimumab plus gp100, 137 to receive ipilimumab alone, and 136 to receive gp100 alone.

Statistical Analysis: Sample size calculation estimated 500 patients with 385 events (deaths) would provide 90% power; Kaplan–Meier curves; Cox proportional-hazards models.

Results

Baseline Data: Patients were well matched according to baseline characteristics across all groups.

Outcomes

Primary: Median overall survival in the ipilimumab-plus-gp 100 group was 10.0 months, in the ipilimumab-alone group 10.1 months, and for gp100 alone 6.4 months. Hazard ratio for death with ipilimumab alone versus gp100 alone was 0.66, p 0.003.

Secondary: There was no significant difference in overall survival detected between the two ipilimumab groups (HR 1.04, p 0.76). The effect of ipilimumab on overall survival was independent of other baseline characteristics. There was a 19% reduction in risk of progression seen with ipilimumab plus gp100 compared to gp100 alone, as well as a 36% reduction in risk of progression seen with ipilimumab alone compared to gp100 alone. The ipilimumab-alone group had the best overall response rate at 10.9% and a disease control rate of 28.5%, while 60% maintained an objective response for at least 2 years. 17.4% of the ipilimumab-plus-gp100 group maintained an objective response for 2 years, and none of the gp100-alone group. Grade 3 or 4 immune-related adverse events occurred in 10–15% of patients treated with ipilimumab, and in 3% treated with gp100 alone.

Discussion

Conclusion: Ipilimumab, administered alone or in combination with gp100, improved overall survival in patients with metastatic melanoma who had undergone prior treatment.

Limitations: The control group of the study was not a dacarbazine-treated group, an observational group, or a placebo, but instead a vaccine-treated group, which, in theory, could have been harmful, thus affecting the results. The difference in median overall survival in the ipilimumab groups compared to the vaccine-alone group was only 4 months, with the best overall response rates of only 6–11%. While a small percentage of patients demonstrated a dramatic response to ipilimumab, the majority of patients treated did not respond.

---

h. BRIM-3 Trial

Improved survival with vemurafenib in melanoma with BRAF V600E mutation.

Chapman PB, Hauschild A, Robert C, Haanen JB, Ascierto P, Larkin J, Dummer R, Garbe C, Testori A, Maio M, Hogg D, Lorigan P, Lebbe C, Jouary T, Schadendorf D, Ribas A, O'Day SJ, Sosman JA, Kirkwood JM, Eggermont AM, Dreno B, Nolop K, Li J, Nelson B, Hou J, Lee RJ, Flaherty KT, McArthur GA, BRIM-3 Study Group

NEJM. 2011;364(26):2507–2516.

SYNOPSIS

Takeaway Point: Vemurafenib improves overall and progression-free survival in patients with unresectable treatment-naïve melanoma with a BRAF V600E mutation.

Commentary: This study assessed the use of vemurafenib, a BRAF inhibitor with activity against the BRAF V600E mutation, in the treatment of metastatic melanoma, comparing it to the only approved chemotherapeutic treatment at the time, dacarbazine. The study found a significant benefit in both overall and progression-free survival with vemurafenib in comparison to dacarbazine. At interim analysis, an independent review board found that survival endpoints had been met, and patients with dacarbazine were allowed to cross over to vemurafenib. Benefits with vemurafenib treatment were seen across all subgroups, including patients with stage M1c disease and those with elevated lactate dehydrogenase levels, both of which typically portend a poor prognosis. There was a 48% relative response rate to vemurafenib, compared to 5% for dacarbazine. 38% of patients receiving vemurafenib required dose adjustments due to toxicity. This study confirmed the use of vemurafenib as a promising therapy in the treatment of metastatic melanoma, and prompted further interest in potential combination therapies and other targeted inhibitors of molecular signaling pathways important in melanoma.

ANALYSIS

Introduction: Approximately 50% of cutaneous melanomas carry mutations in BRAF, and 90% of these are BRAF V600E mutations. Vemurafenib is a potent inhibitor of BRAF V600E. This phase 3 trial compares the efficacy of vemurafenib with the only previously approved drug for the treatment of metastatic melanoma, dacarbazine.

Objectives: To determine whether vemurafenib would prolong the rate of overall or progression-free survival, as compared to dacarbazine.

Methods

Trial Design: Stage 3 multicenter, randomized trial.

Participants

Inclusion Criteria: Patients with unresectable, previously untreated stage IIIC or IV melanoma positive for BRAF V600E mutation, age > 18, life expectancy of ≥3 months, ECOG performance status of 0 or 1.

Exclusion Criteria: History of cancer in past 5 years; metastases to the central nervous system, unless treated for >3 months without progression or need for glucocorticoids; other active anticancer therapy.

Intervention: Patients randomly assigned to receive either oral vemurafenib twice daily or dacarbazine infusion every 3 weeks.

Endpoints

Primary Endpoint: The original primary endpoint was overall survival. Following results of phase 1 and 2 trials, primary endpoint was revised to include overall and progression-free survival.

Secondary Endpoints: Rate of, duration of, and time to response.

Sample Size: 672 patients enrolled at 104 centers in 12 countries from January to December 2010, with 336 randomized to vemurafenib, and 336 to dacarbazine.

Statistical Analysis: Power of 80% to detect a hazard ratio of 0.65 for overall survival with $\alpha = 0.045$, and a power of 90% to detect a hazard ratio of 0.55 for progression-free survival with $\alpha = 0.005$.

Unstratified log-rank test; hazard ratios for treatment estimated with unstratified Cox regression; Kaplan–Meier method.

Results

Baseline Data: Treatment groups were balanced in terms of baseline characteristics including age, sex, race, region, performance status, extent of disease, and lactate dehydrogenase.

Outcomes

Primary: At 6 months, overall survival was 84% in the vemurafenib group and 64% in the dacarbazine group. Median progression-free survival was 5.3 months for vemurafenib and 1.6 months for dacarbazine. At interim analysis for overall survival and final analysis for progression-free survival, vemurafenib provided a 63% relative reduction in the risk of death and 74% of either death or disease progression, compared to dacarbazine ($p < 0.001$). After this analysis, the data and safety board recommended that patients receiving dacarbazine be allowed to cross over to vemurafenib.

Secondary: Response rates were 48% for vemurafenib and 5% for dacarbazine ($p < 0.001$). There was a median time to response of 1.45 months for vemurafenib and 2.7 months for dacarbazine.

Discussion

Conclusion: Patients with metastatic melanoma with BRAF V600E mutation who are treated with vemurafenib have improved response rates, progression-free, and overall survival compared with dacarbazine.

Limitations: Short follow-up; final estimate of survival outcomes still to be determined at the time of study publication. The use of investigator-reported responses rather than an independent review board have the potential to bias the response rates and rates of progression-free survival. Because patients were allowed at interim analysis to cross over to from the dacarbazine arm to the vemurafenib arm, this could alter the rates of overall survival on longer-term analyses.

---

i. MSLT-1 Sentinel Node Biopsy in Melanoma

Final trial report of sentinel-node biopsy versus nodal observation in melanoma.

Morton DL, Thompson JF, Cochran AJ, Mozzillo N, Nieweg OE, Roses DF, Hoekstra HJ, Karakousis CP, Puleo CA, Coventry BJ, Kashani-Sabet M, Smithers BM, Paul E, Kraybill WG, McKinnon JG, Wang HJ, Elashoff R, Faries MB, MSLT Group

NEJM. 2014;370(7):599–609.

SYNOPSIS

Takeaway Point: Sentinel node biopsy has good prognostic value for patients with intermediate-thickness melanoma, but early detection and surgical management of nodal disease do not appear to improve survival in this cohort.

Commentary: This report of the landmark first Multicenter Selective Lymphadenectomy Trial (MSLT-1) has established the prognostic value of sentinel lymph node biopsy (SLNB) in melanoma. Patients with intermediate-thickness melanoma and clinically uninvolved regional lymph nodes were randomized to wide excision plus SLNB versus wide excision plus clinical observation alone. All patients with nodal disease detected by either SLNB or clinical exam underwent anatomic complete lymphadenectomy of the affected basin. In the intermediate-thickness group, 16% had a positive sentinel node, while 17.4% developed nodal metastases at a median of 19.2 months after surgery. The relative equivalency of these rates helped to establish that micrometastases identified at SLNB go on to become clinically apparent disease if not treated. In the primary analysis, there was no significant difference in overall survival between the two groups. However, in a predetermined analysis of patients with nodal metastases at any point, those detected with SLNB had a significantly improved survival versus those detected clinically (62.1% vs. 41.5% at 10 years). The results from this study have established SLNB as the standard of care for intermediate thickness melanoma.

ANALYSIS

Introduction: Regional lymph node management in melanoma is controversial. Routine elective lymphadenectomy without evidence of nodal metastases carries significant morbidity, but prior randomized trials have suggested a survival benefit. Sentinel node biopsy is an attractive intermediate step between full dissection and observation.

Objectives: The MSLT-I sought to determine whether sentinel-node biopsy could be used to identify patients with clinically occult nodal metastases and to compare immediate-completion lymphadenectomy versus nodal observation with lymphadenectomy for nodal recurrence.

Methods

Trial Design: Randomized controlled trial.

Participants

Inclusion Criteria: Patients with localized cutaneous melanomas of Clark level III or Breslow thickness of ≥ 1 mm, or Clark level IV or V with any Breslow thickness. Intermediate-thickness patients (1.2–3.5mm) constituted the primary study group.

Exclusion Criteria: Age <18 or >75 years; primary tumor on the eye, ear, or mucous membranes; secondary primary tumor; additional malignancy within the past 5 years; prior chemo/radiation therapy; immunosuppression; pregnancy; life expectancy <10 years from another cause.

Intervention: Wide excision plus sentinel node biopsy (biopsy group) versus wide excision and postoperative nodal observation (observation group). Observation group patients underwent lymphadenectomy if nodal metastases developed; patients in the biopsy group underwent lymphadenectomy if metastases were seen in the sentinel node. Randomization was stratified by Breslow thickness and primary tumor site.

Endpoints

Primary Endpoint: Melanoma-specific survival.

Secondary Endpoints: Disease-free survival, survival with tumor-positive or tumor-negative sentinel nodes, incidence of sentinel node metastases compared with incidence of clinically detected nodal metastases.

Sample Size: 1347 patients with intermediate-thickness melanomas underwent randomization, with 814 to sentinel node biopsy (805 included in 10-year follow-up) and 533 to nodal observation (522 included in 10-year follow-up).

Statistical Analysis: Sample size calculations after interim analysis estimated 1200 patients were needed for 90% power. Kaplan–Meier survival curves, t-test, χ^2 test, Wilcoxon rank sum, and Cox proportional-hazards model.

Results

Baseline Data: The groups were balanced with regards to tumor site, Clark level, Breslow thickness, ulceration, and age.

Outcomes: At 10 years, 505 out of 805 (63%) in the biopsy group were alive; 326 out of 522 of the observation group (62%). There was no significant difference in 10-year disease-specific survival rates. Disease-free survival rates were significantly higher in the biopsy group (71% vs. 65%, p 0.01). A positive sentinel node was predictive of significantly worse 10-year survival (62% vs. 85%,

$p < 0.001$), and in multivariate analysis sentinel node status, this was the strongest predictor of disease recurrence or death.

Discussion

Conclusion: Biopsy-based staging of intermediate-thickness melanomas provides prognostic information about survival. SLNB does not provide overall or disease-specific survival advantage.

Limitations: Event rates were lower than anticipated, prompting an increase in required sample size at the interim analysis. May have been underpowered to detect survival differences.

REFERENCES

1. Guy GP, Machlin S, Ekwueme DU, Yabroff KR. Prevalence and costs of skin cancer treatment in the US, 2002–2006 and 2007–2011. *Am J Prevent Med.* 2015;48:183–187.

2. American Cancer Society. *Cancer Facts & Figures 2015.* Atlanta, GA: American Cancer Society; 2015.

3. Veronesi U et al. Thin stage I primary cutaneous malignant melanoma: Comparison of excision with margins of 1 or 3 cm. *NEJM.* 1988;318:1159–1162.

4. Balch CM et al. Long-term results of a prospective surgical trial comparing 2 cm vs 4 cm excision margins for 740 patients with 1-4 mm melanomas. *Ann Surg Oncol.* 2001;8(2):101–108.

5. Thomas JM et al. Excision margins in high-risk malignant melanoma. *NEJM.* 2004;350:757–766.

6. Cohn-Cedermark G et al. Long term results of a randomized study by the Swedish Melanoma Study Group on 2-cm versus 5-cm resection margins for patients with cutaneous melanoma with a tumor thickness of 0.8-2.0 mm. *Cancer.* 2000;89(7):1495–1501.

7. Cascinelli N et al (WHO Melanoma Study Group). Immediate or delayed dissection of regional nodes in patients with melanoma of the trunk: A randomised trial. WHO Melanoma Programme. *Lancet* 1998;351(9105):793–796.

8. Morton DL et al. Final trial report of sentinel-node biopsy versus nodal observation in melanoma. *NEJM.* 2014;370(7):599–609.

9. Kirkwood JM et al (ECOG Interferon). Interferon alfa-2b adjuvant therapy of high-risk resected cutaneous melanoma: The Eastern Cooperative Oncology Group Trial EST 1684. *J Clin Oncol.* 1996;14(1):7–17.

Abbreviations

4D	four-dimensional
5-FU	fluorouracil
AAA	abdominal aortic aneurysm
AAST	American Association for the Surgery of Trauma
AAST-OIS	American Association for the Surgery of Trauma-Organ Injury Scale
ABP	acute biliary pancreatitis
AC	doxorubicin and cyclophosphamide
ACAS	Asymptomatic Carotid Artery Stenosis
ACC	adrenocortical carcinoma
ACOSOG	American College of Surgeons Oncology Group
ACS	acute coronary syndrome
ACS	American College of Surgeons
ACS-BSCN	American College of Surgeons Bariatric Surgery Center Network
ACS-NSQIP	American College of Surgeons–National Surgical Quality Improvement Program
ADH	anti-diuretic hormone
AFP	α-fetoprotein
AFS	amputation-free survival
AGB	adjustable gastric banding
AIR	Appendicitis Inflammatory Response
AISP	Italian Association for Study of the Pancreas
AJCC	American Joint Committee on Cancer
ALND	axillary lymph node dissection
ALPPS	associating liver partition and portal vein ligation for staged hepatectomy
ALT	alanine transaminase
ANC	absolute neutrophil count
ANOVA	analysis of variance

APACHE II	Acute Physiology and Chronic Health Evaluation
APR	abdominoperineal resection
ARDS	acute respiratory distress syndrome
ASA	American Society of Anesthesiologists
ASBO	adhesive small-bowel obstruction
ASMBS	American Society for Metabolic and Bariatric Surgery
ASPEN	American Society for Parenteral and Enteral Nutrition
AST	aspartate aminotransferase
ATA	American Thyroid Association
BAP	balloon angioplasty
BASIL	Bypass versus Angioplasty in Severe Ischaemia of the Leg
BCS	breast-conserving surgery
BCT	breast conservation therapy
BE	bilateral exploration
BE	bilateral neck exploration
BM	bowel movement
BMI	body mass index
BRPC	borderline resectable pancreatic cancer
BSA	body surface area
BSX	bypass surgery
CAS	carotid artery stenting
CAVATAS	Carotid and Vertebral Artery Transluminal Angioplasty Study
CBC	contralateral breast cancers; complete blood count
CBD	common bile duct
CDT	catheter-directed thrombolysis
CEA	carcinoembryonic antigen
CEA	carotid endarterectomy
CHF	congestive heart failure
CI	confidence interval
CKD	chronic kidney disease
CLI	chronic limb ischemia
CLND	central lymph node dissection

cN0	clinically node-negative
cN1	clinically positive lymph nodes
CO	crossover
COST	Clinical Outcomes of Surgical Therapy
CPR	cardiopulmonary resuscitation
CRASH-2	a randomised, placebo-controlled trial
CRLM	colorectal liver metastases
CROP	dynamic compliance, respiratory rate, oxygenation, maximum inspiratory pressure index
CRP	C-reactive protein
C-spine	cervical spine
CT	computed tomography
CTA	computed tomography angiography
CTLA-4	cytotoxic T-lymphocyte–associated antigen 4
CVA	cerebrovascular accident
CVL	central venous line
CVP	central venous pressure
DCIS	ductal carcinoma in situ
DDSF	distant disease-free survival
DFS	disease-free survival
DGE	delayed gastric emptying
DISPACT	distal pancreatectomy
DKA	diabetic ketoacidosis
DNR	do-not-resuscitate
DPL	diagnostic peritoneal lavage
DSS	disease-specific survival
DTC	differentiated thyroid cancer
DVT	deep-vein thrombosis
DXA	dual-energy x-ray absorptiometry
EAST	Eastern Association for the Surgery of Trauma
EBCTCG	Early Breast Cancer Trialists' Collaborative Group
EBL	estimated blood loss

ECF	epirubicin + cisplatin + infused fluorouracil
ECG	echocardiogram
ECOG	Eastern Cooperative Oncology Group
ECST	European Carotid Surgery Trial
ED	emergency department
EGDT	early goal-directed therapy
EORTC QLQ-CR38	European Organization for Research and Treatment of Cancer Colorectal Quality of Life Questionnaire
EORTC	European Organization for Research and Treatment of Cancer
ER	estrogen receptor
ERCP	endoscopic retrograde cholangiopancreatography
EUS	endoscopic ultrasonography
EUS-FNA	endoscopic ultrasonography-guided fine-needle aspiration
EVAR	endovascular AAA repair
EVL	endoscopic variceal ligation
FAP	familial adenomatous polyposis
FAST	focused assessment with sonography for trauma
FHH	familial hypocalciuric hypercalcemia
FI	fecal incontinence
FLR	functional liver reserve
FNA	fine-needle aspiration
FNR	false-negative rate
GCS	Glasgow Coma Score
GDA	gastroduodenal artery
GE	gastroesophageal
GERD	gastroesophageal reflux disease
GFR	glomerular filtration rate
GGT	γ-glutamyltransferase
GI	gastrointestinal
GOS	Glasgow Outcome Scale
gp100	glycoprotein 100
GSV	great saphenous vein

HAI	Hepatic arterial infusion
HASTA	HAnd suture versus STApling
HCC	hepatocellular carcinoma
Hct	hematocrit
HDL	high-density lipoprotein
Hgb	hemoglobin
HPB-NSQIP	Hepatopancreaticobiliary-National Surgical Quality Improvement Program
HPT	hyperparathyroidism
HPT-JT	hyperparathyroidism–jaw tumor
HR	hazard ratio
HRQoL	health-related quality-of-life
HSD	honest significant differences
IB	infrainguinal bypass
IBD	inflammatory bowel disease
IBTR	ipsilateral breast tumor recurrence
ICD	intermittent claudication distance
ICP	increased intracranial pressure
IFNα-2b	interferon alfa-2B
IGCSC	Italian Gastric Cancer Study Group
IOPTH	intraoperative PTH
IPAA	ileal pouch-anal anastomosis
IPMN	intraductal papillary mucinous neoplasm
IR	interventional radiology
IRA	ileorectal anastomosis
IRONIC	Invasive Revascularization Or Not in Intermittent Claudication
ISGPS	International Study Group of Pancreatic Surgery
IT	invasive therapy
IT	invasive treatment
ITT	intention-to-treat
IVC	inferior vena cava
JGCA	Japanese Gastric Cancer Association
LA	laparoscopic appendectomy
LA	left atrial
LAGB	laparoscopic adjustable gastric band

LAR	low anterior resection
LCIS	lobular carcinoma in situ
LDS	laparoscopic duodenal switch
LE	limited exploration
LGI	Lower gastrointestinal
LN	lymph node
LO	lumpectomy alone
LOS	length of stay
LR	local recurrence
LRT	lumpectomy with radiation
LRYGB	laparoscopic Roux-en-Y gastric bypass
LS	limb salvage
LSG	laparoscopic sleeve gastrectomy
LSS	limb-sparing surgery
MAP	mean arterial pressure
MBSAQIP	Metabolic and Bariatric Surgery Accreditation and Quality Improvement Program
MCN	mucinous cystic neoplasm
MD	main duct
MEN	multiple endocrine neoplasia
MeSH	Medical Subject Headings
MGD	multiglandular disease
MI	myocardial infarction
MITT	modified intention-to-treat
MODS	multi-organ dysfunction syndrome
MRA	magnetic resonance angiography
MRC	Medical Research Council
MRCP	magnetic resonance cholangiopancreatography
MSLT	Multicenter Selective Lymphadenectomy Trial
MWD	Maximum walking distance
NASCET	North American Symptomatic Carotid Endarterectomy Trial
NCCN	National Comprehensive Cancer Network
NEJM	New England Journal of Medicine
NEXUS	National Emergency X-Radiography Utilization Study

NGT	nasogastric tube
NIH	National Institute of Health
NIS	Nationwide Inpatient Sample
NIT	noninvasive therapy
NNT	Number needed to treat
NOM	nonoperative management
NOTA Study	Non Operative Treatment for Acute Appendicitis
NPO	nil per os
NPV	negative predictive value
NSABP	National Surgical Adjuvant Breast and Bowel Project
NYHA	New York Heart Association
OA	open appendectomy
OHRP	Office for Human Research Protection
OPTX	Occult pneumothorax
OR	Open AAA repair
OS	overall survival
OSTRiCH	Optimizing the Surgical Treatment of Rectal Cancer
PAD	peripheral arterial disease
PAP	primary assisted patency
PCA	patient-controlled analgesia
pCLND	prophylactic central compartment lymph node dissection
PCS	physical component score
PCWP	pulmonary capillary wedge pressure
PD	pancreaticoduodenectomy
PE	pulmonary embolism
PEEP	positive end-expiratory pressure
PFS	progression-free survival
PHPT	primary hyperparathyroidism
pN+	node-positive
pN0	node-negative
POI	postoperative ileus
PP	primary patency
PPI	proton pump inhibitor

PPPD	pylorus-preserving pancreaticoduodenectomy
PPV	positive predictive value
PPV	positive-pressure ventilation
PR	prolonged-release
ProCESS Trial	A randomized trial of protocol-based care for early septic shock
PROMMTT	prospective, observational, multicenter, major trauma transfusion
PROPATRIA	Probiotics in Pancreatitis Trial
PROPPR	plasma, platelets, and red blood cells
PT	prothrombin time
PTC	papillary thyroid cancer
PTH	parathyroid hormone or hypercalcemia
PTS	postthrombotic syndrome
PV	portal vein
PVE	portal vein embolization
PVL	portal vein ligation
QOL	quality-of-life
RECIST	response evaluation criteria in solid tumors
RFS	relapse-free survival
RH	retained hemothorax
RLN	recurrent laryngeal nerve
ROC	receiver-operating-characteristic
RPS	resection of retroperitoneal sarcoma
RRs	risk ratios
RSBI	rapid shallow breathing index
RSI	rapid-sequence intubation
RT	resuscitative thoracotomy
rTAH	radical total abdominal hysterectomy
RYGB	Roux-en-Y gastric bypass configuration
SA	single adenoma
SAPS II	Simplified Acute Physiology Score II
SBO	small-bowel obstruction
SEER	Surveillance, Epidemiology, and End Results
SG	subtotal gastrectomy
SIRS	systemic inflammatory response syndrome

SLI	severe leg ischemia
SLN	sentinel lymph node
SLNB	sentinel lymph node biopsy
SLND	sentinel lymph node dissection
SMA	superior mesenteric artery
SM-BOSS	Swiss Multicentre Bypass or Sleeve Study
SMV	superior mesenteric vein
SNS	sacral nerve stimulation
SOS	Swedish Obese Subjects
SP	secondary patency
SPECT	single-photon emission computed tomography
SSI	surgical site infection
SSO	Society for Surgical Oncology
SSO/ASTRO	Society of Surgical Oncology–American Society for Radiation Oncology consensus guideline
STAMPEDE	Surgical Treatment and Medications Potentially Eradicate Diabetes Efficiently
STAR	Study of Tamoxifen and Raloxifene
SW	standard Whipple
SWOG	Southwest Oncology Group
TACE	transcatheter arterial chemoembolization
TAM	tamoxifen
TASC II	Trans-Atlantic inter-Society Consensus
TBI	traumatic brain injury
Tg	thyroglobulin
TG	total gastrectomy
TIA	transient ischemic attack
TIPS	transjugular intrahepatic portosystemic shunt
TLC	total lung capacity
TME	total mesorectal excision
TNM	tumor, node, metastases
TPN	total parenteral nutrition
TT	total thyroidectomy
TTx	total thyroidectomy
TXA	tranexamic acid
UC	ulcerative colitis

UGI	upper gastrointestinal
US	ultrasound
UTI	urinary tract infection
VA NSQIP	Veterans Administration National Surgical Quality Improvement Program
VA	Veteren's Affairs
VAS	visual analog scale
VascQoL	Vascular Quality of Life
VATS	video-assisted thoracoscopic surgery
VBG	vertical banded gastroplasty
VTE	venous thromboembolism
WHO	World Health Organization
WTA	Western Trauma Association
WW	watchful waiting
XRT	radiation therapy

Index